Nurses' Work, The Sacred and The Profane

NURSES' WORK

The Sacred and The Profane

ZANE ROBINSON WOLF

upp

University of Pennsylvania Press

Philadelphia

103016

Library of Congress Cataloging-in-Publication Data

Wolf, Zane Robinson.
  Nurses' work.

  Bibliography: p.
  Includes index.
  1. Nursing—Social aspects.   2. Ritualization.
I. Title.
RT86.5.W65   1988   306'.46   87-35770
ISBN 0-8122-8104-7
ISBN 0-8122-1266-5 (pbk.)

Second paperback printing 1989

To 7H nurses
and their vice-president
for nursing,
and to Carol Germain,
Renée Fox,
and Florence Downs

Contents

Preface

This book is based on a doctoral dissertation, "Nursing Rituals in an Adult Acute Care Hospital: An Ethnography." It is a study of nursing rituals involving nurses, patients, and other hospital workers who shared experiences when living and working on a medical unit of a large urban hospital.

The nursing staff, including registered nurses, licensed practical nurses, and nursing assistants, as well as patients, physicians, and other hospital personnel were the informants of the study. All names used in the book are fictitious.

I collected most of my data through participant observation techniques, intensive semi-structured interviews, and event analyses. I collected data during the day, evening, and night shifts over a twelve-month period, and most intensively for nine months.

I used the works of Victor Turner, Bronislaw Malinowski, Mary Douglas, Arnold Van Gennep, Charles L. Bosk, Eviatar Zerubavel, Virginia Walker, Willy DeCraemer, Jan Vansina, and Renée C. Fox to frame my study of nursing rituals. Throughout the study, I used the definition of ritual formulated by DeCraemer, Vansina, and Fox: ritual is patterned symbolic action that refers to the goals and values of a social group. Furthermore, as events unfolded I examined and described the explicit or manifest and latent or implicit levels of meaning.

The actions and words of my informants, the medical unit, the objects used in the care of patients, the relationships of actors or informants with each other, and the procedures, routines, and reports of the working nurses were the main foci of data collection for each category of potential nursing ritual studied.

Nurses' work has both sacred and profane aspects. Day after day, nurses participate in the human events of suffering, healing, and dying. Because nurses are intimately involved in these events and because of their caring role, including "laying-on-of-hands" behaviors, it is not surprising that a system of rituals exists. The four nursing rituals that I have identified and described coexist with the technological and scientific aspects of patient care and are part of the fabric of the personal-care tasks delegated by society to nursing over time and assumed and performed by nurses.

I identified three therapeutic nursing rituals through which nurses perform symbolic healing actions that improve the condition of patients: post-mortem care, medication administration, and bathing patients. I identified one occupational nursing ritual through which nurses learn the meaning of what it is to be a nurse: change-of-shift report. By contrast, I did not label patients' admission and discharge procedures as nursing rituals and therefore did not include them in this book. Here I offer a warning. Sections of the book include nurse involvement with some of the most private as well as the most profane aspects of human life.

The study of nursing rituals also identified a pervasive value for nurses, that of doing good and avoiding harm. Nurses passed on their subcultural knowledge about nursing and patient care chiefly by word of mouth and by demonstration.

In the beginning I doubted that anyone in the scientific nursing community would accept my assumption that the American hospital is a quasi-religious or sacred institution. I was pleasantly surprised. I found that others share this assumption and that in many cultures, including our own, health and illness are symbolically located in the sacred domain.

Acknowledgments

I would like to thank my husband, Charles Wolf, and my children, Jessica, Zana, and Kerrin, for their love, patience, and support. My gratitude also goes to my parents, Zana and William Robinson, for their continuous love and encouragement to learn.

Drs. Carol Germain, Florence Downs, Joan Lynaugh, and Renée Fox offered much support and scholarly direction while I worked on my dissertation at the School of Nursing, University of Pennsylvania. I thank them.

I would also like to thank the Christian Brothers, La Salle University, and the Pennsylvania League for Nursing for financial support, and La Salle University Department of Nursing faculty and R.N.-B.S.N. students for listening.

The staff of the University of Pennsylvania Press were most helpful. Special thanks to Patricia Smith and Ruth Veleta.

Nurses' Work, The Sacred and The Profane

I

7H and the 7H Nurses

7H: The Medical Unit

No one ever forgets 7H. [Beth, R.N.]

A large hospital stands in a moderately decayed neighborhood of a major city in the United States. 7H, a medical unit, is situated in this teaching hospital, sandwiched between an orthopedic unit above and a cardiac step-down unit below. 7H is adjacent to three other units on the same floor level: another medical unit to the right and two small units to the left, an isolation unit and a psychiatric unit. 7H nursing staff maintains a good-neighbor policy with these nearby units. Staff visits the other units to "steal" linen, get ice, and borrow medications and central supply items when patient need warrants this. Staff from other units reciprocate with forays into 7H's caches of hospital goods. Requests for permission almost always accompany "begging, borrowing, and stealing" expeditions.

It was July 19, the new graduate nurse and new intern time of the year. The hospital was engaged in a major construction project. So far the construction had had little effect on 7H. The most direct benefit of the construction for the 7H nursing staff was the new parking garage which eased the process of getting to and from work. When 7H's nurses came on duty at 7:30 A.M., they approached the hospital from the parking garage and the outside walkway which threaded through construction workers and equipment. A hard-hat area was adjacent to the main entrance to the

1

hospital. Some of the 7H staff such as Dotty, an L.G.P.N. (licensed graduate practical nurse), entered the hospital here and walked immediately to the coffee shop to buy coffee to sip during morning change-of-shift report.

7H was divided into patient rooms with adjoining bathrooms, a large central corridor, the nurses' station, the utility room, and two offices (Figure 1). The nursing staff typically began each shift from the central location of the utility room and the nurses' station. From here they moved from the corridor to the sixteen patient rooms of the medical unit.

The patient rooms, numbered 740 to 755, were semi-private. Generally the two beds of each semi-private room were occupied. The rooms were small, painted in pastel colors without decoration. A bathroom with a sink and toilet and closets was part of each patient unit. A television was mounted on the wall at a midpoint between the feet or ends of the patients' beds. The wood tones of the headboards and footboards, the bedside cabinet, and the over-bed table offset the functional appearance of the rooms. Ceiling-suspended curtains in off-white were pushed against the wall at the head of each bed. Curtains were used to encircle patients and insure privacy. A large window brightened every room. Often the nondescript window curtains were pushed back to admit a view of low brick buildings. Trees were more visible through the windows of patient rooms on one side of the corridor than the other. So was the construction work. Patients in the "window" beds enjoyed the distraction of the construction activity and the view outside the hospital; patients in the "door" beds enjoyed the diversion of the corridor traffic. The brick buildings were not so interesting.

Traffic "on the floor" was heavy during the early part of the day shift. It is surprising that the hospital staff accomplished their various tasks, considering the continuous movement of staff, patients, and equipment that occurred during weekdays. Traffic was busiest from 8:15 A.M. until after 11 A.M. 7H nursing staff moved through the corridor, sometimes talking to each other about such things as a telephone call to a doctor, a request for a lab study or other diagnostic tests, or a request for change of diet for the dietary department. In the midst of this activity, a medical clerk sat at the

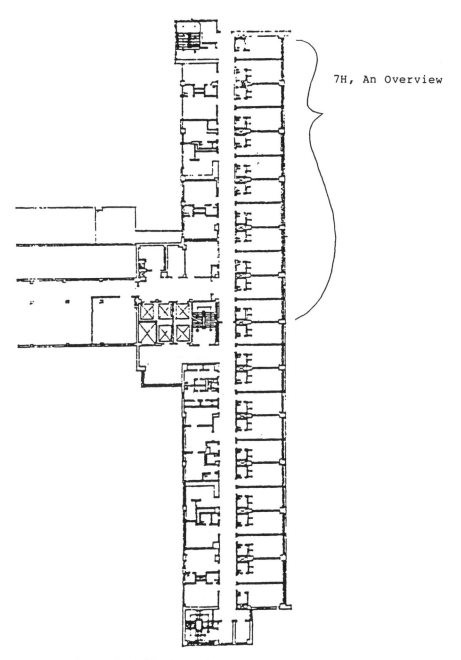

7H, An Overview

Figure 1. 7H, and neighboring unit.

desk in the nurses' station making telephone calls and doing paper work for patients' charts.

Teams of doctors moved through the corridor, going in and out of the patient rooms and animatedly discussing the progress and therapy of patients. Cardiologists assigned to the geographic area of 7H transferred patients from the Cardiac Care Unit (CCU) to 7H. "Rule out" MI (myocardial infarction or heart attack) patients usually spent three days on the unit. The many day shift admissions and transfers of these cardiac cases made patient turnover on 7H very rapid. The longer stays of 7H cancer patients slowed down the turnover rate.

Escort personnel asked 7H staff how patients were to be transported, by wheelchair or litter. The staff worked together to move each patient onto a litter or into a wheelchair, so that gradually the corridor became congested with people and equipment. A housekeeping worker, moving around the staff's feet, dust-mopped the corridor. The diet carts came up on the service elevators, steered onto the unit by pleasant dietary staff. The rattle and aroma of breakfast began. The scurrying of the morning was not haphazard, but nevertheless it was amazing that there was order to morning events on 7H.

The dietary department's job of delivering food was complicated by the "bloods" that had to be drawn while patients were fasting. Laboratory technicians, usually one or two, arranged slips and tubes at the counter in front of the nurses' station before drawing specimens from the patients. At the same time, nurses on each of 7H's four districts made sure that insulin injections were given and that patients were bathed or helped to bathe themselves. During baths, the patient rooms and the hall were warm. The humidity in the rooms increased as hot bath water was drained into basins and the baths began.

Time seemed to move fast in the morning. Change-of-shift report began at 7:30 and lasted until 8:00 or 8:15. Nursing staff moved rapidly and distributed linen when not in shift report. They sometimes started "A.M. care," oral hygiene and bathing, before report. The noise level was high. Staff asked and answered questions about patients and supplies. The younger and more inexperienced graduate nurses discussed problems with the more experienced registered nurses. Nurses asked for help to move patients physically unable to move themselves. Deidre, the nurse manager, acting as a troubleshooter, visited all the patients of her unit to see that they were comfortable and helped her nursing staff with any questions or dilemmas. Jennifer, the medical clerk, answered the telephone and answered questions from the nurses, doctors, and escort and lab personnel who worked around the nurses' station.

On a typical 7H day, three 7H night staff were busy finishing vital signs and weighing patients. Miriam, the permanent registered nurse on nights, counted narcotics and other controlled drugs with Sharon, a new graduate nurse. As more day shift nursing staff arrived, they signed in (and out) on the daily attendance record, which was taped to the shelf in front of the nurses' station. R.N.'s (registered nurses), G.N.'s (graduate nurses), L.G.P.N.'s, and nursing assistants all signed the sheets to document that they had come on duty.

Staff who were sick called the unit by this time. After these messages, Miriam called the Nursing Office with the hope of finding additional staff or "help" for the day shift. Deidre or Kate, the assistant nurse manager, who had earlier assigned nursing staff to specific districts, made adjustments based on staff availability and the seriousness of patient problems. During the times when staff were ill, absent, or attending continuing education programs, or were "pulled" to other units short of staff, the remaining staff complained. When Deidre and Kate were not on the unit, the most senior nurse made patient assignments. Assignments were written on the primary board fastened to the wall across from the nurses' station. When staffing patterns were good, 7H was divided into four geographical districts (see Figure 2). District I included patient rooms 740, 741, 754, and 755; District II, rooms 742, 743, 744, and 745, the closest to the utility room and nurses' station. District III included rooms 746, 747, 752, and 753; District IV, rooms 748, 749, 750, and 751, most distant from the central areas of the unit, the nurses' station, and the utility room.

Morning report started abruptly when Miriam, the night nurse, and nursing staff assigned to each district were ready to exchange

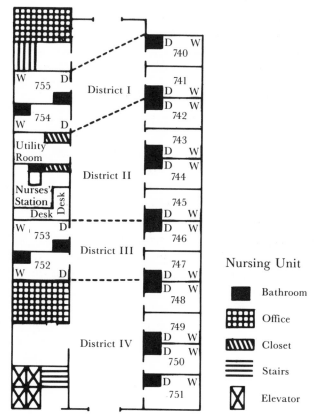

Figure 2. 7H, a nursing unit.

information about patients in each district. Nurses from Districts I and II listened to each other's reports, as did nurses from Districts III and IV. At times the primary nurse of a district had planning sessions with the associate nurse of the same district. The primary nurse's responsibilities included doing paper work, making telephone calls, pouring medications, and giving "direct" care, that is, giving baths and treatments to some patients in her district. The patient load for each staff member was determined by estimates of the physical and psychosocial care needed by patients. The ratio of staff to patients was juggled daily.

When morning report ended, staff moved quickly to complete the hygienic routines of A.M. care and the 8:00 A.M. and 10:00 A.M. medications. The bustle continued through the morning until A.M. care was finished. Beds were made during and following patients' baths. Those needing assistance were fed breakfast sometime after shift report.

When linen supplies, especially the "big three items," pillowcases, gowns, and towels, were low during the early part of the day shift, the morning baths did not begin smoothly, and tension mounted. All of the nurses became upset. When the laboratory technician arrived late, after 9:10 A.M., the nurses complained aloud in the corridor, because many 7H patients could not eat breakfast until the daily FBS's (fasting blood sugars) were collected.

When 7H ran smoothly, the R.N.'s, the G.N.'s, the L.G.P.N.'s, and the nursing assistants moved in an almost serene fashion from checking patients, to calling on the telephone, to pouring their 10:00 A.M. medications. Nurses joked with each other. When the unit was "jumping," the nurses told anyone who listened.

At times, the extra help provided by the nursing students helped the unit run more smoothly. Students were generally assigned to patient care during the day shift. They gave "complete care" to patients requiring a complete bath, treatments, and medications. Even though the students added to the number of staff and the already crowded conditions of the unit, they helped by doing some of the staff's work, and consequently, the staff were more relaxed and even jocular.

Evening change-of-shift report began almost immediately at 3:30 P.M. Fewer nurses staffed the evening shift, since the busiest part of the twenty-four-hour hospital day was typically during the day shift. At the conclusion of report around 4:15 or 4:30 P.M., the evening shift started slowly. Evening shift nurses made rounds and greeted patients. They gave medications. Dinner was served at 5:20 P.M., and nurses fed patients who needed assistance. Next they went to dinner, leaving the remaining nurses to staff the unit.

A few day shift R.N.'s stayed past 4:00 P.M. to finish tasks for which they felt professionally responsible. All of the day shift L.G.P.N.'s and nursing assistants left 7H promptly at 4:00 P.M.

They [L.G.P.N.'s] are out of here at four, unless something is going on like a code. Even then the L.G.P.N.'s try to leave. I won't leave the orders until the next shift. I wouldn't like anyone to do that to me. [Sarah, R.N.]

Generally, by 5:00 P.M. all day shift nurses had left 7H, except Deidre and Kate, who finished discussions about the management of the unit in their office.

By 5:00 P.M., after dinner, Pamela and Ann, G.N.'s, began pouring 6:00 P.M. medications. Often there were many medications to administer and intravenous (IV) infusions to monitor. This complicated the work of the evening shift nurses. Also, there were usually more visitors during the evening shift. A few resident doctors and staff doctors lingered to check on patients and write in charts.

In addition to the nurses and resident doctors on call, other hospital departments worked during the hours of the evening shift. 7H's medical clerk stayed until 9:30 P.M. The Cardiac Catheterization Lab, the Radiology Department, the Chemistry Lab, and the EKG (electrocardiogram) Lab scheduled staff who worked the late evening hours.

The work of the evening shift (referred to as "3–11") involved monitoring IV's; giving medications, treatments, and P.M. care (usually washing the patient's hands, face, back, and teeth or dentures, and changing or straightening the bed linens); and "taking off" doctors' orders from the charts. The unstated rule of three-to-eleven nurses was: "We'll work together, and at nine o'clock we'll be done" (Ann, G.N.). A few 7H nurses who rotated to this shift from the day shift agreed that this rule did not always apply. They found it difficult to work with the two permanent evening graduate nurses because of personality conflicts.

As one R.N. remarked, "Hospitals wake up early, because they never fall completely asleep." After night report at midnight or soon after, the night shift R.N. made rounds on all 7H patients, Districts I through IV. The L.G.P.N.'s, Mary and Denise, checked patients in their districts, I and II, and III and IV, respectively. Miriam, the permanent night nurse, was occasionally joined by a G.N. or another R.N. when the floor was "heavier." Most patients were asleep during this shift. After one peaceful night Miriam commented, "They're quiet for me at night, what can I tell you?"

The night nurses used a flashlight to check sleeping patients' breathing, IV fluid levels, and dressing sites. They bathed incontinent patients as necessary, checked vital signs, completed treatments, ordered medications, and prepared patients for diagnostic tests they would undergo after daybreak.

Incontinent patients, "coding" patients (those patients who suffered cardiorespiratory arrest), patients who "went bad," and confused patients added to the work of the staff by stepping up the pace. For example, once after a particularly noisy and hectic night, Miriam moaned as she finished writing nurses' notes in a chart and left the desk at the nurses' station. When she returned to the station after checking a confused patient, she muttered, "I give up, I give up! A full moon—everybody has been howling all night." Miriam then listened to the voices of two patients vivaciously engaged in conversation and smiled resignedly. She stopped a medical resident who passed the station and reported a patient's elevated temperature. The doctor said, "This is the last time I'll get towels here [for his shower]. It's been crazy." His response to the night that he had just spent confirmed Miriam's response to her experience that night.

NURSES' STATION

The nurses' station was located at the center of the unit, adjacent to the utility room, and visible to patients, visitors, and staff and all other hospital personnel having business on 7H.

Medical clerks, one or two at a time, sat at the front desk of the station, behind a chest-high counter. The counter was always deliberately littered with essential chart forms, booklets, and other printed material important to the unit's work flow, such as, specimen slips, the sign-in sheet, and a telephone directory for patient units.

Along with the utility room, the nurses' station was the central coordination point of the activities of 7H. Hospital personnel, visitors, and patients went to the desk for help, information, and directions. Doctors' orders were written and transcribed there. Telephone calls were placed to answer questions, to identify, and to resolve problems. Although some calls were personal—for example, a nurse might call home to check on a sick child—most were focused by the business at hand, 7H patients. A bulletin board on the wall close to the counter helped the medical clerks remind nursing staff of incoming admissions or transfers to the unit. The nurses' station was also the central depot for incoming and outgoing mail.

When staff walked through the entrance of the station, they faced shelves that held loose-leaf binders containing patients' charts. Anyone could see the room number and door-bed or window-bed designation on the binders, since the print was large. Doctors and nursing staff repeatedly looked for charts missing from the shelves.

Beneath the chart shelves and to the right of the counter stood two medication carts, pushed away from the traffic of the station but always in clear view. Prescription and controlled drugs were kept in the lower drawer of one of the carts. A suction machine and cardiac resuscitation board were stored under the shelves, to the left of the medication carts. This equipment was present in anticipation of a cardiac or respiratory arrest. A locked drug box was also stored on one of the shelves to be used during these emergencies.

On the front wall of the station, next to the utility room and above the medication carts, was an open plastic box where nurses stored drug order slips and narcotic sheets. The primary nurse for each district taped the patient classification sheet on this wall; this reminded day shift nurses to complete the form used to project staffing assignments for 7H nurses.

Along the front of the station to the left of the entrance was a long desk, continuous with the desk behind the front counter. Chairs were pulled close to this L-shaped desk when personnel wrote in charts, filled out slips, talked on the telephone, and answered questions of other staff, patients, visitors, and hospital personnel.

The medical clerks' territory was the desk immediately behind the counter at the front of the station. From this command post clerical staff telephoned hospital departments and doctors, completed paper work relevant to patient charts, and pleasantly greeted anyone who passed the station. (If people were not pleasant, the clerks commented.) Seldom did anyone but the clerks sit in the chairs at the front of the station. Other 7H staff sat in the chairs after the evening clerk left at 9:30 p. m. The remaining chairs in the station were used more by doctors than by nursing staff. There were two telephones in the nurses' station and one on the wall to the left just outside the station.

A wall divided the front part of the station from the back. This wall was originally constructed so that nurses could pour medications free from distractions. However, use of the medication cart as a method of storage and administration of medications changed the area's function to a "nourishment" area. Stock medications were locked in cabinets and other supplies including wound dressings, paper goods, physical examination equipment, food and special nourishments for patients, refrigerated medications and intravenous bags, paper supplies, and nurses' purses and lunches were kept in this back area of the nurses' station.

The sink in the back was used chiefly for handwashing, but nurses also made tea or coffee for patients and themselves at a special hot water tap there. 7H staff stood in this narrow area to drink a quick cup of coffee or tea around 10:30 a.m. Doctors and lab technicians also stopped for a quick, standing-room-only drink of juice, tea, or coffee. As staff took short breaks, they looked out the window to the world outside the hospital.

During the day shift, staff scattered charts on the desk of the nurses' station. Charts that were being worked on were piled high on the front desk. There were drawers beneath the desk that contained paper supplies, old patient charts, and hospital manuals. A small filing cabinet beneath the side desk held medication information used by nurses to teach patients. Above the side desk were shelves holding patient chart forms and textbooks, log books for staff meetings, a worn medical dictionary, the P.D.R. (*Physicians' Desk Reference*), and the *Hospital Policy and Procedure Manual*.

The walls of the nurses' station bore two bulletin boards, covered with printed information and an occasional thank you card from a patient or his family. The printed information included notices about meetings or policy and procedure changes, time charts, and sign-in sheets. Memos notifying staff of changes in departmental services were taped onto the wall. The medical clerks created a "look twice" section where they posted warnings about patients with similar names, to protect them from hospital errors.

The Addressograph stamper, the Addressograph plate holder, cubbyholes for lab slips, and other clerical supplies competed for space at the station. So did the ever-present patient charts which awaited doctors' orders, notes from nursing staff and other hospital personnel, or checks by staff members interested in changes in doctors' orders, taking orders off, and acting on orders. Frequently the station was cluttered and crowded during the day shift. On evenings and nights paper clutter decreased and personnel were sparse.

The following is an example of a typical five-minute period at the station during the day shift.

It is 9:15 A.M., July 27, at the nurses' station. Sharon and Colleen, both G.N.'s, talk on telephones about the transfer of a patient from 7H to a rehabilitation hospital and about a chest X-ray scheduled for another patient. A medical clerk stamps laboratory slips using the Addressograph plate. Another medical clerk, Jennifer, "takes off" doctors' orders from patients' charts, transfers them to the nursing Kardex, and completes laboratory and other diagnostic department forms. She places the charts in the clearly labeled chart holder on the side desk, ready for G.N.'s or R.N.'s to review and check transcriptions of the most recent doctors' orders. Sharon moves from the telephone to a patient's room and returns to the station. She telephones to schedule a carotid flow study. Dan, a laboratory technician, stands at the counter in front of the station. He sorts and labels lab slips and tubes so that he can select the correct tube for the patient for whom a specific blood study is ordered. Deidre, the nurse manager, brings a new G.N. to meet her coworkers. Camille, an L.G.P.N., moves back and forth from the station to her patients' rooms. She stops to fix a cup of coffee for one patient and laughs softly that he was "zonked" (pretending that he was asleep) because he does not want to go to a nursing home.

UTILITY ROOM

The utility room was adjacent to the nurses' station (see Figure 2). It was roughly halfway between the last patient rooms on either end of the unit. To the left of the door was a small linen closet, to the right a supply closet (see Figure 3).

Off to the left inside the utility room was a bathroom, frequented by the nursing staff and a host of hospital personnel including doctors, escort staff, and respiratory therapists. The utility room was cramped, disorderly, and very often dirty. At times the floor was sticky and littered with trash and dust.

An open bedpan hopper, bedpan sterilizer, and cabinets in the back left corner were permanent fixtures of the room. Two trash cans, one for "regular" trash and another, red, for "contaminated" trash only, sat in the back right corner. A movable cart temporarily used for equipment and supplies that did not fit into the cabinets, five to six chairs and a round table, several portable IV poles, a scale for weighing patients, and a bedside commode cluttered the small room. Miscellaneous equipment occupied the corners of the utility room and included boxes and eggcrate (rippled foam) mattresses for patients' beds. The disorderliness was attributable to the limited storage space on 7H. Since the nursing staff had little space to write nurses' notes or take a break in relaxing, spacious surroundings, they used the utility room and tolerated the disorder and dirt.

Two bulletin boards and a small green chalk board hung on opposite walls. Messages to the staff, including policy and procedure changes, equipment information, an ostomy brochure, a stoma measurer for ostomy size, specific precautions from the hospital's infection control nurses, an article on hemolytic anemia, and memos from the nurse who was the patient education coordinator, and similar materials were posted on the crowded bulletin boards.

A memo to the nursing staff from Deidre, about meetings with the psychiatric nurse clinical specialist stood out on one bulletin board. This was one of the newer memos posted. Most were yellowed with time and cigarette smoke. On one wall patient education pamphlets were inserted into plastic slots. Pamphlet topics included diabetes, hypertension, lung problems, heart attack, lupus, surgery, and ostomies. Other signs taped to the wall spelled out R.N. responsibilities for equipment and procedures such as hyperalimentation, Salem sump tube, and Pleur-Evac operating instructions.

A sewage odor permeated the utility room from July through October. The odor came and went as hoppers were flushed in the

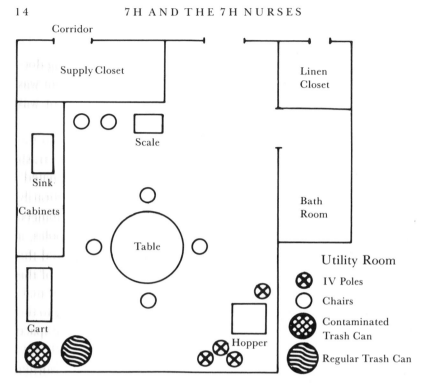

Figure 3. Utility room.

units above 7H. As the hopper bubbled the odor spread throughout the room. Nursing staff concentrated on morning report or
writing their notes on the charts despite the odor. They complained about it, but the plumbing problem was not solved for
months. Deidre felt that the cramped space and the dirt and disorder in 7H contributed to low morale and low self-esteem of the
nurses.

The following entry in the 7H nurses' log book (where staff
meeting minutes were kept) for October 5 confirmed the state of
the unit:

> This unit is a mess. People use things and don't replace them. Don't pick
> up after themselves. This is our unit—we must take care of it and if we
> see someone being sloppy—we should go to that person and tell them
> about the problem. Districts [nurses] now have specific jobs—such as
> cleaning utility room, restocking med cart, etc.

Other comments during change-of-shift report echoed the feelings recorded in the minutes. One nurse said, "That's disgusting," as the hopper erupted during morning shift report. Deidre responded to her frustration several times by taking the cleaning of the unit into her own hands. One day she cleaned the utility room; it was more of a disaster than usual. She found trash in back of the trash cans. The floor man from housekeeping could not have swept in days. He usually swept only around the table in the utility room.

Functions of the Utility Room

7H's nursing staff used the utility room to take coffee breaks or time out from nursing activities, to read charts and articles about patient problems, to look up medications, to take coffee or cigarette breaks, to wait for change-of-shift report to begin, to converse, and to complain.

Periodically the smoke was so thick in the utility room that the nonsmoking staff complained about it. Smoke drifted into the hall during the heaviest smoking times. Since the small window by the hopper provided inadequate ventilation, smoke odor permeated the clothes of all who lingered in the utility room when the smokers were there.

When staff waited in the utility room for report to begin they exchanged accounts of patients' experiences in the hospital or on 7H. For example, Marie, an L.G.P.N., discussed a patient who had "coded" the previous day. The woman, who died, was a former 7H patient. Marie fondly and sadly remembered the patient and her son. "She had a large decubitus [bedsore]. When she went home from 7H, her family knew that she would be in the hospital again."

Most of the time, change in shift took place in the utility room. When there was one R.N. on at night, all four district reports were conducted in the utility room. When there were two primary nurses (R.N.'s) on at night, the reports were given in Deidre's office and in the utility room. Occasionally, the report was given in an office/lab room down the hall from the unit. Because of the limited space in 7H, nurses used space wherever they could find it for their activities and discussions.

Conversations about the nurses' personal lives frequently took place in the utility room, but these chats did not last for long. Staff relaxed for a minute and discussed a new dress pattern, buying yarn, or upcoming holiday plans. Often the staff left coffee or a cigarette unfinished in order to complete nursing care in a patient's room.

The quietest time for the utility room during the day shift was between 8:45 A.M. and 11 A.M. Then staff were busy giving patients clean towels and washcloths for bathing and clean gowns, helping patients bathe, changing beds, administering medications, requesting diagnostic studies, and helping patients eat breakfast by "setting them up" or feeding them. One at a time the nurses might slip into the bathroom or utility room or sit down for coffee. No nurse sat in the utility room very long during a shift unless she was charting nurses' notes or eating lunch.

Staff often complained in the utility room. For example, one day when Marie sat at the table to complete nursing histories with Loretta, a G.N., both complained as they discussed their reponsibility. If the nursing history was not finished by twenty-four hours after a patient's admission to the unit, it became more and more difficult to complete. The policy stated that when a patient was transferred from one unit to another in the hospital, the nurses on the original unit could call the nurses on the unit of admission to finish the nursing care history. This transfer of responsibility did not happen often, but Loretta was annoyed that she had to complete histories that had been started but not finished by other staff members.

Staff also reminisced about 7H patients who had been discharged. Once Marie and Dotty, another L.G.P.N., talked about former or discharged 7H patients. "This hospital is like a revolving door. People are just looking for things so that they'll get back in." They discussed a discharged patient who refused his medications. Dotty remembered that she had asked him why he was in the hospital if he wasn't going to take his medications. "I won't force you, but why stay in the hospital?" Dotty had been blunt with this patient and reported to Marie with some satisfaction that he took his "'meds,' at least that day."

The nurses often consumed coffee and cigarettes as they charted and calculated the patient acuity levels. Occasionally they bought lunch from street vendors outside the hospital and ate in the utility room. One nurse commented that when she ate a sandwich in the utility room, "It's like eating in a toilet." The nurses tolerated the conditions with long-suffering sarcasm, knowing that 7H was targeted for renovation in the next few years.

CONDITION OF THE UNIT

Deidre admitted that 7H was dirty, but, she said, "It's 100 percent improved," and added, about one housekeeping worker, "I had to threaten her with going to the head of housekeeping." Dust and small pieces of paper were still visible in the corners of the nurses' station, the utility room, and patient rooms. The floors needed to be mopped. Spraying and cleaning had failed to eradicate the small roaches that persistently ran around the floor of the nourishment area. Nursing staff tolerated them. They were careful to cover candy or baked goods left on the counter in the back of the station. But at times the roaches seemed to be winning, as they charged the covered food.

OUTSIDERS' VIEW OF 7H

Carol, an R.N. from the "p.r.n. [as needed] pool" (nurses who moved from unit to unit to supplement low staffing levels), was assigned to 7H for several months. Carol said that 7H has had a "lot of problems, a lot":

> This is the only medical floor with only one narcotic drawer [in the medicine cart]. The floor was a mess when I got here. That's why I was put here. It was totally disorganized, a disaster area. It still is. An example, one of the most cluttered utility rooms in the hospital. I knew Deidre on 8W, which was all female at one time and is now leaning to an oncology floor. That floor was a zoo; you never knew what was going on. With Deidre, this floor will be organized. The head nurse [before Deidre] was nice but weak. Before that the head nurse got pregnant and left. . . . Everyone knows that the staffing is poor and that the floor is disorganized. I know Deidre. I think she is good and I expect the floor to stabilize. I was asked to be part of the [permanent] staff, but refused. I wanted to stay part of the p.r.n. pool. When Deidre came, I left the floor. The biggest complaint before Deidre came was scheduling. The last nurse manager had problems.

Carol's comments reflected a hope that the new nurse manager would restore some order to the unit and allay the anger that the nursing staff had felt over unfair scheduling of work hours.

Another 7H outsider, Tressa, described 7H. Tressa's position as a psychiatric clinical specialist enabled her to compare the unit to all the other patient units in the hospital.

> There is a lot of change here. One nurse manager left one and a half years ago. A nurse manager who had the floor closed was not perceived as good. Kate [the assistant nurse manager] has had problems. Deidre, the "hospital hot shot," has high standards. No one has enforced standards on this floor. No permanent R.N. staff, no sense of loyalty, no consistent message from R.N. staff to another. Floats [p.r.n. pool nurses] are competent. L.G.P.N.'s and nurses' aides are the core of the unit. They think, "These new people will leave as others did before."

When Deidre came in as the new nurse manager, she used a "pieces approach" to straighten out 7H's problems. "I wanted to work on the whole, primary nursing [beginning another method of nursing care], but I was forced to work on the pieces." Patiently the new nurse manager dealt with the instability of 7H that was acknowledged by both outsiders and insiders.

7H: The Work

Each shift the most experienced R.N. divided patients among the staff and wrote assignments with an erasable magic marker on the primary board. The primary board was fastened to a wall in the middle of the unit, opposite the nurses' station. Nursing staff names were written beside patient names and room numbers. The names of doctors assigned to patients also appeared on the primary board; medical teams were color-coded by magic markers. All primary board information was written in large print, so that hospital staff could easily identify staff who were caring for 7H patients. The distribution of patients on the primary board helped to organize the day, evening, and night shifts. Nurses knew their own as well as other nurses' assigned patients and the nurses working with them in one of the unit's four districts. Nurses often recorded breaks and lunch times on the primary board.

The unit's patients were divided differently from shift to shift. Nevertheless, nursing responsibility flowed smoothly from nurse to nurse as district assignments were made. Beginning with change-of-shift report, the work of each shift progressed smoothly, barring emergencies. The cycle of work after report included medications, treatments, baths, other direct patient care activities, paper work, and diagnostic test preparations continued.

On the day shift, two nursing staff were assigned to each of the four districts, one primary nurse, an R.N. or G.N., and one L.G.P.N. or nursing assistant. The number of acutely ill patients influenced the distribution of staff. More nurses were given to heavy districts. A G.N. with a few months' nursing experience or a seasoned R.N. was in charge of a district as primary nurse. Each primary nurse worked with an associate nurse, either an L.G.P.N. or a nursing assistant. Since there were eight patients in each of the four districts (thirty-two patients was the maximum unit census), each associate nurse cared for five patients and the primary nurse, three patients. The primary nurse gave medications to patients more often than did the associate nurse, handled many telephone calls to doctors and hospital departments, and processed a large amount of paper work. Generally, primary nurses distributed staff among the patient load according to whether the patient was a "self" bath or a "complete." Patients who required a complete bath were often the sickest.

Unanticipated patient problems arose during the shift and affected the division of work. Patients' conditions worsened and unit activity accelerated. Nurses answered questions from doctors and other hospital personnel. Patients left and returned from hospital departments accompanied by escort staff. Patients were admitted to the unit and were discharged either to nursing homes, extended care facilities, or their own homes. Resident and attending doctors and medical students made rounds, leaving orders in their wakes. Central Supply personnel transported hospital equipment to the unit and removed it after use.

As soon as shift reports and planning sessions were completed, primary and associate nurses scrambled to begin the work of the shift. If the unit was considered short staffed by the Nursing Office, or if Deidre or Kate asked the Nursing Office in person or by telephone for extra help, an additional nurse might be "pulled" to 7H to give medications. This extra help relieved primary nurses of each district and allowed the new graduates to organize other nursing functions. Few nurses were reassigned to 7H once G.N.'s became more confident.

The nurses saw patients frequently in the early part of the day shift because of bathing activities and because medications were given between 8:00 and 8:30 A.M. and between 9:30 and 10:30 A.M. In addition, contacts were frequent when nurses collected different specimens for laboratory analysis and prepared patients to leave the unit for diagnostic tests. Later in the day shift nurses moved patients in and out of bed, gave more medications around noon, carried out treatments, and measured vital signs. Newly admitted patients stimulated more work as doctors' orders were transcribed and executed.

When nurses went to lunch or for a coffee break, or for other reasons left the unit, they asked other nurses to "cover" their patients. Associate nurses and primary nurses within a district usually cared for each other's patients. The nurses scheduled their lunchtimes so that, if possible, there were nurses on the unit who knew the patients of each district.

Whenever 7H nurses "reported off" and "on" the unit, they exchanged information about the current status of patients. For example, Beth, an R.N., reported off to Marie, an L.G.P.N., before leaving for lunch. She warned Marie about a patient who had recently returned to the unit after a brachial arteriogram and reminded her to check vital signs and watch the arterial puncture site for bleeding. Beth also told Marie of another patient's tachycardia (rapid heart rate) and added that he had received medications, digoxin (a cardiac drug) and Lasix (a diuretic), which were already working. Nursing responsibilities were maintained shift to shift with seasoned R.N.'s answering for less experienced nurses and for the L.G.P.N.'s and nursing assistants. The most experienced R.N. on the day shift oversaw the nursing work of G.N.'s, L.G.P.N.'s, and nursing assistants. The G.N.'s on the evening shift did not usually work with a seasoned R.N. The evening supervisor supplied them with help and information when necessary. Miriam, an R.N. of two years' experience, was often alone on the night shift with two L.G.P.N.'s. She relied on the night supervisor for solving unusual problems.

When day shift officially ended after evening shift report, the two G.N.'s working that evening made rounds with associate nurses who were either L.G.P.N.'s or nursing assistants. Each G.N. and L.G.P.N. or nursing assistant greeted patients and their visiting families in their rooms and mentioned that they would care for the patient that evening. The G.N.'s checked the IV fluid remaining in the patient's IV bag to compare the amount of fluid left with the amount identified during report. The nurses noted which patients were not in their beds or rooms and checked whether they were having a diagnostic test in another hospital department. At the same time both nurses made specific observations on patients, such as checking the fingernail beds (circulation) of a patient with a recent skin graft and heavily bandaged arms, or the breathing of a patient who had had a tracheostomy (artificial opening into the airway with tube insertion). Ann, a G.N., admitted that she especially checks on "whether the patients are breathing and mention[s] that I'll be on [duty] during the evening."

During the night shift, Miriam, the permanent night shift R.N., or a substitute R.N. made rounds on all 7H patients, the whole floor. The nurse used a flashlight, since the corridor lights and many of the lights in the patients' rooms were off. Two L.G.P.N.'s made rounds on the patients in their assigned districts. They also used flashlights to observe the breathing patterns of sleeping patients, IV fluids levels, or postcardiac catheterization or postoperative dressing sites. Most of the patients were asleep. Those awake might ask a question, request a pain medication, or greet the night nurse.

Frequent observations on patients continued throughout each shift as nurses checked IV's or bathed, medicated, and comforted their patients. Nurses continued to share nursing work and information about patients throughout the twenty-four-hour nursing day.

THE NURSING STAFF

From July to April the permanent nursing staff of 7H consisted of twenty-nine people classified according to different nursing categories. The six R.N. staff consisted of Deidre, nurse manager; Kate, assistant nurse manager; Miriam, primary nurse or charge nurse on night shift; Beth, primary nurse on day shift; Sarah, per diem nurse and primary nurse on day shift (more or less permanently assigned to 7H); and Tammy, primary nurse on day shift.

The nine G.N. staff included Colleen, Sharon, Ann, Pamela, Loretta, Chris, Suzanne, Cecile, and Meredith. Some of the new nurses came to the unit in May or June; others started late in the summer and in the early fall. All graduate nurses became R.N.'s after passing state board licensing examinations while working on 7H. Most passed by mid-September. The few who failed the examination at first passed the February examination.

The eleven L.G.P.N. staff included Marie, Dotty, Camille, Denise, Nancy, Mary, Wanda, Pat, Elsie, Leslie, and Mabel. Marie, Dotty, Camille, and Elsie worked the day shift most often. Nancy and Wanda worked the evening shift, and Denise and Mary, night shift. Leslie and Mabel were permanent staff for a short time after leaving the CCU and were awaiting positions in the cardiac step-down unit, then under construction.

Rachel, Caroline, and Betty were nurse's aides or nursing assistants for 7H. Kathy was a student nurse associate who worked during the summer and weekends as her college schedule permitted. Demographic information on the 7H nursing staff, excluding the student nurse associate, is included in Table 1.

Deidre, R.N.—Nurse Manager

Deidre was born in Ireland and later emigrated to the United States. She began her nursing career as a nurse's aide (two years), and an L.G.P.N. (five years), and then she worked as an R.N. for thirteen years after graduating from an associate degree nursing program. Deidre's association with the hospital began when she was hospitalized in the Intensive Care Unit following a laminectomy. After her recovery she started working in the hospital as an assistant head nurse on another medical unit. Deidre came to 7H knowing that the unit was "a shambles." Morale was at a low point. The former nurse manager had permitted work schedule inequities to persist. Deidre brought hope to the long-tenured core of 7H staff, Marie and Camille, the L.G.P.N.'s, and Caroline, the nursing assistant. Kate, an assistant nurse manager for over two years, had been unsuccessful in reducing unit problems.

The law of nursing for Deidre was, "Pitch in and provide the best care that you can. You have to do the best you can." Deidre expressed her feelings about nursing as she told of a patient who had recuperated after being shot in the head during a robbery. "Inch by inch she progressed during a long hospital stay. She came back later to the hospital for a cranial plate insertion. Two years later she returned to the hospital to have a baby. Now, there're the rewards of nursing." Her sense of responsibility was so strong, that during the night she once drove to the hospital in the middle of a snowstorm. "My husband thought I was crazy but admired my determination." Deidre frequently gave A.M. care or distributed medications when staffing was poor.

Deidre took her responsibility as nurse manager seriously. There were occasions when she did not sleep because she was worrying about 7H errors. Her first concern was for the patients. She missed the control that went with the role of head nurse after the hospital introduced the position of nurse manager. She felt that she had been better able as head nurse to delegate responsibility and evaluate nursing care. Now as nurse manager, she regretted the frequent management meetings, patient care problems resulting from insufficient staff, and work of evaluating G.N.'s and other nursing staff.

Deidre enjoyed caring for patients and often gave direct patient care when she saw the need. She confessed that her tendency "to do" might hinder the development of G.N.'s, since they needed to demonstrate their developing abilities. Other staff respected this tendency. Another R.N. proudly described Deidre to a doctor, saying that Deidre "does everything a nurse does." A medical clerk pointed out to the same doctor that Deidre, "pinch hits when the staff and patients need it."

Considered by many to be a hospital "hot shot" with very high standards, Deidre came to 7H as a favor to the associate vice presi-

TABLE 1. 7H NURSING STAFF: DEMOGRAPHIC DATA

Name	Age	Sex	Race	Nursing Category	Basic Program	Religion	Predominant Shift Worked	Years in Nursing	Time on 7H
Deidre	38	F	W	R.N., Nurse Manager	Nurse's Aide to L.G.P.N. to Associate Degree	Roman Catholic	Days	20	10 months
Kate	28	F	W	R.N., Assistant Nurse Manager	Diploma	Roman Catholic	Days	7	2 years, 4 months
Miriam	25	F	W	R.N., Primary Nurse/Charge Nurse	Bachelor of Science	Jewish	Nights	2	2 years
Beth	52	F	W	R.N., Primary Nurse/Preceptor	Diploma	Episcopalian	Days	9	1.5 years
Sarah	35	F	W	R.N., Per Diem Primary Nurse/ Preceptor	Diploma	Jewish	Days	11	9 months
Tammy	26	F	B	R.N., Primary Nurse	L.G.P.N. to Associate Degree	Baptist	Days	4	4 years
Colleen	24	F	W	G.N. → R.N., Primary Nurse	Nurse's Aide to L.G.P.N. to Associate Degree	Roman Catholic	Days	6	1 year
Sharon	24	F	B	G.N. → R.N., Primary Nurse	Bachelor of Science	Baptist	Days	1	1 year
Ann	29	F	B	G.N. → R.N., Primary Nurse	Associate Degree	Baptist	Evenings	1	1 year
Pamela	24	F	B	G.N. → R.N., Primary Nurse	Bachelor of Science	Baptist	Evenings	1.5	1.5 years
Loretta	23	F	B	G.N. → R.N., Primary Nurse	Diploma	Baptist	Evenings	1	9 months
Chris	22	F	W	G.N. → R.N., Primary Nurse	Bachelor of Science	Roman Catholic	Days	1	1 year

Name			Age	G.N. → Primary Nurse	Bachelor of Science	Roman Catholic	Days	0.33	4 months
Meredith	F	W	45	G.N. → Primary Nurse	Bachelor of Science	Roman Catholic	Days	0.33	4 months
Marie	F	B	46	L.G.P.N., Associate Nurse	Diploma	Methodist	Days	14	14 years
Dotty	F	W	54	L.G.P.N., Associate Nurse	Diploma	Roman Catholic	Days	2	2 years
Camille	F	B	30	L.G.P.N., Associate Nurse	Waiver	Baptist	Days	25	25 years
Denise	F	B	33	L.G.P.N., Associate Nurse	Diploma	Muslim	Nights		3 years
Nancy	F	B		L.G.P.N., Associate Nurse	Diploma	Buddhist	Evenings	6	5 years
Mary	F	B		L.G.P.N., Associate Nurse	Diploma	Baptist	Nights		
Wanda	F	B	42	L.G.P.N., Associate Nurse	Diploma	Baptist	Evenings	20	3 years
Elsie	F	B	29	L.G.P.N., Associate Nurse	Diploma	Pentecostal	Days	5	3 years
Leslie	F	W	33	L.G.P.N., Associate Nurse	Diploma	Roman Catholic	Days and evenings		3 months
Mabel	F	B	46	L.G.P.N., Associate Nurse	Diploma	Methodist	Days and evenings	28	4 months
Rachel	F	B	56	Nursing Assistant	Public School Program, Certificate	Baptist	Days	14	14 years
Caroline	F	B	49	Nursing Assistant	Hospital Program, Certificate	Baptist	Days	24	24 years
Betty	F	W	59	Nursing Assistant	Hospital Program, Certificate	Greek Orthodox	Evenings	14	10 years

Arrows indicate that during the course of data collection (1 year), the G.N.s passed the State Board of Nurse Examiners' licensing examination. All of the names are pseudonyms.

dent for nursing. Deidre promised that she would stay from June to February of the next year but ended her employment at the hospital in late April, two months longer than promised.

Initially Deidre seemed very discouraged by 7H. She felt that the high noise level of the floor was "unbelievable." She thought that the inadequate, disorderly space demoralized the nurses and contributed to their inability to value what they did. She instituted "acknowledgment meetings," where she encouraged nursing staff to take credit for helping patients and fellow staff members.

Deidre described her recently assumed nurse manager position on 7H:

> Mostly I manage incident reports. Time [scheduling enough staff to cover the patients] is erratic; over 80 percent of my time is spent finding staff to be here. There is no "professional" nursing. I am working on safe care with meds and treatments. They [the staff] are only interested in getting the bath done. There are a lot of missed treatments. The staff is just getting to know me. There is some backlash or muttering after I come down on them. . . . One patient didn't have a [nurse's] note [written on the chart] for eight days!

Later, Deidre admitted:

> [The people in] the Nursing Office only look at the numbers [of staff scheduled to work on a particular shift]. I work hard on staffing and keep in touch with the per diems. Today the Nursing Office pulled staff scheduled to work four to twelve and told them to report to another unit.

When coming into the utility room one day in early August to discuss the district assignments for the following three days, Deidre commented on staffing problems and acknowledged with chagrin that management "isn't like the textbooks." She hoped to staff the unit sufficiently to insure that there would be enough nurses working to provide "continuity of care." Deidre stated ruefully that she "spent the summer looking for help" and "was operating on faith all summer" juggling the permanent and p.r.n. pool staff so that patients were covered.

Deidre had been plagued by the staffing problem. When the unit was short-staffed, patients and nurses suffered. At one point in September, Deidre resorted to creating a new assignment sheet to improve the ratio between staff and patients. She completed the form for use the following Monday. Later as she awaited the staff's reaction she "wondered whether the sheet was insulting." Using the time or work assignment schedule as a guide, she assigned one R.N. to each district and listed the number of patients both for the R.N. primary nurse and for the L.G.P.N. or nursing assistant who served as associate nurse. Clearly Deidre felt this designation of patient assignments to the staff was necessary, since the L.G.P.N.'s and aides had been complaining that the number of patients assigned to them was excessive. The new R.N. staff were apologetic to their associate nurses about the change in patient load, but they felt relief about having less direct patient care to deal with. Some of their other duties included ordering equipment and scheduling and preparating patients for diagnostic tests. The assignment sheet dramatized some of Deidre's management problems. The L.G.P.N.'s resistance to a change in assignment emphasized the existing L.G.P.N.-R.N. conflict, which was illustrated by the following L.G.P.N. law: "R.N.'s have to get their hands dirty. They have to get into the shit to prove themselves to the L.G.P.N.'s and nursing assistants."

As the nurse manager, Deidre's responsibility to 7H required a twenty-four-hour, seven-days-a-week commitment. Deidre soon became aware when the staff had problems on any of the three shifts. She directly questioned the staff involved in any current problems in an open, yet firm manner. When errors increased and patient safety was jeopardized, she was like a persistent bloodhound, eager to document the problem by witnessing the staff's performance at work, and working thereafter to correct the situation. For example, she brought Pamela back to day shift from evenings for closer supervision by a more abundant R.N. staff because of her persistent difficulties in organizing patient care.

In late October, Deidre had difficulty with the clinical performance of Denise, one of the L.G.P.N.'s on night shift. Denise was sullen and tended to make her own, arbitrary, decisions about what needed to be done. Even her fellow L.G.P.N., Pat, hinted that Denise was difficult to work with. After talking to Denise about her concerns and those of Miriam, the night nurse, Deidre decided to work the night shift with Denise as her associate nurse.

Deidre became the primary nurse and Denise the associate nurse of Districts III and IV. Deidre indicated that she wanted Denise to see her as a working nurse. They worked successfully together through the night. Deidre wanted the hall lights on at 4:45 A.M. to do the baths of the "preop" (preoperative) patients, which the night nurses called "morning care." Although Denise did not want the lights on, Deidre insisted, because she "had a sense" that something might go "wrong." Denise and Pat divided the patients by assigning themselves to rooms. By the time Deidre reached the last room she found a patient with diffuse chest pain, neck pain, and diaphoresis (profuse perspiration). The patient had not bothered to call a nurse. Nurses moved rapidly to evaluate the patient's chest pain since MI was a likely possibility. A medical resident was summoned. EKG's (electrocardiograms) were taken and IV's and medications started.

Deidre talked about how her preoccupation with this very ill patient enabled her to understand the difference between the role of an R.N. and the role of a L.G.P.N. Denise kept doing the tasks throughout the chest pain episode. Deidre planned ahead, responding to her premonition. This helped her and the doctor to stabilize the acutely ill patient. Deidre acknowledged that L.G.P.N.'s did deal with more "dirty work" than the R.N.'s, but the R.N.'s had to prove themselves equally capable of doing dirty work and capable of much more. R.N.'s had a more global, less task-oriented picture of the unit than did the L.G.P.N.'s.

Deidre mentioned that the L.G.P.N.'s and nursing assistants were more time bound by the hours of the shift and the limits of their responsibility. The R.N.'s stayed to finish their work. "Yesterday both Tammy and Sarah stayed overtime," completing their responsibility to patients before they left.

When Kate took a short vacation in late September, Deidre felt her absence acutely. Managerial work piled up as Deidre filled in when patients' needs, an insufficient number of staff, and G.N. inexperience combined to create potentially unsafe nursing care conditions. In February when Kate decided to leave 7H and her position as assistant nurse manager for a staff nurse position in the CCU, Deidre worried. When Deidre had her days off, no middle management level R.N. would be present to answer the questions of the staff. Deidre left a list of her whereabouts on days off so that staff could call her when in need.

Because of the poor state in which Deidre found the 7H staff at the beginning of her tenure as nurse manager, and because of her swift realization that some of the 7H nursing care was unsafe, Deidre saw herself as a dictator. She was authoritarian periodically, out of necessity, but regretted that she had to be. She rationalized her policies of standard-setting by referring to the rules, policies, procedures, and job descriptions published by the hospital.

Another time, while Deidre cleaned the utility room, which was more of a disaster than usual, she complained that the utility aide and housekeeping workers did not do their jobs adequately. "Maybe I'm going to become a dictator," she said. And later: "As it is, I act like a glorified nurse's aide, picking up after everybody." Referring to the G.N.'s she added, "We're still in our infancy here." In time Deidre felt more hopeful about 7H. She pointed out that staffing patterns had improved and that therefore more R.N. positions had opened up. But she remained fatalistic:

> New graduates come for a year, and they go to the suburban, smaller hospitals. They don't have time to integrate within the institution. They burn out faster. The average day and the amount of expectations—we do set them up to be discouraged. . . . Look at this Performance Review [R.N. performance evaluation form]. I think it's a lot. The form is very complex; it is used at six months and at a year [to evaluate the new nurse]. Kristen [the clinical director of nursing of 7H and other units and Deidre's immediate superior] has me doing the evaluations on the new graduates three months after employment to give the nurses an idea of how she is [*sic*] progressing.

By October, Deidre saw more improvement, but problems continued. When her morale was lowest, she sought comfort in her previous successes in nursing and took pleasure in describing the gradual improvement of another unit under her management. Hospital staff attributed the success of that unit to Deidre. "They didn't need me at the end. They could solve problems independently." She was especially proud of the breast cancer program she developed and the strong patient education focus of the unit. Deidre, "the hospital hot shot," had high standards for herself. She measured her success by the improving level of nursing care given by her staff.

In addition to the week-to-week problem of staffing 7H with nurses around the clock, patient scheduling problems thwarted Deidre. She described how in a single day one patient might be scheduled for laboratory studies as well as an EEG (electroencephalogram) and a radiologic study. No department other than nursing considered the patient's reaction to these studies. Each day primary nurses moved rapidly from report to check on the patients and next telephoned the radiology department to determine when a study was scheduled and whether a laboratory "slip went down" to request a blood specimen. If time conflicts arose among the different diagnostic tests, the primary nurse had to absorb the problem, getting caught between departments that vied for the patients at the same time. In addition, doctors who ordered diagnostic tests became irate when scheduling problems inconvenienced them. If a diagnostic test was cancelled because of scheduling conflicts and a patient had to stay an extra hospital day, the hospital could be refused financial reimbursement for that day.

Along with the nurses, the medical clerks were annoyed by the problems associated with scheduling diagnostic tests:

> We have trouble with same day scheduling of diagnostic studies. All of them [doctors] try to get the patient scheduled in one week. Utilization Review Staff checks charts, asks questions about diagnostic tests, and calls the attending [physician] to warn him or her. Benefits are cut off if hospital bed [use] is not justified by testing.

Nurses and medical clerks realized the importance of diagnostic tests for the patient. But it was difficult for new G.N.'s to master the interpersonal and logistical skills of scheduling. Deidre was aware of their lack of confidence and worked to help them. Sometimes, in order to relieve the work load of the G.N., she would "do" a district or be the primary nurse for eight patients in four semiprivate rooms. When she cared for the patients on one district, she had trouble staying in the district because of her more global view of 7H. She felt committed to and responsible for the total unit.

Deidre was anxious for my opinion about whether the unit had improved during my time on 7H. "Was anything different in the new graduates?" she asked me. Colleen, for one, seemed happier and more secure. Before this, she hadn't been "sharing her frustrated feelings" with Deidre. Pamela also had improved after being rotated from the evening back to the day shift for close observation. She had made medication errors when working the evening shift. Deidre needed reassurance that the G.N.'s were gaining skill, even though she acknowledged that some of the staff saw her as the enemy.

Deidre went on the evening shift in order to determine how the unit was being managed with Pamela and Ann, both G.N.'s, in charge. There had been complaints of poor care by patients and by other nurses rotating to that shift. Pam and Ann were boisterous at times. Their behavior this particular evening was somewhat subdued. They knew they were being evaluated. Both seemed to resent this, Ann more than Pam. When the evening laboratory technician came to draw some blood specimens and asked why Deidre was on this shift, the medical clerk answered for both of the new graduates, "She's playing 'I spy.'" In one sense, this was true, since Deidre found it necessary to check on the nurses. Her responsibility to the 7H patients extended over twenty-four hours.

Pam made a medication error by administering IV fluids incorrectly. Deidre felt that patient safety was at risk. Deidre's sense of responsibility to the patients overrode her annoyance at being perceived as a dictator or spy. The following example illustrates her sense of responsibility.

Despite the fact that she wondered which was the best management style, "pure management versus the mixed role, where the nurse manager moves in and out of the patient care situation," Deidre chose to practice the mixed role. She did not want to be the "authority" all the time and wished that the nurses shared the responsibility of the unit with her: "It's their unit. The nurses should communicate better with each other. If someone is upset about something, share it. It won't change otherwise." Nevertheless, Deidre used her authority to change the method of staff assignment to districts, to assign different unit-wide jobs to each district, and to change the way change of shift report was handled. The change to district assignment and the addition of specific jobs for each district persisted longer than the change of shift report modification, which was openly resisted and quickly abandoned. Deidre felt that these changes would prepare staff for the time when she would leave her temporary position as nurse manager. "They know I came here on a temporary status. I told them yesterday that I want them to be able to function without me."

Deidre consistently supported her staff. One day she realized that Sharon, a G.N., had more than her share of work in the early afternoon. Deidre helped her and interrupted report to tell Sharon that some of her work was taken care of.

> DEIDRE: The bed's ready in ICU [Intensive Care Unit].
>
> SHARON: Oh, really? Great. Do I have to go down there and give report?
>
> DEIDRE: We'll handle it.
>
> SHARON: Oh, O.K. I was gonna say, if I do, I better go get the charts—I'd have forgot [sic] what went on today.
>
> DEIDRE: No, we took care of it and Colleen gave an excellent report.

Not only did Deidre support the G.N.'s, but she also kept abreast of her new nurses' problems by evaluating how they were managing and helping them as they worked. She also encouraged the nursing staff to help each other. Deidre's commitment to patients, family, and staff emerged frequently. On one occasion Sharon, a G.N., admitted during a change-of-shift report that she wanted to delay calling a patient's family when he had chest pain a second time. They were "all over the unit" the last time the patient "went bad." Deidre warned Sharon that there would be more problems from the family if they were not called.

Another example illustrates Deidre's interest in the well-being of patients. A recuperating patient was transferred from ICU to 7H. He was recovering from Guillian Barré Syndrome and required a pulmonary toilet (tracheal aspiration) and chest physical therapy every two hours. Deidre told a resident that the patient's wife was very upset. She could not afford private duty nurses, since she had exhausted her financial resources. Deidre wondered if the hospital would pay for the private duty nurse by absorbing the cost since 7H nurses could not give the required care to the patient. She called the nursing administration office and the attending physician. Deidre achieved success after exerting her influence. She also moved the patient to another room, 744, directly in front of the nurses' station. This increased the possibility that staff would be more available to him and would check on him frequently. Private duty nurses cared for the patient and eventually he was assigned to primary or associate nurses.

Deidre continued to set high standards of nursing care. When the staff openly complained about a very ill and very annoying patient, Deidre arranged for conferences with the psychiatric nurse clinical specialist so that the staff could begin to work out their anger about this demanding woman. Even though some of the L.G.P.N.'s expressed doubt about the benefits of these conferences, they went along with Deidre's request that they attend the conferences.

When there were very difficult patients, Deidre insisted on kindness. Once a patient told Deidre that she was mistreated. Deidre quickly identified the nurse as Ann, a G.N., and immediately informed her that patients were not to be mistreated; she would "not have it." Nurses' first responsibility is to give considerate patient care. The patient who complained was an elderly, obese, stroke victim, admitted with a pulmonary embolus to 7H from an extended care facility. The patient's urinary frequency plagued the nurses on each shift. She was on and off the bedpan "constantly." Deidre helped Ann and the other staff deal with the problem by having them offer the bedpan frequently to the patient. Deidre bathed the patient during the day shift in order to spend time with her. She helped the patient prepare for discharge to the extended care facility by arranging for the physical therapist to help the patient walk. Up to this time the physical therapists had only helped the patient to stand when she went for her physical therapy treatments. By giving direct care to this patient, Deidre helped the patient and earned the respect of those nurses who respect other nurses who can "do." She also prevented the patient from having an unpleasant hospital stay.

Worry and anger about a medication error led Deidre to regret showing her anger to staff on another occasion and to state, "Maybe I overreacted. I talked to my husband about it last night; I hardly got any sleep." When medication errors proliferated in late September, Deidre discussed this and other issues at the next staff

meeting. To heighten staff awareness, she Xeroxed an article entitled, "Medication Errors to Avoid" and posted it in the utility
room on the bulletin board so that nurses read it while waiting for
shift report and during coffee breaks.

Deidre's concern about a serious medication error forced her to
talk about the problem to all of the medical residents on 7H. She
explained the problem and reminded them of their responsibility.
She asked them to check the medication Kardexes and determine
if medication orders were transcribed and the drugs given to the
patients. The residents defended themselves and the 7H nurses by
telling Deidre that both the nurses and "the doctors were working
hard." While Deidre agreed, she reminded them of their legal responsibility with medications. "It's theirs as well as the nurses," she
said. The doctors knew about the large number of medication errors on the unit. They promised that they would check the medication Kardexes. Deidre next reminded them to look for responses
to the drugs ordered: "Don't you look for these responses?" Doctors, like nurses, get caught up in the doing of tasks. Deidre understood this pressure, but the medication errors seriously disturbed
her since patient safety was at stake.

Deidre's sense of responsibility to patients and her commitment
to "modeling" good nursing care for the 7H G.N.'s and other staff
was manifest. At times she suspended her management functions.
For example, she put off writing the first evaluations for her G.N.
staff: "How can I pull them off of the unit [for evaluation and discussion of performance], when they are thinking of patient care?"
Instead of interviewing them in her 7H office, she reviewed their
performance by looking at competencies over lunch in the em-
ployees' cafeteria.

Deidre's worries about the unit and her sleepless nights caught
up with her, and she was hospitalized herself at Christmastime with
a viral infection. She had worked out the staff's Christmas and New
Year's holiday schedule so that each staff member would have a
long stretch of days off. The staffing pattern was "bare bones." Staff
knew that only their *death* would be an acceptable reason for absence from the unit. Deidre's admission to the hospital highlighted
how sick she must have been since she broke her own rule of unit

coverage. She was ill again in February and periodically had recurrent fevers during the early spring.

Deidre was disturbed by her illness since missing work was a serious offense. It was imperative that those nursing staff who were scheduled for work report as scheduled. Nurses called in sick in order to alert the remaining staff. Frequently the nurse who took the sick call reported to others, "——— called in sick today and she really sounded sick," as if to justify the absence with a "more than a cold" excuse.

As nurse managers, Deidre and Kate were required to show intolerance to staff absences. Staff absenteeism directly affected one of the unit's major problems, staffing. The nurse manager and assistant nurse manager were required to counsel staff with an obvious pattern of absence. Periodically they conferred to determine which staff required counseling or warning. At one meeting they reviewed the records of attendance of a nurse's aide, two L.G.P.N.'s, and two R.N.'s. Deidre explained the counseling/warning policy to Kate and rehearsed possible responses of the staff who were called in for a conference. A yellow sheet filed in a staff record meant that the nurse manager had "spoken to you; you know my feelings and my expectations." A green sheet was a warning for termination: "I'm warning you, you'd better comply." If a staff received one green sheet, she would be subject to termination of employment. "The first step is suspension; after that, termination." Deidre and Kate were both intolerant of nurses who repeatedly feigned illness. Kate remembered one "horrendous weekend when two staff" did this and she could not get help: "It was awful."

When Deidre talked about her time commitment to 7H, she described it as short-lived, since she had taken the nurse manager position as a temporary assignment. She held a real estate license and admitted that in ten years she would like to have her own real estate office. She would also enjoy taking humanities and business courses. As she discussed her plans, she again reminisced about her success on the oncology floor and asked for my confirmation of the positive changes happening on 7H or how the new G.N.'s had "blossomed." As patient safety improved and error decreased, Deidre was able to recognize that she had made a positive impact on 7H

for the patients and the staff. At other times, when she faced medication error, staff absences, poor housekeeping, and poor staffing,
along with her recurrent illness, she was negative: "It sounds
funny; it almost seems as if there is an evil spirit on the floor in that
office. I'd like to bomb it and start from scratch."

During one of her low periods, Deidre told me that she thought
that she was going to stick to her original commitment and leave
the nurse manager position in February. Instead she stayed until
the end of April. She was exhausted. "The list [of problems to be
brought up at the staff meeting] gets longer. I said to myself today,
'What would happen to 7H if I died?' It would go on. 7H wouldn't
end." At that realization, Deidre told me that she went to bed that
night finding some comfort in the ongoing character of 7H.

Deidre was a nurse who relied on her ability to care for people,
using traditional and nontraditional modes of therapy. She saw
herself as an almost inconspicuous role model for the G.N.'s and
quietly encouraged them to avoid relying on pain medications
alone to take care of patients' pain, adding, "Not that I would with-
hold pain medications." To illustrate her approach to patients, she
told a story about a renal patient with hypertension and headaches.
She was cautious about using pain medications alone:

> In nursing in our society, I believe that we have to do something physical
> with people, in order for them to see us as helping, while we may be
> doing emotional care at the same time. With this lady, I applied a cool
> washcloth to her forehead and gently massaged her [indicating the tem-
> poral area of her head]. Her blood pressure came down and her pain
> went away.

Deidre next described her interest in using laying on of hands and
touch. She was cautious in her use of this therapy and did not force
her ideas on her staff. Her approaches to patients came out gradually as I came to know her.

Deidre described how she helped another patient by teaching
him to use a visualization technique. His surgery was cancelled because his platelet count dropped. The night before the scheduled
surgery, he had chest pain that did not respond to 20 mg. of morphine. Deidre talked to the patient about what he was thinking.
Twenty years before he had been divorced; he was thinking of all
the bad things he had done, as if he were dying and needed a life

review. She asked him if he had anything in his life that he did that relaxed him. "Deep-sea diving," he responded. Deidre spent twenty minutes with him recreating the deep-sea diving experience. Subsequently he had no pain. The next day his platelet count rose and he told Deidre later that he repeatedly reviewed this deep-sea diving experience after she left him so that he could relax.

When I discussed with Deidre the subject of nursing rituals and my idea of the hospital as a quasi-religious institution, she responded with recollections of some "codes," when patients were resuscitated: "Sometimes, the code went so smoothly, everything went well, and the patient died. Other times, the code went all wrong, there was delay, and the patient lived. I've often wondered, do we ever do any good?" She suggested indirectly that it might be out of the hands of hospital staff and in God's.

Deidre told another story. One night she called a doctor after having taken a patient's vital signs, which were stable. But she had a "sense that something wasn't right." She told the doctor that he would probably think she was crazy; he agreed. He said, "What do you want me to do?" She said, "I don't know." Forty-five minutes later the patient "paced" or "coded." The doctor told her she was a witch. (In this hospital, the call for respiratory arrest used to be "pacemaker" along with the patient's room number. Later the word "paced" changed to "coded," that is, the patient was said to have paced or coded.)

Kate, R.N.—Assistant Nurse Manager

Kate, a twenty-eight-year-old registered nurse, was the assistant nurse manager of 7H from November to February. She worked as a primary nurse on the unit before her promotion. Kate had seven years of nursing experience before graduating from a hospital school of nursing.

Kate was a 7H nurse for two years and four months before Deidre became nurse manager. She described the former head nurses of the unit: Monica was an "autocrat" who efficiently managed the unit. The "floor ran well" during her tenure and the staff "were crazy about her." There was a "chasm" between the time Monica resigned and her former assistant assumed the head nurse

position a few months later. She resigned and was replaced by a
head nurse of the "old school." Julia, the new head nurse, confided
to Kate on several occasions that it was difficult for her not to wear
her nursing cap in the hospital when many of the nurses in the
hospital stopped wearing their caps at work. Julia was a "laissez-
faire" leader who was unable to say no to her staff. For example,
during the holiday season many staff requested both Christmas and
New Year's Day off. Julia scheduled according to their desires, and
Kate, the assistant head nurse, had to work both holidays.

Kate welcomed Deidre and was relieved by Deidre's fair approach to management. She was pleased that the hiatus in nursing
management created by Julia's resignation was filled when Deidre
took the position of this respected nurse manager. Kate happily
ended her tenure as the unit's highest nurse in authority.

Kate was a slim, wide-eyed, earnest, hard-working, and clinically
competent nurse. She acknowledged that management was not her
"cup of tea." Her lack of confidence as a manager was evident when
she had to set standards or correct staff infractions of policy. Her
confidence and skill as a nurse emerged at the patient's bedside as
she pitched in and helped the staff with different patient problems.
Beth, another R.N., regarded Kate's clinical skill with open awe.

Before Deidre's appointment as nurse manager, Kate staffed 7H
with R.N.'s and L.G.P.N.'s from the hospital p.r.n. pool. According
to Kate, the unit was closed, that is, it stopped admitting patients,
when an ineffective nurse manager failed to raise patient care standards. After that nurse manager left, 7H was reopened and Kate
was overwhelmed with its many problems.

Kate was a self-conscious assistant nurse manager even after
Deidre came to the unit and stability was reestablished. While she
performed well as a clinician, she yearned for a career in decorat-
ing. One day she blurted out a story from her nursing student days
that illustrated her views of nursing authority: "When I was a student I was thrown out of school because I took care of a leukemic
patient when I had a cold." Kate was very upset by the incident and
the way the nursing instructor and head nurse had treated her.
Even though she was permitted to return to the school of nursing
as a student, the pain of her mistake remained with her years later.
The incident affected her reaction to being observed; she admitted

that she was often uncomfortable when anyone watched her at work. Consequently she hated to observe and evaluate other nurses as assistant nurse manager.

Despite Kate's discomfort with her present job, Kate was not only an excellent bedside nurse but also a competent manager able to solve managerial problems such as narcotic count irregularities, staffing problems, and graduate nurse orientation to 7H. Kate finally decided in December to leave 7H and transferred to a CCU staff nurse position. After Kate announced her decision to leave, she felt that the nurses on the unit were "pretty good about my transfer," and she wondered if they would miss her. She imagined that they were treating her more like a human being, "getting on my case" or teasing her. She looked forward to her CCU staff nurse position, "Even though I'll have to get used to rotating again."

Before Kate left 7H, the staff had a party for her in the utility room. They served lunch and gave her gifts. Kate looked happy. She left 7H in February, spent some time as a staff nurse in the CCU, and then transferred to per diem nursing work because there was less shift rotation. While working among three hospitals as a per diem nurse, Kate changed her mind about becoming a designer and enrolled in travel agent's school.

Beth, R.N.—Primary Nurse and Preceptor

Heavyset and with dark hair and smiling eyes, Beth had a soft, gentle voice. Her internal standards of professional nursing behavior were high. Day after day she moved rapidly into and out of the patient rooms of her district, District I. She was a "nurse's nurse"—the kind of nurse another R.N. would be pleased to have take care of her husband, mother, or child. I repeatedly observed that Beth's nursing care was considerate and expert.

Beth was easygoing until she encountered violations of her standards. One incident illustrates her high principles. She disagreed with Sarah, another R.N., over how to fill in the patient classification sheet, a patient acuity instrument used by the Nursing Office to determine staffing patterns. "Sarah does it differently. I try to remember that the purpose of it is to determine staffing needs. I fudge on the numbers, but. . . ." Beth felt justified in making adjustments. She went on to say that she confronted Sarah with her difference of opinion: "I'm getting angry. It's part of growing up as a nurse, I guess." Beth acknowledged that she felt uncomfortable that several nurses witnessed the disagreement with Sarah, but she also felt that her approach to completing the classification form helped 7H get more nurses to give patient care.

Beth was a preceptor for several of the new G.N.'s who arrived at different times. She took great pains with their development and helped Chris, Cecile, and Suzanne gain independence as nurses. If another R.N. stepped in and gave information to a G.N. that differed from what Beth had said, she was annoyed and somewhat possessive. She was always available to the G.N.'s and also oriented them to the evening shift.

Beth was in constant motion. Rarely did she sit in the Utility Room to take a break. If she did sit there, she checked patient charts, wrote nurses' notes, or showed a G.N. some of the record-keeping duties of the primary nurse of a district. Beth's routine nursing work illustrated the typical duties of a primary nurse (R.N.) on District I. After morning report at about 8:15 A.M. on a typical day, Beth checked the medication Kardex to see if there were any insulin injections or other medications to be administered at times that were not routine. Since she had already checked on her patients on rounds while waiting for report between 7:30 and 8:15 A.M., Beth moved to get bed linens from the cart in the hall and walked into her district's patient rooms.

After getting help to move a patient up in bed, she responded to an alarm sounded by the electronic IVAC pump, which controlled the flow rate of intravenous solutions. She left the patient's room to retrieve an IV bag containing Heparin from the medication refrigerator area in the back of the nurses' station. She reentered the patient's room, started a new IV bag, and reset the IVAC pump.

Beth rapidly checked on the other patients in her district. She prepared and gave pain medication to a patient. Mixing the narcotic with Vistaril, she next recorded the narcotic on the narcotic flow sheet and wrote on the medication Kardex that both medications had been given. A team of doctors was in the patient's room, so on returning to the room, she asked them about the intravenous Heparin drop rate. She spoke softly to the patient before injecting him with the pain medications. Agreeing with Beth's advice, the patient decided to wait until after his pain subsided to bathe himself.

Beth left the patient who was in pain and went into another room. She bathed her "complete" patient first, as she worried aloud about patients who needed to be fed breakfast. That day she was the only nurse on District I. Usually Marie, L.G.P.N., was her associate nurse, but it was Marie's day off. Beth moved in the district among the four rooms and seven patients. One bed was empty. Later Beth learned that an amputee patient who had coded on 7H and moved to CCU would be transferred back to occupy her empty bed.

After completing most of her patients' A.M. care, Beth picked up the zippered pharmacy bag, which was full of recently ordered medications after it had been left during the morning "drop." At 10:15 A.M. she checked the yellow medication order slips against the medications in the bag. After putting the drugs in drawers on the unit's two medication carts, she began "pouring meds" for the patients in her district who were scheduled to receive 10:00 A.M. medications. While she moved to the four rooms of the district and administered medications, she checked and flushed a patient's blocked IV tube, explained to another patient why she was listening to her heart, and helped a patient to move up in bed. Beth spoke directly to patients when giving medications. "Now take this medication, Mr. Roberts. It's your heart medication." She recorded the medications given in the Kardex.

Interrupted by a telephone call about her transfer patient, Beth next ordered a continuous suction machine from Central Supply and asked a volunteer to get it. Going into a patient's room to answer a light, she reset the IVAC pump that was controlling the IV heparin infusion. She checked another patient in a different room, pulled the curtain back, and emptied a bedpan. Returning to the medication cart in the hall, she closed the Kardex: 10:00 A.M. medications were completed.

Beth walked into the nurses' station and found a patient's chart that needed to be checked for doctors' orders. Signing off a new IV order, she placed the chart on the shelf on the wall of the nurses' station. Beth remembered to call Respiratory Therapy and order a

venti-mask and oxygen set-up for her patient who was being transferred to 7H from CCU. She checked more doctors' orders, completed the patient classification sheet for her district, and sent a
volunteer to the IV lab for a patient's recently ordered IV.

Since Beth was the only seasoned R.N. on 7H that day, she answered the new graduate nurses' questions about IV medications,
the timing of IV's, etc. She called CCU to ask for a nursing report
on her transfer patient. When it was time to go to lunch, she talked
with Sharon, G.N., about the patients in her district and the transfer patient who would soon arrive.

After lunch, Beth checked in each room to see how her patients
were doing. She received report from Sharon about her district
and Sharon's district. When Sharon left to go to lunch, Beth
checked orders again and signed them off. She wrote nurses' notes
in a patient's chart.

A patient's son came to the nurses' station to ask Beth whether
his mother had a fractured pelvis. She checked the Ortho consult
(orthopedic consultation) form in the patient's chart and answered
affirmatively. She then agreed to give his mother Percocet for pain
and prepared the medication at the medication cart. She helped
her patient take the medicine with water.

Meanwhile the transferred patient arrived from CCU. Beth took
his vital signs, checked his IV, checked his Foley (urinary catheter),
and put his venti-mask on at 40 percent oxygen.

Later Beth poured 2:00 P.M. medications at 1:30 P.M., beginning
with the patients in room 740D. Leaving tablets with the first patient, she moved to the next room and poured medications for a
patient who complained about not having anything for arthritis.
She looked for pain medication orders in the Kardex and told the
patient to chew the tablet she gave her. She moved to the next patient who sat in the corridor on a geri chair (a high-backed chair on
small wheels with a movable, waist-level tray that supported the
patient's arms). Giving him water to drink with his medications, she
listened to Sharon describe how he had "scrounged" food while
Beth was at lunch. He was a diabetic. She talked to Sharon about
his diabetes and explained why he should not have had additional
food. Beth finished giving her 2:00 P.M. medications and moved
the medication cart to District II for Karen. It was 1:55 P.M.

Later Beth applied a dry sterile dressing to the gangrenous toe of her diabetic patient. She continued to check her patients and write nurses' notes on each patient's chart. Her responsibility to the district ended around 4:00 P.M., after she gave change-of-shift report on her district for the evening shift nurses. She frequently stayed after 4:00 P.M. to complete unfinished business.

Beth was modest about her nursing skill. She extolled the clinical skills of Deidre and Kate, seeing herself as much less able. Once she beamed as she described a compliment from Gloria, the staff development instructor, who commented on her "clear, good nurses' notes." She was obviously touched and very pleased by the recognition. Patients openly praised Beth for how good she was to them.

Sarah, R.N.—Primary Nurse, Per Diem Day Shift

Sarah was an assertive, independent, efficient, sure and expert nurse who had eleven years of nursing experience. She worked on 7H for several months while new G.N.'s were learning the ropes of the medical unit.

Sarah was skillful and tenacious in identifying and solving problems, whether they were patient problems or nurse problems. If Sarah disagreed with nurses, patients, doctors, nursing students, or other hospital personnel, she told them. She did not pay attention to bruised feelings but consistently acted self-confident and businesslike. Sarah also had a good sense of humor.

When there were nursing students on the unit, Sarah delighted in teaching, correcting, and praising them. "I like to work with students," she admitted. When a group of students prepared to finish their clinical experience on 7H, Sarah called them to a meeting in the utility room. She thanked them for the care they gave 7H patients and shared her memories of her capping ceremony twelve years ago. She described her vivid recollections of lighted candles and a recitation of the Florence Nightingale Pledge. She ended her meetings with the students by admonishing them to have a good vacation: "You'll need it next year."

Sarah, like Beth, valued the patient involvement and decision-making aspects of her nursing role. She disliked seeing suffering and worked to ease pain. When asked what she thought important when she admitted a patient to the unit, Sarah replied with her perspectives on nursing:

> I zero in on things pertinent to their diagnosis, phlebitis of the leg, first time in the hospital, any social or emotional problems; I think about whether they will have any problem going home. I like to know it right away. I like to make care very personal. I imagine it is one of my relatives. I know their name and they know mine. I try to make them comfortable, orient them to their room, introduce them to their roommates. I get the family involved right away, especially with a stroke patient. Range of motion exercises and decubitus problems. Sometimes this is limited because the family can't come in during the day. I encourage the family to do, continue to do what they have been doing at home. Sometimes they don't want to do it, they need a break. I can understand that. I like the patients to know I'm around; I check on them if I hear in report that they have had an uncomfortable night. I'm not the kind of nurse who can't empty a bedpan. I enjoy nursing.

Sarah consistently used time before A.M. care and after morning change-of-shift report to have a short but very detailed planning conference with the associate nurse or nurses on her district for that day. She reviewed the patients' diagnoses, medications, and diagnostic studies. She identified patient problems and equipment problems for the L.G.P.N.'s or nursing assistant with whom she was working. She openly expressed her feelings, whether positive or negative. At times she threatened to write incident reports when a hospital department such as Pharmacy balked at her requests.

Sarah resented being told what she should do as a nurse. Once Deidre reminded all the nursing staff sitting in the utility room during afternoon report to "yellow out" the Kardex notation when a diagnostic test was done. Sarah was annoyed; she took care of details independently and did not appreciate reminders. She had been a head nurse before leaving her staff position to have her first child.

Sarah's attention to detail encouraged her to complain about the failure of the new G.N.'s to complete the bedside chart forms. Deidre encouraged Sarah to use peer pressure when she saw this problem: "It isn't ratting. We have to know so that the floor runs smoothly."

Sarah saw herself as an expert nurse. For example, on one occasion she discontinued a patient's "neuro" checks on the Kardex. The attending doctor discovered this the following day and wrote his order again. When Sarah learned during report that the doctor had been annoyed, she responded quietly and confidently when discussing this with the reporting nurse.

Sarah was a clinically competent nurse, solicitous toward patients and attentive to detail. She was a preceptor to two G.N.'s and helped other nurses care for patients in other districts when the work load of the unit demanded. Her reporting of relevant details to other shifts was exemplary. Her relationships with other nursing staff were good, despite the fact that her direct approach unnerved some staff. All respected her, including the doctors and other hospital personnel. When the G.N.'s had gained some experience and the staffing pattern of 7H had improved by the early winter, she went to other units in the hospital since she was a per diem or hospital pool nurse.

Tammy, R.N.—Primary Nurse, Day Shift

Tammy worked on 7H for a few years, first as an L.G.P.N. and later as an R.N. after her graduation from an associate degree nursing program. Tammy had a more easygoing relationship with the L.G.P.N.'s and nursing assistants than did the other R.N.'s. Dignified and quiet, Tammy frequently solved problems using few words. Her sense of humor was gentle and her kindness to patients ever present. Although she could be firm with patients if they were pulling on an IV when confused or getting out of bed unsteadily and unaided, she was always respectful.

One day Tammy entered Room 740, where an elderly man, Sam George, was in a Clinitron bed (a pressure relieving bed) and his roommate was in a regular hospital bed. She greeted Mr. George and the other patient and checked the drop rate of an IV bag. Mr. George was noticeably upset. He was gesturing and muttering, "Son of a bitch." His speech was difficult to understand, since words in his sentences were out of order. Nevertheless, he communicated very effectively as he moved his eyes, hands, head, trunk, and legs. His extreme state of frustration held Tammy's attention. She listened and tried to calm him. "Sam, don't get upset,

calm down." It took a few minutes for Sam to stop his tirade.
Tammy learned that earlier in the day he had accidently spilled a
urinal on the floor. A doctor had made him feel bad about it; Sam
was embarrassed and did not "want that doctor to come near him."
Sam also had a bowel problem. Tammy comforted him. She touched
him, talked to him, and tried to ease his embarrassment. Tammy
demonstrated patience and gentleness with all of her patients.

Miriam, R.N.—Primary Nurse, Night Shift

Miriam, a B.S.N. (Bachelor of Science degree in Nursing) graduate
with two years of experience, preferred the night shift because her
husband also worked nights. Tall and attractive, she never stopped
working, either checking on patients or doing paper work. Her
clinical skill was well established and evident in the nursing care she
gave to her patients, in her skill with change-of-shift report in the
morning, and in the fact that the unit ran smoothly as the day shift
staff took over the nursing work of the night shift.

Miriam had no trouble expressing whether her night was "crazy"
or not. When she scurried to finish her shift's work after a difficult
night, she would mutter, "I give up, I give up!" After a quiet night
she said, "They sleep for me. What can I tell you?" Miriam belongs
to that group of hospital personnel who believes in the loony effects
of a full moon on patients. She used the advent of a full moon
to explain why 7H suddenly "went crazy." She was superstitious.
When talking about death and post-mortem care, she said, "Death
comes in threes—it always happens like that and with the full
moon."

Miriam worked well with her night staff, despite the previously
mentioned L.G.P.N. problem. Her humorous approach to difficult
situations was pleasant to behold. She enjoyed telling hospital "war
stories." She laughingly warned nurses about a resident doctor who
was "the biggest pincher in the hospital—even he would admit it."

Miriam contributed to the stability of 7H. She supported the new
G.N.'s during their orientation to the night shift. Frequently when
a new nurse gave report, Miriam asked if there was anything unfinished or if she could help in any way. Most often she acted without
asking and then reported completed tasks. In addition, her posi-

tion as permanent R.N. on the night shift insured the other R.N.'s of less rotation to that shift. Miriam kept in close contact with Deidre and often sat and conferred about problems in Deidre's office after morning change-of-shift report ended.

Graduate Nurses

Graduate nurses came to 7H at different times during the first year of their professional practice. Pamela came first in February. After her orientation to the day shift, she staffed the evening shift. She was a graduate of a B.S.N. program but had difficulty passing the State Board of Nurses licensing examination. She finally passed the examination but had some difficulty adjusting to her new primary nurse duties. For months her change-of-shift reports were tentative, lasted longer than did those of other nurses, and lacked the factual specificity that the nurses receiving the report required. Pam was obviously embarrassed about this and admitted that she needed to do better. When asked specific questions during report, she was unable to respond with accurate, in-depth answers. She made a few medication errors when she was primary nurse on the evening shift and was moved back to the day shift for a more extensive orientation by Deidre. Her lack of experience and difficulty adjusting were addressed when a seasoned R.N. once again served as Pamela's preceptor.

When asked in November how she was progressing with giving medications and organizing nursing care, she replied:

> Things are much better. I'm faster [administering medications]. Me and Wanda [L.G.P.N.] were talking about how much I improved since February. I gave out 6 P.M. meds, did a few other things, and cleaned up two [incontinent] patients. It was hard at first. When I was on nights during orientation and had to pour [medications] for the floor, the meds plus the IV's nearly made me cry. I could just about manage it.

Most of the time Pam was jovial and pleasant, but at times she was impatient and brusque, probably because of her lack of confidence.

Ann, a recent graduate of an associate degree program, came to work on 7H in the summer. Ann was older than the rest of the new graduates. She had been a secretary in a now-defunct company.

She said she had loved her previous secretarial job in the small business, but its closing had led her to consider a nursing career.

After her orientation to each shift, Ann worked as a permanent primary nurse on evenings. Ann's adjustment to evenings on 7H was smoother than Pam's. Her more mature and poised approach to life helped her handle difficult situations easily, even though her nursing knowledge and clinical skills were far from perfected. Ann was able more easily to accept the fact that the L.G.P.N.'s on evenings, Wanda and Nancy, were much more clinically experienced than she.

At times Ann was boisterous in the corridor of 7H and occasionally abrupt with patients. After one incident of alleged insensitivity to a patient who required frequent help on and off the bedpan, Deidre corrected Ann openly and quietly in front of other staff in the utility room. Ann had laughed at an elderly, confused patient who had been incontinent of stool and who had smeared the stool all over herself and her bed. While some of this humor may have been a response to anxiety by an immature nurse who worked on a poorly staffed shift, it was nevertheless difficult to avoid judging her action as cruel or at best insensitive.

On the whole Ann was pleasant to staff and patients. Her manner was soothing and reassuring. It was obvious at times that she had favorites among her patients; during change-of-shift report she discussed "cute" and "nice" patients. Ann did not enjoy being observed by Deidre or anyone else. The fact that she made a medication error once was very embarrassing to her. She preferred not to discuss it, even though I assured her that "just about every nurse" makes these errors.

In early spring, Ann left 7H to work in another large teaching hospital. Deidre did not understand how she got the job, since she had not requested a letter of reference from Deidre. Deidre admitted that her letter of reference would not have been favorable.

Both Ann and Pam freely admitted that they preferred the usually steady, more relaxed pace of the unit during the evening shift. Although the work required that they keep moving through the evening hours as they gave medications and treatments, took vital signs, cleaned incontinent patients, and gave P.M. care (washing patients' hands, faces, and backs and giving back rubs), they enjoyed their freedom from the surveillance of the nurse manager and assistant nurse manager.

Meredith was a G.N. who came to 7H in the late summer. During the time that Meredith was oriented to the day, evening, and night shifts over the summer and into September, it became progressively evident that she was having considerable difficulty performing her nursing duties safely. Again and again she was overtly nervous, especially when she conducted change-of-shift report for oncoming nurses. Her reports were long and full of superfluous comments.

The nursing staff each reacted differently to Meredith's difficulty. Since she frequently laughed nervously during report and often omitted mentioning important facts specific to the care and diagnostic studies of the patients, staff listening to report in the utility room became restless. Although most listened patiently, the L.G.P.N.'s and Ann were obviously impatient. At times Ann's tone of voice bordered on mockery.

Deidre, along with the staff development instructor and Sarah, Meredith's preceptor, worked hard to support Meredith and to ease her adjustment. Nevertheless, medication errors and other problems forced Deidre to counsel Meredith to resign her primary nurse position on 7H. Meredith left in September, about two months after beginning her employment. Her departure for a community hospital was announced by Deidre in a staff meeting. Another G.N., Chris, seemed upset at this, yet Deidre reassured her that the decision to leave 7H was a mutual one.

Loretta, a graduate nurse from a diploma program, worked on evenings after her orientation to all three shifts. She worked hard, seemed never to stop moving, was very quiet, and seemed to adjust more rapidly to the demands of her primary nurse position. One evening, before shift report, staff noticed that Loretta, very slight and of thin build, was getting thinner. She said, "That's what this place will do to you." She admitted that during this first year of nursing work she had contracted many viruses.

Chris, a graduate of a B.S.N. program, was an energetic nurse and hard to pin down in discussion. Uncomfortable at being observed, she used a variety of reasonable excuses to get away, such as having to check on a patient. Once she admitted that being observed made her feel that she was back in school again. Chris was obviously very organized and self-possessed as she moved about the unit as a primary nurse.

Deidre thought that Chris was a definite asset to 7H. Chris was extremely gentle and considerate with her patients. She apologized once when she felt that her nursing care was not up to her own standards. She explained that she did not feel very well because of a viral infection. Chris initially planned to stay on the unit, but when other G.N.'s asked for transfers within the hospital or resigned, she joined the exodus and moved to a critical care unit in the hospital in late spring.

Suzanne came to 7H in September. She was preceptored by Beth, who became increasingly happy with the consistent manner in which Suzanne learned and demonstrated her primary nursing duties. Suzanne was slow, factual, dignified, and quiet. She smiled quietly and frequently as she successively mastered the many aspects of her job.

Cecile came to 7H in November after having worked in another hospital as a new graduate. Deidre spent considerable time interviewing her deciding that Cecile would "fit in well" with the 7H staff. Cecile's clinical ability improved over the next several months. Yet for Cecile as well as for the other new G.N.'s, the adjustment was not easy. An example illustrating the difficulties of the adjustment occurred in February, when Cecile was working nights.

Miriam, the permanent night nurse, was having difficulty with an L.G.P.N. who ignored her repeated requests to suction the airway of a patient on a ventilator. Cecile had a hard time on the night shift during the time that this problem persisted. Because of Miriam's preoccupation with the L.G.P.N. problem, Cecile had a difficult orientation to the night shift. After morning change-of-shift report, an exhausted Cecile spent over an hour talking with Deidre and Miriam about how to manage the shift better. The next night and several nights thereafter, Cecile delegated more work to her L.G.P.N. associate nurse.

Sharon graduated from a B.S.N. program before taking her staff nurse job on 7H. She was not new to this hospital. As a senior nursing student she had spent time doing "heavy" patient care on another unit. Beth described her as "savvy." Despite her obvious clinical abilities, Sharon also experienced the frustrations of the other G.N.'s. 7H was not usually a quiet floor. A high level of activity characterized each shift, especially days.

In late July, when talking to a resident doctor about who should eat some cake left for the staff by a patient, Sharon was assertive: "I deserve the cake. I'm the one who came here [to 7H] in this mass of trouble and confusion."

Not all of the G.N.'s were lucky enough to have a preceptor, because there were not enough R.N.'s on the 7H nursing staff. To fill in some of the gaps, a staff development instructor systematically checked on the skills of the G.N.'s. To ease the new nurses' adjustment to the role of R.N., the staff development instructor developed a special program about conflict management and emphasized medication administration and documentation or charting.

Sharon adjusted well to 7H. She made it "look easy" as she moved day by day as primary nurse. Camille, an L.G.P.N. associate nurse who worked consistently with Sharon on District III, obviously respected her. When Mabel, another highly skilled and hard working L.G.P.N., came later in the fall to work with Sharon, she too respected Sharon's ability. Ann wistfully teased Sharon that she never sat still. Sharon was serious and determined. She frequently double-checked facts, and had little time for levity. Patients approved of her care. For example, a patient once commented, "She's the best," as Sharon gave her medications.

It was evident in September that Sharon, like the other neophyte nurses, was just beginning to learn the routine of 7H. The R.N.'s helped them by instructing, clarifying, and helping with patient care. Sharon was respected by the staff for learning faster than many. In October, after one of Sharon's patients had "coded," Deidre asked Kate how Sharon had performed during the stress of the resuscitation efforts. Kate reported, "She was in control, she was out of control. I think she went home feeling good. You know, she never 'bagged' [inflated a patient's lungs with the help of an Ambu bag] anybody?"

Deidre responded, "You know, you forget how little they [the G.N.'s] know; it's amazing. Sometimes it's no wonder that there are errors; it's been horrible this week."

By late winter, Sharon decided to leave 7H for a critical care unit.

She and Colleen, another G.N., arrived at their decisions to leave the unit about the same time. Colleen, a nurse's aide for a few years and an L.G.P.N. for three years, graduated from an associate degree nursing program when she was twenty-four years old. She was extremely independent and held high standards of care for herself and for the other staff of 7H. Colleen preferred solving problems independently when she had patient and district problems. Frequently Colleen worked in District IV, with Dotty as her L.G.P.N. associate nurse. Both worked very well together and respected each other's commitment to good nursing care and to reporting to each other the details of the patients in their district. Colleen's standards were evident by her reaction to a patient who told her, as she washed his back during A.M. care, that no one had washed his back in three weeks. She said that she could not believe it, but she did believe it. She was unhappy with 7H.

Colleen showed her frustrations openly. At one point in early August, she stomped around the utility room when she came on evening shift to discover that she would be the only R.N. on 7H with one L.G.P.N. Two of the nursing staff had been pulled to another floor. Deidre hastily arranged to get another staff to come to work. Agreeing with Colleen, Deidre said, "She doesn't think it's fair to her or to the patients." Deidre shared some of Colleen's frustrations with the unit and tried to help her by improving the work schedule and putting pressure on the housekeeping department to clean. She appointed Colleen to a nursing committee whose purpose was to study some of the problems that beset the nurses, such as how many times they had to call the X-ray Department and the lab to follow up on scheduled diagnostic tests. Colleen planned to air her thoughts at these meetings.

Identifying her unhappiness with 7H, Colleen said:

> Deidre wants me to stay, because things will get better. I don't like the lack of communication and work among the L.G.P.N.'s of 7H. I worked on patient care a lot when I was an L.G.P.N. I don't like the level of nursing care on 7H. It's a disgrace. I was amazed at how good the L.G.P.N.'s were who were transferred from CCU. . . . When I came to this hospital, I applied for a position on a pediatric unit. Instead, I was placed on 7H. I hope that I will be able to transfer within the hospital. I hear from the per diems that this floor is known for poor nursing care. Tensions on the floor are running high.

Colleen's high expectations of her own performance were illustrated in a respiratory arrest situation described by Deidre. Once when Colleen went back for an extra look at a patient, she found her choking on prunes and helped remove the food. The patient next experienced chest pain and suffered a respiratory arrest. The doctors inserted a CVP (central venous pressure line) and inadvertently caused a pneumothorax (collapsed lung). Colleen actively participated in the team's resuscitation efforts during this crisis. After it was over she had a difficult time accepting how well she had performed. She worried about her other patients even though Tammy covered Colleen's district during the code.

The G.N.'s showed the strain of their first professional nursing jobs. They often appeared tense and tired during the first six months. Some of them were better adapted, or were, according to Kate, "cutting it better," than others. One resigned for a job in a smaller hospital. Another was moved back to days from evenings for "shadowing" (close observation and direction by an experienced R.N.).

Even after passing the state's licensing examination and officially becoming R.N.'s, the recent G.N.'s admitted that they were still upset about their lack of knowledge. In the following example, these feelings were evident when they talked about a medical diagnosis, lingular infiltrate:

PAM: I'm going to look it up, though, because I want to know, too.

SHARON: Me too.

PAM: I'm embarrassed when I don't know a diagnosis, but. . . .

KATE: Oh, come on!

SHARON: We can't know everything. That's how I feel. . . .

The new R.N.'s lack of knowledge and their limited clinical skill as a group contributed to the R.N.-L.G.P.N. problem that awaited them as they began their careers on 7H. Almost always, Kate or Deidre assigned a new nurse to be the primary nurse of one of the districts. Even though they had been preceptored by more experienced R.N.'s, they still encountered problems being in charge of a district where most often the associate nurse was an L.G.P.N. with many years of clinical experience.

Thus the new G.N. who became an R.N. in September or February had to make decisions about patient care and management of a district. These decisions, tentative at first, gradually became more sure. The new R.N.'s divided the work among the staff and soon learned this skill well. They were constantly aware that any sudden change in patient status could ruin their well-contrived plans. Their uncertainty was evident.

The seasoned R.N.'s were a source of knowledge and support for the new nurses. Deidre most often arranged the staff's work schedule so that one experienced R.N. was available to the new graduates. However, there were shifts when this was not possible. Then the G.N. relied on the nurse managers and assistant nurse managers from neighboring units. In addition, there was a director of nursing, an administrator of a few units, and a shift coordinator on evenings and nights who were sometimes called when answers were not found among the available nurses.

Licensed Graduate Practical Nurses and Nursing Assistants

Camille was a heavyset L.G.P.N. who had just celebrated twenty-five years of employment at the hospital. All of these years were spent caring for the patients of 7H. She was quiet-spoken, patient, and gentle. Her sense of humor was light and infectious. She moved constantly as she worked the day shift, walking stiffly with her arthritis. She was a woman of strong religious faith who never said an unkind word and who occasionally admitted that her hypertension medication made her a little dizzy. On one occasion, Camille mentioned with pride that she was pleased with how well Sharon, a new R.N., was doing as the primary nurse of a district they commonly shared. It was evident that this hard-working L.G.P.N. thought that Sharon worked hard also.

Marie, an L.G.P.N. with fourteen years of experience on 7H, was a slim, skeptical, sarcastic woman. Marie had most patient situations under control and little of what happened on 7H surprised her. This is not to say that Marie had few comments. On the contrary, she spoke often, sharing her perspectives with anyone who caught her sardonic, terse comments in the utility room. Her sarcasm, which was usually tinged with humor, might lead some to think that she did not care. Marie did care, but one would never guess it listening to her complain about "complainer" patients in the utility room. She had a hard exterior but soft interior. When caring for patients, Marie was patient, competent, gentle, and matter of fact. Her nursing style emerged most clearly one day as she cared for a confused, difficult patient who had caused the staff much consternation. The patient was very upset that day and repeated self-deprecatory remarks. Marie corrected him saying, "Would I spend time with you [if you were not worth it]? You're worth it." She patiently walked him down the hall so that he could have a tub bath and washed his hair. Marie also enjoyed reminiscing about former patients who came back to 7H or were admitted to other hospital units.

Exuding an air of "I'm not surprised at anything that happens here," Marie had seen everything and was quiet, and for the most part patient, about the lack of change on 7H. When Marie was angry about unit or patient problems, however, she vented her emotions in the utility room. For example, one day she expressed anger at the utility room hopper odors, but she never raised her voice when she complained. She also dramatized the poor conditions of the hospital by recounting a story about rats and mice in the coffee shop. Nevertheless, she continued to work on the same unit despite physical conditions and a succession of head nurses, nurse managers, and new G.N.'s. When told about the administrative promise that 7H would be renovated she stated, "When I come in all bent over on a cane—they've been talking about renovating for years." Marie's devotion to 7H may have been due to her view of the unit as an old, predictable, sometimes difficult friend.

It was clear that Marie knew the hospital and many hospital personnel well. She greeted people cordially who came to 7H, whether to visit or to work. She planned to stay on the unit, though there would be job opportunities in the new hospital building now under construction.

Dotty worked on 7H for the two years following her graduation from an L.G.P.N. program. She was a middle-aged nurse who set high standards of patient care. The patient came first with Dotty. She worked well with the new G.N.'s and especially appreciated the skill of Colleen, who was often her primary nurse.

When confronted by a difficult staff-relations problem, Dotty would discuss it straightforwardly. There were new graduates that Dotty preferred not to work with. She made this clear to Deidre. Dotty's love was nursing. She thrived when she cared for people. Dotty planned eventually to take high school chemistry in order to seek admission to an R.N. program of studies, because, she said, "I love this profession. I think it's wonderful."

Nancy, a slim, attractive L.G.P.N., worked the evening shift permanently and only rarely rotated to the day shift. She was eloquent, saucy, and intelligent—a woman with high expectations of herself. Anyone who failed to perform her job well as either an R.N. or an L.G.P.N., Nancy did not respect. She knew how to work the hospital system and the unit system. Her nursing assessment abilities and clinical skill with patients were respected by her primary nurse. Nancy's insights, suggestions, and comments about patients were obviously well received by all of the nursing staff during evening and night change-of-shift report.

Two other L.G.P.N.'s were transferred to 7H in October, Leslie and Mabel. They came from CCU and awaited new positions in the soon-to-be-completed cardiac step-down unit. Leslie and Mabel, who described themselves as "displaced persons," were both expert L.G.P.N.'s. They were upset with the types of patients and heavy patient care load of 7H and were depressed about the oncology patients for whom they now cared. All of the nursing staff, particularly the permanent L.G.P.N.'s, were very impressed with Leslie's and Mabel's clinical skills, especially their ability to read EKG's. The new L.G.P.N.'s constituted both a stimulus and a threat, and as a result of their coming, both "new" R.N.'s and "old" L.G.P.N.'s improved their performance.

Leslie's pride in her nursing care was reflected in the following incident. A middle-aged woman, in the hospital because of lumbosacral pain, kept complaining to Leslie and asking for pillow adjustments and back massage. She told Leslie that she did not believe that Leslie gave her Tylenol for pain. Leslie was incensed by the patient's disbelief and lack of trust in her. She prided herself on her honesty and excellent patient care.

Mabel also gave expert, compassionate patient care and respected her patients' rights to make choices about their nursing care. Because of her expertise in patient care, Mabel delighted many of the 7H staff when she shared the same district with them as associate nurse. The permanent L.G.P.N.'s started to pour medications more frequently after her arrival, since she frequently gave medications to her patients. In addition, Kate complimented Mabel on the clarity and the abundance of assessment findings included in her nurses' notes. Despite the staff's warm reception, however, Mabel was upset by the unit's oncology patients, most likely because she hated to see their pain. Mabel also had other regrets:

> You never get the chance to read patient charts on the medical floors as you do in CCU. There you know a great deal of information about the patient through the help of the thoroughly completed Kardexes [used at change-of-shift report]. Here, on 7H, the nurses did not have time to read charts.

Both Leslie and Mabel commiserated about working on 7H and waited longingly for the time when they would be transferred to the cardiac step-down unit. Soon Leslie was moved to a neighboring medical unit because they needed more staff. In late winter, both Leslie and Mabel transferred to the newly built cardiac step-down unit. Mabel was relieved to go back to cardiac care and said, "You know when they're dying down there. You have the monitors." On 7H she had had a dying cancer patient who, as Mabel fed her orange sherbet, asked her, "Am I dead yet?"

Mabel's skill and compassion were missed. In early February, before she left, the nursing staff regretfully celebrated her transfer and the departures of Leslie (who had departed earlier) and Kate with a party of coldcuts, salad, and cake. The 7H staff teased the departing nurses, especially Mabel, about missing them and not coming back: "You leave us; don't come back."

Betty was a middle-aged, buxom nursing assistant who was permanent evening shift staff. She never stopped bustling about the unit and was constantly working in her patients' rooms. Very intense and perfectionistic about her job, Betty disapproved of the boisterousness of the younger, evening shift nurses. Betty explained how she worked in the later part of the evening shift:

> After my 8 P.M. vital signs I begin getting my patients ready for bed by changing sheets, washing incontinent patients (I give a partial bath),

straightening sheets. . . . I call it P.M. care. . . . Yes, I do backrubs. Cer-
tainly, I have my standards. I always ask the patients if they want a back-
rub; it's their choice. . . . Look at the room; there are supplies for the
next shift.

Betty nursed her patients in the old fashioned way. For her a patient was always right and a nurse should always be professional.
She was the only staff on 7H who still wore a nurse's cap. Betty
thought that nursing was a vocation, a calling. She insisted that
there had to be something of God involved in nursing care and that
the devotion to human welfare had to be there.

Both the L.G.P.N.'s and the nursing assistants held their time-
worn niches on the unit. The R.N.'s respect for the L.G.P.N.'s and
nursing assistants was particularly noticeable during change-of-
shift report. Nancy, Camille, Mabel, Dotty, Marie, and Elsie freely
contributed information that was well received. In addition, the
R.N.'s had their preferences to work with certain L.G.P.N.'s and
nursing assistants in their districts because their expertise made the
shift "go easier."

Many of the nursing staff of 7H have not been described. Those
who were described were chosen because they were primary or secondary informants who effectively characterized the unit. The
complete list of 7H's nursing staff is found in Table 1.

L.G.P.N.'S AND R.N.'S: DIFFERENCES IN ROLES

During the time of my study, L.G.P.N.'s and R.N.'s worked reason-
ably well together on the unit. They sometimes had problems, and
some of their problems stemmed from the fact that the new R.N.'s
had less clinical and life experience than did most of the L.G.P.N.'s
and nursing assistants. A lunchtime discussion with two L.G.P.N.'s,
Dotty and Camille, elicited from Dotty the practical nurses' interpretation of how the new R.N.'s saw them:

> Some of us are old enough to be their mothers. They don't like to tell us
> what to do. Besides that, they are inexperienced. They stay at the hos-
> pital for not even a year. They get restless and look around for some-
> thing else to do. The L.G.P.N.'s stay [on 7H] year after year. I don't think
> that this hospital will ever get rid of its L.G.P.N.'s.

Both of these L.G.P.N.'s were sensitive to the fact that they wielded a lot of power by virtue of their persistence and experience. As Camille said, "I just keep going and doing."

Situations often developed on 7H that pointed out R.N.-L.G.P.N. role differences and difficulties. For example, after a series of G.N. and R.N. medication errors, Deidre instituted a medication-order chart check to be completed by primary and associate nurses at the end of each shift. Deidre was adamant about this check, but did not get cooperation from the L.P.G.N.'s. Marie responded to Deidre's dictum and simultaneously clarified the boundaries between the R.N. and the L.G.P.N.: "Lots of time I see the orders before the primary nurse [R.N.], lots of times. I won't babysit the charts" for the newly graduated R.N. This was Marie's way of telling Deidre and the experienced and new R.N.'s that the orders were the R.N.'s domain, and that they were on their own.

Another example emerged when Beth let a blood transfusion run for over four hours, thus inadvertently violating hospital policy. Marie did not offer sympathy to Beth over this error. Instead she said, "R.N.'s should think like R.N.'s. No blood should hang over four hours." Once again Marie delineated the difference between the roles of the R.N. and the L.G.P.N.: the higher status of the R.N. brings more responsibility.

NURSING STAFF ESPRIT

Both R.N.'s and L.G.P.N.'s worked hard as primary and associate nurses in the four districts of the unit and cared for the unit's cardiac, cancer, other medical patients, and occasional surgical patient. Temporary nurses from the p.r.n. pool complained about the heavy work load of 7H patients and criticized the nursing care they witnessed. As part of the 7H staff, Beth felt that an esprit de corps was missing among the nursing staff. She therefore doubted, on one occasion, that nursing care planned for one of her patients would be followed from shift to shift:

> Even though I write it on the Kardex and remind them in report, I can't be sure that it will be done. The patient with the excoriated perineum says, "No one does it like you do."

The patient's perineum was healing, but with inconsistent follow-up; Beth believed that her work would have been in vain. Beth wished that the nurses would join together for more concerted patient care efforts.

Some of this lack of mutual effort was related to the persistence of staff behavior that maintained the status quo. The staff's resistence to change was evident in their reactions to a new policy of patient coverage and assignment designed and instituted by Deidre. The policy was included in the nursing staff's log book for October 5:

> Log Entry #18: New policy: associate nurses [L.G.P.N.'s and nursing assistants] are now distributing linens and answering lights while primary nurse takes report. Primary nurse will evaluate load and make assignments accordingly, then give report to associate nurse. Starting tomorrow A.M., one district of P.N. [primary nurse] and A.N. [associate nurse] will take report. P.N.'s will exchange reports when time is available or if something significant is going on.

Nancy, a powerful L.G.P.N., sabotaged Deidre's policy. Deidre confronted her and tried to convince her that the policy would provide more support to the new G.N.'s and reduce the stress of their growth period. Deidre also hoped that this policy would reduce R.N. turnover. Nevertheless, Nancy opposed the policy and persisted in taking fewer patients than the new R.N. assigned her. She left Ann, a recent G.N., to "pick up" the uncared for patients. Eventually the new policy was ignored by all of the staff.

Deidre knew that the unit was in an uproar because of staff relations. She set six-month goals and committed herself to shaping her staff, including R.N.'s, L.G.P.N.'s, and nursing assistants. She planned to spend more time with the stronger-willed L.G.P.N.'s, Marie (day shift), Nancy (evenings), and Denise (nights). She was not surprised that a lot of "backbiting and ratting" was going on among the staff. Deidre initially saw the new policy as a way to move toward primary nursing, a newer method of twenty-four-hour patient care responsibility and planning.

Despite, and perhaps because of, the staff's abandoning the change of assignment policy and of Deidre's delaying primary nursing, 7H moved into a period of relative tranquillity in November and into December. Parties, a pollyanna, and better staffing patterns were planned for the holiday season. Inexperienced R.N.'s became more confident and began to look for different jobs within the hospital.

OTHER HOSPITAL PERSONNEL

Medical Clerks

The medical clerks of 7H wielded their power skillfully. Their territory was well established. They sat at a desk in front of the nurses' station dressed in blue uniforms to distinguish them from nursing and other hospital personnel. The medical clerks no longer reported to the nurse manager. They had their own beeper-carrying supervisor, who wore a blue lab coat. She in turn reported to a unit manager. Deidre resented the fact that the medical clerks were not under her managerial jurisdiction. Her resentment was obvious, for example, when she tried unsuccessfully to determine which clerk's initials were written on a doctor's transcribed order. She felt that the head clerk was trying to sabotage her authority, and she had evidence of two orders on which clerks had incorrectly followed through.

Jennifer, the head clerk, was slim, attractive, and quiet. Most of her working hours were devoted to the patients' charts. She repeatedly transcribed doctors' orders from the chart to the nursing Kardex and laboratory and other departmental forms. She checked on patients' scheduled appointments and reported this information to the primary nurses. She called departments to track down misplaced or delayed reports of diagnostic studies. She thinned charts and added to charts. She also alerted the busy R.N.'s when charts piled up and awaited R.N. signatures confirming that doctors' orders were noted and clerk transcriptions accurate.

Jennifer and Pamela, another medical clerk, worked together at the desk when the unit was really busy. Pamela also worked as clerk on a neighboring unit. Louise, the evening shift clerk, came about 12:30 P.M. and worked until 9:30 P.M.

The clerks were pleasant to all who came to the desk. They appreciated those personnel who greeted them cordially. Often they would direct questions to the nurses and doctors. They could be very helpful to the R.N.'s when they shared their knowledge about which departments handled unusual diagnostic tests. Frequently the R.N.'s and other nursing staff, in an effort to reduce error, helped the clerks decipher some of the doctors' writing.

The tensions in 7H increased during the fall as the number of medication errors increased. Both the nurses and the clerks complained about doctors who either wrote illegibly or failed to "flag" orders. At other times, the nurses blamed some of the problems with medications on the medical clerks and nurse–medical clerk relations worsened. One day, for example, Colleen complained about the clerks during shift report: "And they [the doctors] cut back on her Lasix. Damn it. I don't believe they [the medical clerks] didn't take this order off." Medication errors and the details of medication orders were a constant source of frustration to the nurses. Eventually, however, medication errors decreased and working relations among the nurses and medical clerks improved. The R.N.'s were pleased that the clerks handled a lot of the unit's paper work and thus freed them for more time with patients. Nevertheless, the presence of the medical clerks added to an already complicated patient care system.

The pressures of 7H affected all of the people who worked there permanently. The nurses did not always notify the medical clerks when most of the nurses closeted themselves in the utility room for a staff meeting. Pamela expressed her displeasure about this oversight and asserted her importance by complaining once when a staff meeting was in progress.

Overall, the working relationship of the medical clerks and the nurses was pleasant. They shared parties and snacks, laughs and sorrows on a unit that was difficult most of the time.

Laboratory Technicians, Volunteers, and Escort Staff

Dennis spent more time on 7H than did any other lab technician. He was always friendly and easygoing. In the morning he greeted the medical clerks and nurses and stopped in the back of the nurses' station for a quick cup of coffee. After his coffee, he prepared the blood tubes, stickers, and lab slips with patients' names. He was skillful and almost always "got the veins," as he moved from patient to patient.

During the summer months a high school student from the neighborhood around the hospital worked as a paid volunteer. The nurses used her as a messenger and sent her to different departments to pick up equipment or IV's. Most often she made beds, checked patient identibands (identification bracelets printed with name, hospital number, and other data), and inserted signs in the slots over the patients' beds. She dressed in street clothes and a pink jacket, as did all volunteers.

Another volunteer, a middle-aged woman, was a 7H regular. She came to the unit one day a week, week after week, moving in and out of patients' rooms as she made beds and ran errands for nurses and patients. She was quietly cherished by the staff.

Escort staff, easily recognizable in their dark blue jackets, moved to and from 7H transporting patients by wheelchair or stretcher to different departments for diagnostic testing or surgery and returning them to their rooms. The nursing staff had their favorites among the escort workers. These were the ones who gently helped the nurses move cancer patients with bone pain from bed to litter to bed again with the least possible suffering.

Often escort staff tracked down nurses in the utility room during report or found them in other patient rooms. Nurses and escort personnel worked together to move patients back into bed. Many of the escort staff were considerate of the exhausted patients but resented the time it took for the nurses to stop other patient care to assist them. The escort staff kept up a quick pace of rapid patient transport in the hospital so that diagnostic testing, physical therapy, and operating room schedules could be maintained.

Patients

Patients wore bedroom attire, including pajamas, night gowns, or short, open-backed patient gowns that left back and buttocks exposed if the patient or nurse was not careful. At admission, patients had identibands placed on their wrists. Most nurses called patients by their first names. Often they asked patients permission to do this.

Patients stayed in their rooms, unless they left the unit for diagnostic testing or other business related to their hospital stay. Sometimes a few patients visited a small lounge that was shared with the patients of the neighboring medical unit. Most 7H patients preferred their rooms and were too ill to move far from their beds.

Confused, elderly patients were seated in geri chairs and rolled by the nurses into the corridor to help stimulate their orientation to reality and to help the staff keep an eye on them. For example, one patient with Alzheimer's disease was kept in view in the hall because he had flushed paper towels down the toilet in his room and caused plumbing problems.

If a patient or family member appeared frequently at the Nurses' Station, the medical clerks and nurses became annoyed and labeled such a person "a pain." The patients were expected to use the electrical call bell attached to their bed rail or bed sheet when they needed assistance. The operation of this device was explained at admission by a staff member. Some call bells were more pressure sensitive than others and were given to weaker patients. A light over the patient's room signaled the staff at the same time the patient pressed on the electrical cord.

In general, patients seemed to think that 7H was a good unit. For example, Florence James, a sixty-year-old, mildly obese black woman with severe cardiac problems and diabetes, spent several weeks on 7H. She liked the unit and was proud that she was Pamela's first patient as a new nurse. "I love this floor," she said. "[There are] some good nurses on this floor. They are really compassionate."

7H received many patients admitted with cardiac problems. Cardiologists were allocated a certain percentage of 7H beds. This affected the patient turnover rate, since the turnover of cardiac patients was rapid. "Rule out" (R/O) MI patients, in for a three-day stay, balanced the workload with the long-term 7H patients. In addition, there were cardiac catheterization patients, oncology patients, a few orthopedic and general surgery patients, and patients with other medical diseases. Ventilator-dependent patients also came to 7H after having survived the therapeutic efforts of the critical care units and vacated critical care beds for more acutely ill patients.

Patients who could move around easily were labeled "walkie talkies" by R.N.'s during report. In some ways, younger and more alert patients were treated differently from older patients. It was as though the staff was more personally threatened by the combination of youth, alertness, and disease.

The nurses arranged small birthday parties for patients. For example, they arranged a modest birthday party for an eighteen-year-old with a card from the staff, a slice of cake from the dietary department, and a song by the nurses. The staff were unhappy because the hospital did not send a whole cake for everyone to share.

The 7H nurses were critical of how other nursing and medical staffs handled patients on other hospital units. The term "dump job" was common to hospital personnel. It referred to patients with little hope of recovery and who were abandoned by family and to some extent by the health care delivery system. 7H nurses patiently cared for these patients and often resented the various hospital therapies that "kept them going." On the other hand, should a doctor discontinue a routine IV, the nurses would balk. The nurses could not bear to "dump" a patient on their unit by stopping the fluids and limited nutrition that an IV offered.

Miriam told Marie and Beth a "dump job" story during change-of-shift report:

COLLEEN: Excuse me, Miriam, did you get a Donna Brown in 743 Window?

MIRIAM: No we didn't; she coded last night right before she was supposed to come down.

COLLEEN: O.K.

MIRIAM: I've got a good story for you on that one. [Amused.]

MARIE: They were going to send her down here?

MIRIAM: Oh, yeah. They were yelling and screaming and Pamela . . . said, "We're tying up loose ends; we can't take her until 11:15 [P.M.]." 11:25 code blue 8H! And Phyllis said, "Oh God, I haven't. . . ."

BETH: It's horrible, isn't it?

MARIE: Oh, God, suppose that escort had her.

MIRIAM: They said they wanted her off 8H. She's a screamer. Because she's a screamer, they figured they didn't want the noise up there. It was disturbing the other patients.

BETH: Because we've got screamers here!

MARIE: But that's not fair to Deidre and us down here.

MIRIAM: I know! I agree! So what happened was. Wait till you hear the best part. They ran the code. The supervisor goes up there. They still want to move the lady down here! The nurse says, "How soon can we get her down to 7H?" She [the supervisor] said, "She's either staying here or going to ICU." The lady's intubated and everything up there.

BETH: That must have been a new nurse to give a request like that.

MIRIAM: All I know is they were pretty hot up there.

BETH: Somebody's coded, they can't move them.

MARIE: Oh, why not? [Sarcastically].

MIRIAM: Why not? [With amusement.]

MARIE: This is a garbage can, so why not?

MIRIAM: [Laughter.] True.

BETH: You're not going to allow them to become garbage down here.

MIRIAM: Yes they are, yes they are.

MARIE: That's all they put down here.

MIRIAM: The rejects.

The 7H nurses respected and enjoyed patients as well as complained about them. One type of patient who invoked disrespect was the abuser of alcohol or drugs. The nurses especially feared the violence of DT's (delirium tremens, alcohol withdrawal) because they had heard stories about nurses who were physically harmed by patients. The following is an example of how 7H nurses approached an alcoholic patient.

Loretta, a new G.N., went into a patient's room. Wanda and Marie, L.G.P.N.'s, followed. The patient was lying sideways on the bed. He looked almost ready to put his head between the side rails. He was elderly and disheveled with an ecchymotic (bruised) area around his one eye with swelling that caused his eyelid to close. The nurses discussed the doctor's refusal to write an order for Haldol (a tranquilizer). The patient was so agitated that they retied his arm restraints and moved his water pitcher out of reach. "He's a Houdini," Loretta said. He kept complaining about having to go to the bathroom (urinate) even though each nurse told him to go to the bathroom through his tube. He was confused and afraid of wetting the bed. He did not realize that he had a Foley (urinary catheter) in place. While the nurses did not touch the patient roughly, the tones of their voices revealed attitudes of disrespect. This patient consistently caused the nurses to worry about how he might harm himself. He pulled his Foley out, nearly strangled himself with IV tubing, and frequently pulled his IV out of his arm. He spat on Elsie, one of the L.G.P.N.'s. While the nurses were amused at some of his antics, they were also worried and annoyed. Their ambivalence was evident as they tolerantly and impatiently spoke of him during report.

The nurses also expressed tenderness toward their patients. An elderly patient was admitted to 7H from the Emergency Room with myxedema (hypothyroidism) and cervical neck fractures of cervical vertebrae C4 and C5 caused by an accident. She had swallowing difficulties and was very anxious. The patient asked Tammy to kiss her. When Tammy did, the patient said, "Then I can die." The nurses were afraid to turn this patient; her cervical fracture had been unstabilized for twenty-four hours. They were afraid that bending the patient's neck would result in "killing" her, in spite of the immobilizing collar she wore. The patient told Miriam, the night shift nurse, and Beth and Cecile, the day shift nurses, that she was afraid of dying. The nurses did not disagree with her, but talked with her and gently bathed her, turning her from side to side. 7H nurses' caring was seen most often in their soft voice tones and in their remembering the details that patients requested.

In general, patients seemed to think that 7H was a good unit. Many thanked the nurses at discharge. Some left flowers, candy, or food. Families mailed cards and notes to the unit. These were posted on the bulletin board in the nurses' station for all to see. The nurses delighted in these visible acknowledgments of their work. All the staff shared the food. Some ex-patients returned to the unit for what the nurses called "remember me" visits.

The 7H nurses, patients, and hospital staff coexisted and shared part of their life on the unit. Their perspectives provided a social context for this study of nursing rituals. The complexity of the unit's social life is evident in the descriptions of this section. These descriptions are a stage on which are embedded the descriptions and explanations of the nursing rituals studied.

II

The Nursing Ritual of
Post-Mortem Care

This chapter includes descriptions and analyses of the shared experiences of patients, families, and staff with the resuscitation dilemma and post-mortem care. The resuscitation dilemma, or "code/no code" decision, provides a context for the discussion of post-mortem care. 7H nurses did not give post-mortem care to dead bodies. Instead, they cared for patients they knew both before and after death. This chapter also contains a brief discussion of the tradition of post-mortem care by American nurses and also includes recollections by 7H nurses of dying patients they had cared for.

Dying and the "Do Not Resuscitate" Dilemma

7H nurses confronted dying and death as they worked, but dying and death disturbed them and disrupted the patterns of the unit. 7H nurses participated in the dying and deaths of some of the patients who came to their medical unit. They often predicted deaths. Some deaths surprised even the most experienced staff member.

Patients, families, and nurses shared the death crisis. Doctors arrived when called, confirmed, and left the death event. Nurses anticipated, confirmed, and participated in the after-the-end activities. Families suffered throughout the dying and deaths of their loved ones.

All of the deaths that occurred on 7H involved the dilemma of whether or not "to resuscitate." The Category III, DNR (do not resuscitate) predicament appeared innocuously in the R.N.'s change-of-shift report:

751W. Mr. Price with septic shock. Category III, DNR. Vital signs × 3. No problems on him. Venti-mask. The man is NPO, changed to liquid. No gag reflex yesterday. IV 80 drops per minute. 450 credit till 9 A.M. Another bag in back. Had a culture of his decubiti in E.R. Attempted to suction him. He fought it. He has a deviated septum. He's pinky. He has a mini neb. Check the start date on his Sustacal. He's so thin, he has no meat. I've never seen anyone so thin in my life.

The DNR, Category III phrase refers to a decision made by a patient and family to prevent resuscitation efforts by hospital staff in the event of cardiac or respiratory arrest. Because the phrase was usually surrounded by other abbreviations and the contracted language nurses use during change-of-shift report, it is difficult to detect from the reports the struggle that always accompanied the patient and family decision of Do Not Resuscitate.

Resuscitation actions have become nursing care measures. The nurses on 7H wrestled with resuscitation decisions. Without a doctor's order not to resuscitate, the nurses were afraid not to act. They equated inaction with letting someone die without nursing care. The 7H nurses' rule about what to do in the event of cardiac and respiratory arrests, the events that called for resuscitation, was: Resuscitate Everyone Who Does Not Have a *Do Not Resuscitate* Order.

In the following situation, the nurses are instrumental in obtaining a DNR classification for a patient whom they discuss during an evening change-of-shift report:

751 Window: Padula with her left CVA [cerebrovascular accident]-infarct. I just . . . we just made her a DNR. I told Dr. Fischer, we have to get a code [status] in her because . . .

Right.

She was ready to kind . . . she's not doing good back there. So the husband was here at the time, so I said [to the doctor], "Quick go in there and talk to him" you know, and see. And at first the husband did refuse. He wanted her on a respirator and he didn't care. But then they explained that once she went on a respirator she would never come off, and that there is damage to the brain so they . . . it's all signed in the progress notes and everything.

Uh huh.

Her Salem sump is still in, and it's clamped. It's not [connected] to anything. She had a feeding tube in with her Isocal at 80. You have a credit of, last time I looked at 3, was 300 . . .

She get a S & A [sugar and acetone urine specimen] on her?

Yeah, it was +3 and negative. O.K. I suctioned her twice today. She is so thick with mucus. It is so gunky. But it just runs out of her nose. I went out there and like the whole pillow, I mean was soaked with the stuff. And besides, just suctioning her, how much I got out. She's really going through. . . .

Um hum.

I asked Dr. Fischer about putting that Venti-mask back on because that'll at least break up her secretions 'cause those secretions we can't get up; so he said he would evaluate that and talk with his res, . . . you know, the senior about that. Since she was a DNR, he didn't see why we should do that. I have to get new IV's put in so they're both now in her, I think, right hand.

They're both in her hand, one hand?

Yep. I think that's the only place they could get them. Her insulin now, she's a DNR, they want no coverage on her. They D/C'd [discontinued] all her blood work, her daily fasting sugars and everything. Because her sugar for me was 215 and I asked him, they want her covered, and they said no. . . .

She was out for 3 P.M. [blood sugar]

Yeah, that was her 3 P.M. . . . I mean that was her fasting and she's out for 3 P.M. Her BUN [blood urea nitrogen] and creatinine, 41 and 1.5. Hemoglobin and hematocrit, 11.8 and 36.1. O.K. She's on hematest stools which I forgot to do. She did have three stools for us today. Her hydralazine, her pressure was 120/90.

This discussion during shift report demonstrates the nurses' position. They thought that the patient was "going bad" and was likely to code. They did not believe that the patient should be subjected to the therapeutic assaults of their efforts and the resuscitation team's efforts. They warned the doctor of the impending event and encouraged him to approach the patient's husband. A "DNR code status" was obtained, recorded in the doctors's progress notes, and signed by the patient's husband (see Figure 4). The nurses felt more secure after they had received family permission not to initiate resuscitation efforts in the event of cardiac or respiratory arrest. Without this signed permission, they feared litigation.

Progress Notes   DNR Class III

2/1   6:50 P.M. Mr. N. A. is not to be resuscitated or
       receive any type of CPR. In addition, no other
       heart medications or special treatments are to be
       undertaken. The patient is DNR Class III.

Nurse's Signature   Doctor's Signature

                           Patient's Wife's Signature

Doctors' Order Sheet
2/1   1. DNR Class III
       2. D.C. Isordil

Doctor's Signature

Nurse's Signature

Figure 4. Example documentation of "Do Not Resuscitate Decision"
on patient chart: Progress Notes and Doctors' Order Sheet Entry.
2/1 = date; D.C. = discontinue.

When a patient was classified as a DNR, certain therapeutic
actions were abandoned. Blood sugar coverage with insulin was
stopped along with other blood studies. The more basic life support measures of nutritional and fluid intake were maintained,
however, with a Sustacal feeding through a gastrointestinal tube
and through IV's which were restarted after other "lines" infiltrated. Doctors continued to "round" on dying patients and write
orders. Nursing care continued. Nurses bathed, fed, checked

breathing, monitored IV's, watched, and talked to the patients who waited for death.

Some patients were aware that death was imminent; others were not. When one of these slowly dying patients was "dumped" by his family, the 7H nurses became his most frequent source of contact with other people. For example, for weeks Marie cared almost exclusively for a dying patient during the day shift. Beth, as primary nurse, was also a major caretaker. Irving Stern, who was ninety years old, lay in bed with his eyelids half closed, aware of no one, restless and occasionally "rammy" (moving around in his bed in an erratic manner, taking his patient gown off), but most frequently moving little, moaning seldom. His face was a reddish blue color. According to an elderly man who visited Mr. Stern, the patient had been a pleasant man before his illness.

Mr. Stern breathed "on his own," without a respirator. His family agreed to make him a DNR, Category III. Marie had not seen them visit during the day and did not know if they visited in the evening. She resented and disapproved of their absence, especially his daughter's.

Mr. Stern was admitted to 7H with a stroke. He came from a semi-independent residence for the elderly. Recently he had had several episodes of fluctuating low blood pressures and some apneic periods which led the nurses to the conclusion: "Oh, God, he's gonna go!" Despite these problems, he lived and was able to take a small amount of nutrition by eating a pureed diet and "keep open" IV fluids. Then, over the course of two weeks, his health declined further. He stopped eating. He received no medications "except an occasional shot of Haldol." His respiratory rate was erratic at times. Rapid mouth breathing dried his lips and tongue. The doctors inserted a nasogastric tube for feedings and arranged for his discharge to a nursing home. At mid-September, he was abruptly discharged from 7H and the hospital to a nursing home.

The morning of his discharge, two hospital transport personnel (EMT's) came to transport him to a nursing home. His feeding tube was in place. Marie complained about the transfer. She thought that the patient "looked terrible." "Well, nothing can be done," she said sarcastically. She knew he was leaving to die. Deidre and Marie helped the EMT's get him onto the transport litter. Marie plugged in the nasogastric feeding tube and removed the INT (IV access). The EMT's asked Marie to sign the sheet releasing Mr. Stern. Marie used sarcasm to hide her outrage and feeling of impotence. She said she hoped "they," the hospital, would not bill her. Both Diedre and Marie were surprised by the early arrival of the hospital transport. They had no time to react to and stop Mr. Stern's discharge. The next morning during the change-of-shift report, the nurses discussed this event:

MIRIAM: He was so close to going, they didn't have no right to ship him out.

BETH: You mean he died?

MIRIAM: Of course he died. Stern made it to the nursing home.

BETH: God, That's so sad.

MIRIAM: They wouldn't let him in [the nursing home], and they put him back on 8H. He died around 2:00 [A.M.] They called me. They [8H nurses] said, "I hear you have a dead body for us." I said, "No!"

As soon as the EMT personnel brought Mr. Stern to the nursing home, the nursing home staff there "took one look at him" and sent him back to the hospital. The nurses felt sad, guilty, and disgusted that a ninety-year-old man was shuttled back and forth between institutions just before his death.

This incident dramatizes the unintentional abandonment by the hospital and its utilization review board of a DNR patient and the breakdowns in communication between nurses and doctors. The attending physician had been pressured by utilization review. He arranged a transfer of which the nurses were unaware. The transport personnel came early on the morning shift, surprising Marie, who interpreted the situation as, "They don't care about this man. Didn't everyone know how ill Irving was?" He had been ill for days and close to death before, so why was it necessary to discharge him to a nursing home that particular day? The hospital needed the bed. "Nothing much" was being done for him. In this sense the hospital was an abstract agent concerned only with optimum bed use, and the 7H staff, represented by Marie, felt powerless to remind the abstract institution about a patient's vulnerability. The "nothing much" that was being done for him was care by the nurses on a twenty-four-hour basis. They bathed, fed, turned, and talked to Irving Stern while waiting for his death.

The nurses consistently applied their rule of "everyone is a code, except those who are DNR's." Patients surprised them at times when they "didn't have a chance" to get a DNR code status from the family through the doctor, such as in the following example given at morning change-of-shift report. The patient was a cancer patient who was dehydrated:

> MIRIAM: She woke up and she was like . . . she looked like she coded for a second. [Nervous laughter.] Because . . . 'cause she did stop breathing momentarily. I yelled . . . you know I yelled for help and she, you know, she started [breathing] right back up. Her pressure today was 128/70. [Laughter.] I mean, it scared the life out of me! I mean, she really scared me. I talked with Dr. Leonard and he put her . . . made her . . . just made her a Category III.

> SARAH: Oh, she is?

> MIRIAM: He just wrote us an order. He wrote it in the progress notes. He has discussed it with her husband, but he has not signed the. . . .

> SARAH: The husband hasn't?

> MIRIAM: Yeah. He hasn't signed the progress notes as of yet.

> SARAH: But it's documented in the progress notes that it was discussed?

> MIRIAM: Um hum.

> SARAH: All right, we have to have him sign. . . .

> MIRIAM: Yeah, I know. I hope she doesn't code until he gets in. All right. Yeah. 'Cause he's. Dr. Leonard had said that he discussed it with him. He said, you know, the husband decided not to make her a no code . . . to do everything possible, but if she had cardiac or respiratory arrest to just let her go, you know, doing for her. But he did write it in his progress notes if you can read his scribble.

The nurses had a conflict; they knew that it would be uncaring to resuscitate the patient, but they also recognized that legally their inaction could be questioned. Starting resuscitation would be morally offensive to them. They worked in a gray area. The husband had to sign, soon. In the event of an arrest, the nurses knew that the ultimate decision about whether or not to code rested with them, since most often they diagnosed the arrest event, called the "Code Blue," and initiated resuscitation efforts.

A DYING PATIENT, THE DNR DILEMMA, AND HIS POST-MORTEM CARE

The following report illustrates many aspects of dying and death on 7H. The patient was an emblematic example of the slow agony that some dying patients experience.

BETH: [7]41 Door: Blocked? [Since the patient in the room was seriously ill, dying and on a respirator, the room was "blocked" or "screened." No other patient was admitted to this semi-private room until his death.]

MIRIAM: [7]41 Window: Harry Bowman with COPD [chronic obstructive pulmonary disease]. Still had a 45 percent trach collar on. Vital signs have been stable on him. His color does not look as good today. He looks a little bit weaker; says he doesn't feel as strong today. Everything's been stable on him. She [night shift private duty nurse] suctioned him and didn't get too much, secretionwise, from him. She just got enough to do a Luken's sputum [sterile aspirated respiratory specimen] on him.

BETH: Is it grayish?

MIRIAM: Yeah. But she said it's a little bit thinner this morning than it was yesterday. It's not as congested today. He's out for a chest X-ray today.

BETH: He's still not having loose stools?

MIRIAM: Harry? Not that I know of.

BETH: He had been.

MIRIAM: She [private duty nurse] didn't give me anything. That's the report she gave me. He was medicated once for pain . . . for whatever kind of pain.

Harry Bowman, a man in his sixties, had been in the hospital since May. Most of this time was spent in and out of ICU. He stabilized to the extent that the doctors decided to transfer him again to a regular medical floor with private duty nurses caring for him on a twenty-four-hour basis. Intensive care beds were always in demand. This forced doctors to use beds in critical care units for patients with a better chance of recovery.

The nurses thought that Mr. Bowman was a "lovely man." He did not complain about his chronic suffering. He endured it. Often he turned his face away from the door at the entrance to his room. He looked toward the window and at the wall beneath the window. He was alert to his situation and his surroundings, a fact that made his lingering death seem particularly hard for him, his family, his nurses, and his doctors.

The 7H nurses seemed to respect Mr. Bowman's day shift private duty nurse, Melinda. This was unusual, since as a rule staff distrusted private duty nurses who came to the unit. (Melinda was forty years old, a diploma graduate from the hospital's nursing school who had entered nursing school after she had her children.) Melinda was in constant attendance to Mr. Bowman and his family. When he did not need her caring skills she made coffee for his wife and son. She was upset by the fact that her patient decided that day, August 2, that he did not want to be on his respirator. However, he had been on the respirator over the night hours from 10:00 P.M. to 8:00 A.M. and for many days before that.

While Melinda was preparing coffee in the nourishment area for Mr. Bowman's wife and son, she responded to a question about how her patient was doing. It was unusual for her not to "try" with a patient. "He's tired," she said. He made an "active" decision. "He wants to die." She was teary-eyed and cleared her throat.

I explained to Melinda that I was studying post-mortem care. My question, her patient's decision to die that day, and the fact that it was August triggered tragic memories for her. She explained that her sister had been murdered the previous year. She cried and apologized for crying. "It's August. My sister was murdered. Her throat was slit." Melinda, the youngest and strongest family member, had identified the body. She also had told her father about his daughter's death because she was afraid that his neighbors would tell him. It was on the television news that day. She cried and apologized again.

Melinda went on to recount some details of her personal tragedy. Her sister's son had found his mother at home, dead and under the bed. Her father saw the news about the murder on television, yet his deafness had prevented him from knowing that it was his daughter.

Melinda digressed from the story of her sister's death and talked freely about nurses, about dying and post-mortem care, and about the acts of covering the faces of dead patients and wrapping dead patients in shrouds. She discussed what she did when one of her patients died. She said that she says an "Our Father" (the Lord's

Prayer) and added: "When I close their mouth and cover their face, I say it's final. Every time I see a dead body, I think of her [my sister]. I think that some of these life experiences make us more sensitive.

Melinda thanked me for listening and left the utility room. Mr. Bowman's wife and another relative were standing in the hall next to room 741. They looked as if they had been crying. Melinda was in the hall standing at the medication cart. She prepared an injection, 5 mg. of morphine sulfate for Mr. Bowman's pain. She went into his room and I followed her. Four of his family sat at the bedside.

Mr. Bowman was obviously in respiratory distress. He sat in bed in a semi-reclining (semi-Fowler's) position. Melinda said, "I have an injection for you, Harry, to make you more comfortable." Mr. Bowman refused, motioning her away with his hand and head. Melinda left the room, tears in her eyes. She wasted the drug, injecting it into a trash bag. Mr. Bowman's son had refused to let Melinda give breakfast to his father. It was difficult for nurses to stop trying, as Melinda said, to stop offering pain medication and food. Food was a very ordinary means of keeping patients alive and relief of pain through narcotics offered some comfort to Mr. Bowman.

The nurses and doctors needed a "do not resuscitate" order to disconnect Mr. Bowman's ventilator. Apparently no written permission had been obtained by the doctors to discontinue this life support. Connection to the ventilator was equated with prolongation of Mr. Bowman's life.

Mr. Bowman's son soon talked to a physical therapist about suctioning his father's tracheostomy (surgical opening into trachea). The therapist, who had come to Mr. Bowman's room to perform routine suctioning and chest physical therapy, and to check the ventilator, agreed to stop suctioning. She spoke to Chris, primary nurse for Mr. Bowman's district, and asked her opinion about discontinuing the chest physical therapy. Chris hesitatingly agreed that it should stop.

Later, Melinda sat at the nurses' station and wrote nurses' notes in Mr. Bowman's chart. She looked very worn, as though she had been through an exhausting time. She said Harry was "so-so. It's hard to say (when people will die). I'm not the type to fuss around. I could change his top sheet. I washed his face and put his teeth in and gave him a cold drink. I don't know what else to do. It's hard on us not to do something. That's the way we're trained to do."

Melinda's Nurses' Notes:

8:00—Received pt. [patient] very lethargic. Breathing is very poor. Pt. c/o [complained of] difficulty in breathing. Blood gases drawn. Refuses to go back on ventilator; states he wants to die. Does not want to go back to ICU. Refuses all futher treatment.

9:00—Pt. made DNR by Dr. Thomas with consultation of family.

10:00—Refused sedation. MSO$_4$ [morphine sulfate] as ordered by Dr. Thomas. Refused 10:00 meds.

10:30—Chest PT [physical therapy] not done. Visited by wife, son and immediate family members. Suctioned one time.

Mr. Bowman's son came to the nurses' station and asked, "Can anyone handle a kind of special request?" His father wanted a Dixie cup of ice cream. Melinda said she would be happy to get it, but his aunt wanted to get it, so Melinda sent her to the coffee shop. Later Sarah checked on Mr. Bowman and reported, "Harry's enjoying his ice cream; we got him ice cream." She smiled in delight.

During the shift, Melinda and the family moved in and out of the dying patient's room. Melinda was concerned. Mr. Bowman was hungry for more air. If the nurses and the doctors increased the oxygen liter flow rate, respiratory depression would result and the patient would "go to sleep" or die. Mr. Bowman was more alert and talking, a noticeable change since his decision to come off the ventilator. Beth, Deidre, and Melinda discussed Mr. Bowman's decision. They were ambivalent about it.

Melinda felt that Mr. Bowman was doing a little better in the early afternoon but that it was becoming harder for him to breathe. The family worried about getting a private duty nurse for Mr. Bowman for the evening shift. They had cancelled several private duty nurses, as evident in the following change-of-shift report.

Morning Report, August 2:

The family was not pleased with her performance because they didn't . . . she didn't suction him as often . . . she didn't think he needed it, and the family was, you know, saying he should be suctioned more often and this type of thing. . . . She was like the third or fourth one [evening private duty nurse] I've seen this week alone.

Mr. Bowman's family asked Melinda to stay over into the evening shift. She planned to. When Melinda gave Chris her afternoon report on Mr. Bowman, it became clearer that he, his family, and his nurses were just waiting for him to die. Death was coming slowly:

Afternoon Report, August 2:

CHRIS: [7]41 Window: Is Mr. Bowman. Mr. Bowman today decided to stay off the ventilator. He's refusing . . . you know, he's not taking any meds. He's just. . . .

PAMELA: What are they doing for him?

CHRIS: Just waiting for him to die. You know, he just feels that's his. . . .

CHRIS: They can't do it.

PAMELA: So Harry refused. . . . Oh, and he refuses medications and everything?

CHRIS: He's not taking any meds, no. He doesn't want them. He even had morphine ordered and he didn't want it.

PAMELA: Oh, he never said. . . .

CHRIS: It's getting more difficult for him to breathe now, so he did have a mini-neb [a medication to open his respiratory tract] and that helped him, but that's about all he's doing. He doesn't want any kind of chest PT. They came up to do an X-ray and he doesn't . . . he just doesn't want anything. He just wants to go. He's real ready. His whole family's here and the private duty nurse is willing to stay for a couple of hours. And she's going to try and get the night private duty nurse to come in a couple hours early 'cause the evening private duty, there is none. So, you might have him for a few hours. . . . Apparently the family didn't like her and she wasn't . . . you know, they weren't pleased with her performance and I don't think she was pleased with them, so it's just . . . she's not coming back.

PAMELA: Oh, O.K.

CHRIS: O.K., but he is alert. You'd be surprised at how good he looks. He looks better, I think, than he did this morning. They did gases [blood gases] on him, but I haven't even checked the results, but I'm sure they're not too good.

PAMELA: O.K.

CHRIS: O.K. That's about it for him. His O_2 [oxygen], I think, is set at 50 percent. So you know the story for him. I don't know how long he'll be around.

PAMELA: I didn't think he'd make it. . . .

Mr. Bowman decided the next morning to rescind his "no resuscitation" decision.

Morning Report, August 3:

MIRIAM: [7]41 Window: Harry Bowman with his respiratory failure. He's now a Category III, which he made himself yesterday. However, the way the progress note's written, he did not want to be in . . . put on a ventilator again. No heroic type measures. Well, the man started having respiratory pain. His . . . Dr. Thomas went in and talked to him, and told him he could have either some pain meds, put on the ventilator, or both. He decided to go back on the ventilator and take the pain meds. The son was very annoyed with the doctor for putting him back on the ventilator because it went against everything they had just signed for release yesterday. So as far as the DNR or Category III status, what I was told is if he had a cardiac arrest, let him go, but if he starts showing respiratory distress, you've got to do what you can for him. But just see if they want to put a clarification on that today. You know, it's like a total turnaround from what was there before. Mrs. B.'s [night supervisor] really upset about it, and knowing the man the way I do, when he starts to get hypoxic he's not real rational, so I'm wondering if, you know, even though the son signed it, you know, who's going to have the final say in this, the patient or the son at this point, because it looks like it'll be an ongoing battle. . . . The son's feeling all along has been "do everything for my father." If he doesn't like the way the nurse is doing it, he says he wants more, more, more type thing and the father decided he doesn't want all the stuff yesterday and the son went along and signed. . . .

CHRIS: Is he taking his meds?

MIRIAM: Yes, he is taking his meds. The guy's back on the ventilator. . . . He started taking meds in the evening. . . .

CHRIS: If I were his family, I'd be upset, too.

MIRIAM: I mean, you did it like a total 180 turnaround from what he was saying yesterday. . . . I don't know . . . he seemed, he just seemed like, "I'm ready, I don't want any more," you know it's too much. . . . They increased his Percocet [pain medication dosage].

After morning report it was obvious that the intern, Dr. Thomas, was concerned about supporting Mr. Bowman's decision to go back on the ventilator. He explained the situation to his senior resident. The more experienced doctor wanted to talk to Mr. Bowman's son.

He saw trouble brewing since the patient decided to rescind his DNR decision. Mr. Bowman's son was very unhappy with the intern's and his father's decision to go back on the ventilator.

Melinda was back on the day shift. She followed the doctors to Mr. Bowman's room and waited to hear what they would say on rounds. Melinda sat in a chair beside Mr. Bowman's bed, holding his hand and drinking coffee. She smiled, looking very comfortable. She looked more at peace with herself. Mr. Bowman was lying in bed. His tracheostomy was connected to an MAII ventilator. He looked weak, yet somehow at rest. His glasses were on and his head was turned toward Melinda. His eyes were closed and he was pale. None of his family was in the room. The No Visitors But Family sign remained on the open door.

Melinda talked later about the events of the previous evening. She had stayed until 9:30 P.M. At one point Mr. Bowman joked to his wife, who was feeding him: "I'm trying to go, and you're feeding me." He had had chest pain the previous evening; despite the Percocet, his pain had intensified. Melinda called the doctor and eventually the decision was made to put him on the ventilator. Melinda gave him another narcotic. Mr. Bowman's son became angry with the doctor; Melinda was upset. Should she have discouraged the move back to the ventilator? She was unsure. She stated that "comfort and hope" were part of her reasoning.

Despite having slept well, Melinda said that she was exhausted. She was troubled by the "on the respirator" change but thought that Mr. Bowman was mentally alert and able to make his decision. That morning the father and son had a long talk. The doctors wrote orders to disconnect the respirator and put the tracheal oxygen collar over Mr. Bowman's tracheostomy. Morphine sulfate was ordered to make him more comfortable.

Melinda wondered aloud how often an alert patient made an active decision to be disconnected from a ventilator so that he could die. Perhaps the fact that he was not dying fast enough was disturbing to all, patient, family, and staff.

Mr. Bowman had obviously convinced the nurses and doctors to connect him to the ventilator. The attending physician came to 7H to check on Mr. Bowman. He decided that the move back to the ventilator was a mistake. He ordered the ventilator discontinued and morphine sulfate 5 mg. q 2–3h p.r.n. (every 2–3 hours as needed).

When Sarah and Melinda were asked who would disconnect the ventilator, they said that Respiratory Therapy (technicians) would. Both nurses seemed very uncomfortable about performing this death-inviting action. Sarah knew Mr. Bowman from other units where she had worked that summer. She enjoyed him as a patient. No one on the staff disconnected Mr. Bowman from the respirator for hours after the doctor's order was written.

Melinda went to lunch and Chris, District I's primary nurse, "covered" Mr. Bowman. During that time, a respiratory therapist came to 7H to disconnect Mr. Bowman from the ventilator. His family sat with him. Chris was with him and asked him if he was ready to be disconnected. Mr. Bowman held up his hands in a gesture that communicated to Chris, "I don't know."

The respiratory therapist did not want to disconnect the patient from the machine in front of the family. The whole situation about disconnecting the ventilator was becoming more complex and troublesome to the family and the nursing staff. Melinda wanted to keep Mr. Bowman comfortable and told him this. She offered him morphine within the specified times of the medication order. She told the nursing staff that Mr. and Mrs. Bowman retained their sense of humor and thus relieved the tension of their dilemma. Melinda admitted having a hard time staying in the room with Mr. Bowman. She reflected on her nursing care and said that the quiet time she had with him that morning made her glad.

The next morning's report on Mr. Bowman revealed an increasingly complex situation.

Morning Report, August 4:

MIRIAM: [7]41 Window: Bowman. He's basically the same. . . . He was medicated twice for pain. Now, it's a goofy order the way his pain med's written. It's written morphine sulfate, 2 to 10 mg. every two to four hours p.r.n. So what we've just been giving him is 2 mg. That's holding him. . . . [Miriam worried about giving him too much morphine as much as his having severe pain. Too much morphine could have depressed his respirations and hastened his death.]

BETH: That's IM [intramuscular route]?

MIRIAM: IM. What was I going to say?

BETH: You just gave him some meds.

MIRIAM: Yeah. During the evening shift, his son kept coming out and asking for it and wanted to know why he was in such severe pain. During the night he was holding his chest, even though he wasn't complaining. She medicated him once. . . . He has a 50 percent trach collar on and he's been tolerating that well. Sounds gunky. His secretions are a lot looser. She [night private duty nurse] already sent a sputum which is there for the lab. Has an IV which is a 500 cc bag of D5W, O.K. Now, whoever hung it yesterday, hung it at 40 rather than 20, so we slowed it down. She presently turned it off, so probably they're going to end up discarding it. There's about 100 left in the bag. It might be slightly less than that. And she already paged the IV nurse to take a look. He's out for a Theophylline level, and other than that, he's been the same. He has a small decubitus on his buttock or . . . which I think is more to the left, front. It is oozing a little bit of bloodyish type material.

Mr. Bowman had been disconnected from the respirator the day before by a respiratory therapist. None of the family members witnessed this.

Melinda continued to care for Harry Bowman and prepared his morphine. She hastily wasted 5 mg. of a 10 mg. tubex syringe. Standing at the medication cart, she explained what she was doing. Mr. Bowman was having more pain. His respiratory secretions were thicker; he had more "fluid." As Melinda spoke, Mr. Bowman's son came out of room 741 to speed Melinda in her injection preparation. He was visibly anxious. Melinda hurried into the room with the pain medication.

Later, in the utility room, she mentioned that he would probably "go" from pneumonia and pulmonary edema. His pain had increased. His son had been in the room since 7:30 A.M. It was time for him to go to work and he wanted someone to be with his father. Melinda sighed a lot and seemed very tired. Yesterday at lunch she had said, "I can't wait until this case is over."

Shortly thereafter the IV nurse went into Mr. Bowman's room. She had been told to "restart" the IV in case the nurses and doctors needed one. The son waved her out as she entered the room. The

IV nurse found Beth, District I's primary nurse. Beth went into the room. She came out and told the IV nurse not to start the IV. If they needed a line (IV) later, they would get it.

In the early afternoon, Melinda came out of 741 to Beth, who stood at the medication cart. "Beth, I just suctioned up part of his lung; I think he's hemorrhaging." She had suctioned the respiratory secretions through his tracheotomy tube. She had inadvertently suctioned a piece of bloody tissue, which she held in a paper towel. Beth called the resident, asking that he check Mr. Bowman. Melinda went back to the room and stroked his head. The patient was unaware of Melinda's fears about the suctioned piece of lung tissue.

Mr. Bowman continued to decline for the next several days. Both private duty nurses and regular 7H nurses continued to care for him. Mr. Bowman died several days later. Death had come slowly for him. He had been on and off the ventilator. His nurses and doctors had waited patiently and had witnessed a sad and exhausted family waiting for a much loved man's end.

The 7H nurses, along with Melinda, performed Mr. Bowman's post-mortem care. Chris, a new R.N., commented, "His family wouldn't leave." She did not think that a religious need kept them a long time at the bedside. "It just seemed as if they had to sit with him awhile before they could leave." When asked why the nurses were eager to start the post-mortem care, Chris said, "I think that we had someone else [a new patient] coming into the room."

After Mr. Bowman's family left, Chris said that Beth, Melinda, and she gave him post-mortem care. "Beth helped me because I hadn't done it before." "Three of us did it; it was a joint effort." Beth described the events before and after his death.

> I remember telling them to be careful about the way they turned him. He exsanguinated. The blood would just pour out of his mouth. I was with him. He was foamy, just brand new blood, It clotted just there. It just happened quickly. The wife was glad he waited until she came. It was a long time before we did the post-mortem care. The son and wife were there. His breathing changed, so I got the doctor before he expired. We cleaned him up [after the bleeding]. The family stayed awhile. They had a hard time letting go. He got better and got bad, got better, got bad, when the ventilator was on the last time. The family was angry. A lot of times before they [patients] die, they don't have much pain. It

recedes before the end. I see other patients in the hospice program, about a day before they die, they don't want the pain medication, even if they die.

It was a gentle time, he'd been there for so long. He'd been a gutsy person, just remembering him as a person. We went over it, how he went, how his family was taking it.

Beth described her approach to post-mortem care after thinking about Mr. Bowman's death:

A lot of times when I do post-mortem care, I treat them as if it's my family. My son died at home with the family; he was 14 and had cancer [spinal cord]. [Beth cried at this.] I didn't know that's what I was doing, but I was. [In a flood of tears and memories, Beth recalled her son's death and identified the fact that she treated any dead person as family during post-mortem care.]

Sometimes you joke—it depends on who the people are [who die] and who you are with. The spirit of whoever is there is in the room. The spirit stays by the body awhile. He's too nearly gone. As though he's still there.

After the body is wrapped, the nurse calls Escort. The escort staff come with a stretcher. The patient is moved in the shroud onto a stretcher. The stretcher is covered with a sheet, the slide rails are up, so no one can see the dead person.

When Beth was asked if she was protective of the way the body is handled by the escort workers, she said, "If they yank it over, I get angry. If they treat the body like a piece of meat, I find it disrespectful. I like to use the draw sheet to move them over," that is, to lift them from the bed to the stretcher.

Beth described the usual way post-mortem care was given:

With the Jewish patient, you don't cross their arms. With patients of other religions, it is customary to cross the arms and tie them. You have to check the name tag to be careful about this. [The religion would be stamped with other identifying data, on the tags attached to the toe and shroud.]

In response to a question about whether there are any particular parts of the body you cover first or last, Beth replied:

I always cover the head last. It's the center of who the person was, the most distinguishing part. There's a reluctance to cover the face, putting off accepting death. Who wants their face to be covered with plastic? [Figure 5]

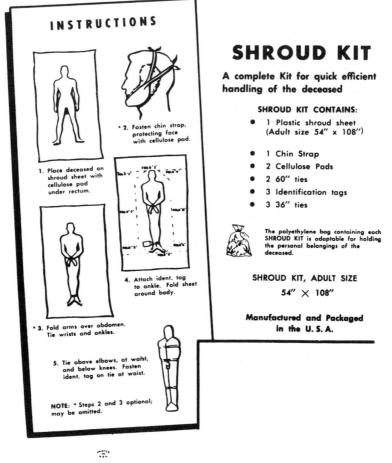

INSTRUCTIONS

* 2. Fasten chin strap, protecting face with cellulose pad.

1. Place deceased on shroud sheet with cellulose pad under rectum.

4. Attach ident. tag to ankle. Fold sheet around body.

* 3. Fold arms over abdomen. Tie wrists and ankles.

5. Tie above elbows, at waist, and below knees. Fasten ident. tag on tie at waist.

NOTE: * Steps 2 and 3 optional; may be omitted.

SHROUD KIT

A complete Kit for quick efficient handling of the deceased

SHROUD KIT CONTAINS:

- 1 Plastic shroud sheet (Adult size 54" x 108")
- 1 Chin Strap
- 2 Cellulose Pads
- 2 60" ties
- 3 Identification tags
- 3 36" ties

The polyethylene bag containing each SHROUD KIT is adaptable for holding the personal belongings of the deceased.

SHROUD KIT, ADULT SIZE

54" × 108"

Manufactured and Packaged in the U. S. A.

Figure 5. Shroud kit insert.

When the commercially manufactured, disposable morgue packs were purchased by the hospital, nurses complained about the plastic shrouds. They preferred the traditional cloth shrouds. They were softer and had less of a tendency to rip. Beth agreed that using the plastic material was offensive and said that she felt that she was doing a "good job" with post-mortem care when she was, "taking care of them till the end. Seeing them off, a tender fare-well." Beth added an afterthought:

Another part of the body I hesitate to wrap [in the shroud] is the hands. Sometimes, I partially wrap the body, leaving the head out. But I've thought about leaving hands out. What if the family member doesn't want to kiss the dead person, but to hold their hand? Touch is impor-tant. Hands are how we greet people or say farewell.

Chris, an R.N., described her first experience with post-mortem care with Beth as her preceptor:

About Mr. Bowman. I knew he was really sick that morning. I went to lunch even though I didn't want to, because Beth told me to. He died when I was at lunch. I was disappointed. I know that sounds ghoulish, but I never saw anyone die before.

Beth helped me, because I had never done post-mortem care. Beth was there; I was still being oriented, so it was all right for her to be shadowing me. I wanted to do post-mortem care for the experience. It wasn't eerie or gruesome. He had a peaceful death. Beth said he was ready for it. He was done suffering. It was a good feeling I had when we went into the room. It was hard for me to believe it was just a body, because I'm a Catholic, and we believe that the soul or mind went else-where. I was real gentle when I washed him [he had blood on him, because he had hemorrhaged], as if I would hurt him. Did you know that with Jewish patients, you don't cross their arms? He was Jewish. His wife wanted to come in again, so we wrapped him [in the shroud] to the axilla.

It had been a crazy morning. I had to ask him if he wanted to come off the ventilator. That was the hardest thing I've ever done, asking him to come off the ventilator. [Chris took him off the ventilator for the last time.]

It was selfish that I wanted to be with him when he died and to do his post-mortem care. His dying was a sort of buffer for me; against some-one and their family who wasn't ready for death. His was a smooth mo-tion of events. Everyone accepted the fact.

I had a friendly relationship with him. It's funny that I was not exactly excited about doing it, the post-mortem care, but do you understand what I mean?

Chris wanted to experience a patient's death, "handle" the death, and do a post-mortem care. She thought that Mr. Bowman's antici-pated and accepted death would help her prepare for future deaths. Those future patients and families who found death very unacceptable could be supported by a nurse with some experience. She seemed to want to be a brave nurse, courageous in the face of death. Since Beth was still preceptoring her, it was acceptable that Beth help her do the post-mortem care.

When patients did not die as predicted and continued to live as if by will, 7H nurses became disturbed. One patient's situation illustrates a nurse's response to this kind of situation.

Mary Lloyd was not ready to die. Mabel said she was not in a "calm position." The nurses were upset since this woman would die soon from cancer and leave an eleven-year-old child for her older daughter to rear. The nurses needed emotional support in dealing with her death, Mabel asserted. The day-in-and-day-out care of a dying patient was exhausting.

Mabel was one nurse who admitted how trying the care of the dying was. Before transfer from 7H to the new cardiac step-down unit, Mabel stated that she loved cardiac care. "You know when they're dying down there. You have the monitors," she said. The data available from the cardiac monitors helped the cardiac nurses predict and prevent death with a bit more certainty than the nurses on 7H could because 7H patients were rarely connected to cardiac monitoring systems.

Patients with cancer and with chronic obstructive pulmonary disease died slowly. The perception that the deaths of 7H patients were less easy to predict than the deaths of cardiac patients who were monitored could have been a technological delusion. The technology might have helped the nurses feel more confident that they had early warning signs of death and that therefore they could help prevent death.

The 7H nurses readily recognized evidence of dying and death. The ability to identify the harbingers of death was part of their clinical knowledge. They learned to look for: dull, glazed eyes; dilated pupils; mottled, pale, and blue tinged skin; blood pressure that "bottomed out"; heart rate irregularities; respiratory irregularities such as Cheyne-Stokes respirations; and increasing coolness of hands and feet and legs. Finally, absent heart sounds and stopped respiratory movements confirmed death, as did the technological evidence of a flat EKG.

DNR: "DO NOT RESUSCITATE"

When a patient's "code" or resuscitation status was classified as DNR, Category III, extraordinary means of therapy ceased. The definition of extraordinary means was not explicit. Clues about the kinds of nursing care still given to DNR patients were evident in nurses' change-of-shift report discussions:

MIRIAM: [7]51 Door: Lacey with CHF [congestive heart failure]. He's a DNR, number 3. He's on a 2 gram sodium diet, fluid restricted diet, fluid restricted to 1200 cc. They put a CVP [central venous pressure] in yesterday and did you know that they did the IV line open?

SARAH: They gave him 900 cc. in what, forty-five minutes?

MIRIAM: Twenty minutes.

SARAH: Twenty? Oh. So he wanted to go [die] real good after the 900.

MIRIAM: Yeah, he has rhonchi and rales [abnormal lung sounds] in the lung. His BP runs 70/50 to 80/50 and I got only 50 cc output. . . .

DOTTY: Don't you think that's a good idea to have a Clinitron? Even though he's a DNR, at least a DNR, make him comfortable.

SARAH: Well, it's just probably there are people who need it more than he does that aren't DNR's, like the quads or other people, you know are gonna walk out of here. I think they need it more. If it were a choice between him and a young guy that needed a Clinitron bed, I wouldn't give it to him. Anyway.

MIRIAM: He might not be with us long enough to have a Clinitron bed. . . .

SARAH: Is he alert at all, or awake?

MIRIAM: He's awake, but I don't think he's oriented.

Clinitron beds are pressure relieving and reduce the negative effects of bed rest on a patient's skin and deeper tissues. There was a limited number of these beds available in the hospital. Sarah's response to Dotty revealed that patients who were considered salvageable, who had some hope of survival, were given therapy and equipment considered extraordinary for the DNR patients.

The "do not resuscitate" status was often mentioned by the nurse giving change-of-shift report. Most frequently, it was handled matter-of-factly.

Afternoon Report:

[7]48 Door: Anna Landry in with the CA [cancer] and insulin overdose. She's on I & O [intake and output], S & A's, which was trace, negative for us. She's a DNR, III. Force fluids with her. She has a Foley in. Fasting blood sugar done at 6. O.K. Nothing really on her. She's still the same.

DNR PATIENT WHO RECOVERS

For one patient a resident obtained a DNR permission from a family and viewed the permission as a kind of trophy. The patient had been recently admitted to Room 755 Window. She weighed about eighty pounds. The resident, a small, flamboyant woman, spoke on the telephone to the employer of the patient's son. She urged the employer to tell the son to call the hospital, on an urgent matter related to his mother's health.

Mabel Thomas lay in bed with an IV running. Dehydrated and malnourished, she did not appear to be aware of her surroundings. She was septic. Her temperature was 38°C (normal is 37°C) in the Emergency Room. Marie took her temperature and found it to be 37.1°C. Sharon adjusted Mrs. Thomas's IV flow rate. The resident came into the room and explained that she did not want to "defibrillate this lady because [resuscitation] would crush her chest and kill her," but that until the son signed the DNR permission, resuscitation efforts might have to be made.

The resident told Sharon to call her "slowly" if the patient was dying. This delayed code was called a slow code; the staff would slowly initiate resuscitation. The resident continued to speak, obviously upset about Mabel's condition:

DOCTOR: How do these nursing homes do this?

SHARON: They may come to the nursing home in poor condition.

Marie took Mrs. Thomas's blood pressure. She palpated it at 80. In a few minutes, while some of the nursing staff were in the utility room, the resident announced, with obvious satisfaction, "Just so everybody knows, there's a DNR in Room 755W; I just got it from her son." This telephoned permission gave the resident the security of knowing that in the event of impending death, resuscitation efforts would not be initiated, but permission needed to be written in the patient's chart.

The nurses were glad to hear of the son's decision. They were left with nursing a frail woman who was near death. However, Mabel Thomas gradually began responding to Marie, Beth, Sharon, and the other nurses. She did not eat well but was helped by the IV's and antibiotics.

Eventually a surgeon inserted a gastrostomy tube into her stomach for nourishment through tube feedings. Mrs. Thomas became more alert and periodically conversed with the nurses. Miriam, the night nurse, said, "She's so cute; she holds a conversation." She became a favorite of the nurses and was discharged to the nursing home. Mrs. Thomas escaped death and her DNR–no hope label. She represented a 7H nursing success story. When she left 7H, the nurses worried about how she would fare in the nursing home.

PATIENT WHO "CODES," IS RESUSCITATED, AND "COMES BACK":
A FULL CODE

Peter Jones, sixty-three years old, was admitted to 7H for pain control. His eyes were expressive and reflected long suffering. His hair was gray and his face was angelic. He had been in severe pain for several months.

Afternoon Report:

[7]50 Door: Is a new admission that came in. His name is Peter Jones. He apparently, a couple of months ago had a prostate. . . . CA of the prostate and now they think it's spread to his spine. He has severe back and shoulder pain. He wears a brace. He's been at home. They haven't gotten him out of bed and he's done no walking because of the pain. He says he has no feeling from the knee down. Then he changed his mind and said from the waist down. But his wife said he feels you, but he just can't use his legs or anything like that. He doesn't stand or walk or anything. The brace is off him now. He's in bed, resting comfortably. He was complaining of severe pain when he came so I called the doctor. He came up and . . . he's still here workin' him up. I just gave him two Percocets 'cause they couldn't. . . . I called down Pharmacy and they couldn't get the hospice mix [hospice mixture, i.e., morphine sulfate in solution] for us right away. So they wanted to give him something. So I gave him two Percocets and when I went back on my rounds now he said that it . . . he really feels better from the two Percocets.

What's this CA of the spine?

Possible CA of the spine. . . .

> He lost like 35 pounds in the past couple of weeks. . . . He doesn't eat
> very well he said. He gets very nauseous. He's got a very poor appetite.
> He used a Texas catheter [condom-like appliance attached to a uri-
> nary drainage system] at all times.

Later the doctors determined that Mr. Jones's prostatic cancer
had metastasized to his right hip, and his spinal cord was compressed from the spinal metastasis. Mr. Jones's pain was eventually
fairly well controlled with the hospital's morphine hospice mixture
and Percocet. His nurses obtained an electric bed and had a trapeze
put on to help him move himself in bed. They worried about his
sacral skin "breaking down" with a bedsore, so they moved him
onto an electric Clinitron bed.

Gradually Mr. Jones became more comfortable and began to
take Sustacal liquid food supplements between meals during the
day when he could manage to drink them. He was fairly immobile
in bed and allowed the nurses to bathe him when his pain abated.
He began to go to radiation therapy. The nurses started to predict
his fate, "I don't think this man is gonna make it out of here. I think
he's gonna be with us till the end."

At one point during shift report one night, the nurses dramatized the severity of Mr. Jones's pain by their unwillingness to move
him after he returned from X-ray therapy:

> When he returned, he had so much pain in his shoulders . . . that his
> partial bath has not been completed . . . and he's laying on the sheets
> that he went down to X-ray therapy in, but he did not want us to
> move him.
>
> As soon as he got back, he got his morphine again and his fellow
> [nursing student] just gave him his Percocets. So I don't know if the
> pain's ever gonna go away enough for him to want . . . the sheets to be
> taken off. They're still smooth underneath him.
>
> His cervical collar . . . because of the severe cervical pain he was havin',
> they ordered it for him.
>
> And all I did, I went in to him—this was mid afternoon after he'd
> been back like an hour and a half and I went in and I said, "How ya
> doin?" And he went [sigh], "Don't talk to me."
>
> He's in a lot of pain so he might not even want you to touch him
> tonight.

Sometimes Mr. Jones preferred that no one touch his shoulder and warned the nurses to avoid jarring the bed. The nurses were afraid to move him, his pain was so chronic and intense in spite of the narcotics he was given every two hours. They respected his limits and did not force their care on him. Instead, they waited for his permission to move him.

7H nurses also worried about Mr. Jones's hemoglobin level; it dropped consistently over the weeks of his hospitalization. He was a Jehovah's Witness and opposed on religious grounds to receiving blood transfusions. When the doctors ordered Imferon, an injectible iron medication that they hoped would raise Mr. Jones's hemoglobin, the nurses were upset. Often patients complained of pain from these deep intramuscular injections. The nurses debated the wisdom of giving the medication. But, the patient refused the injection to the nurses' relief, since the pain of turning him over to receive the injection in the buttock and the injection itself were too much for him.

> He refused it last night. . . . So I just wrote refused [on the medication Kardex].
>
> O.K. You didn't give it to him today—we don't have to give it to him tonight, do we?
>
> No, he's just refusin' it. We can't force it on him.

Mr. Jones's hemoglobin continued to drop, 8.2 to 7 to 5.5 (normal for men is 13.4–17.6 Gm%). He was taking oral iron medication three times a day. This iron supplement and his radiation therapy decreased his poor appetite even more.

Abruptly one afternoon, Mr. Jones stopped breathing. He had never been designated as a DNR, Category III.

At 3:00 P.M., Colleen ran out of Mr. Jones's room. She called a Code Blue on this patient with metastatic prostate cancer. Mr. Jones had lain for weeks on his Clinitron bed, hardly changing his position in bed, and rarely being moved by nurses and escort personnel except to go to X-ray therapy for radiation treatments.

The full code "ran." At least twenty people, including doctors, nurses, an anesthesiologist from the resuscitation team, medical students, and a respiratory therapist descended on his room. Both

Deidre and Kate were off duty that day, so the nurse manager and the assistant nurse manager from the adjoining medical unit came to support Colleen through her and Mr. Jones's ordeal.

Collen used an ambu bag to ventilate Mr. Jones's lungs. A doctor compressed his sternum. A suction machine, defibrillator, and a drug box were moved into the room. The EKG machine, documenting cardiac activity, ran continuously. Finally, Mr. Jones began to "breathe on his own"; he had pulses.

As soon as Mr. Jones responded to resuscitation efforts, most of the hospital staff left the room. Sally, the nurse manager from the adjoining medical unit, Colleen, Camille, an anesthesiologist, and a medical resident remained. The room was a shambles, crowded with equipment. Worst of all, Mr. Jones's face exhibited fear. He looked to the left, frightened and restless. Colleen took his heart rate, blood pressure, and respiratory rate. He was breathing so rapidly on his own, without the ambu bag, that the anesthesiologist and the medical resident decided not to intubate him.

Mr. Jones's attending physician entered the room, reporting that he could not reach the family to request a DNR permission. Without the family's permission, the decision to resuscitate held, in the event the patient "coded" again.

The medical resident was in and out of the room. Sally and Colleen stayed in the room with Mr. Jones, discussing his restlessness and their fears that he would "go out" again. Sally wanted him sedated; his fright and restlessness were upsetting. Colleen went to find the resident and returned to complain, "All of the doctors have left the floor; the nurses alone are running the code and taking care of this critical patient."

Mr. Jones continued to look over his shoulder with terror in his eyes. His pupils were dilated. He raised his shoulders and head off the bed. He moaned. He had never moved like this previously. His pain had always been so severe that the staff had moved him with extreme gentleness. Sally discovered that the resident ordered Haldol for Mr. Jones's restlessness. She disagreed with this and discussed it with Lynne, her assistant nurse manager. They talked in Mr. Jones's presence about their unit's business, stopping occasionally to say, "Mr. Jones" or "Hon, please don't move like that. Calm down." They had restrained his wrists because of his restlessness.

He was full of strength, pulling his trunk and head off the bed. Colleen was surprised that he was so strong, because his usual behavior was immobility. His restraints were necessary, since the nurses thought that he might pull his oral airway out and his oxygen mask off.

Eventually Sally convinced the resident to order Demerol (narcotic analgesic) instead of Haldol (tranquilizer). Sally thought that Mr. Jones's cancer pain relief was more important to care for than his restlessness. The relief nurse came so Colleen could give afternoon report on her district. Colleen chose an unusual place for report, an unoccupied patient room. Colleen and Ann were laughing, on the verge of tears and hysteria, at Colleen's code description. Colleen said she had yelled for a stethoscope, forgetting that she had one around her neck. She laughed when she said, "He didn't get his bath today," or his 4:00 P.M. medication, Percocet. All listening to Colleen's report, Ann, Dotty, and another L.G.P.N., recognized the stressful intensity of Colleen's experience with Mr. Jones.

Sharon came into the room complaining about the attending physician's less-than-considerate behavior. Mr. Jones's wife had come as usual for her afternoon visit. She was confronted by a dramatically changed situation. Sharon was upset with the doctor. "Do you believe it? He wouldn't even come onto the floor. What humanity." The doctor asked Mrs. Jones for "do not resuscitate" permission over the telephone. She agreed to it.

A few days after the code, the nurses wondered why Mr. Jones remained in the hospital. His pain was managed better. His family could resume taking care of him at home as they had before his admission to 7H. The nurses were still afraid "to touch him. You're afraid to hurt him." They thought he would die soon. The DNR permission relieved them of the responsibility to resuscitate him the next time he had a cardiac and/or respiratory arrest.

A week after Mr. Jones's arrest and code, the nurses had stopped mentioning the event during change-of-shift report. They all knew about it, but no one mentioned it. Mr. Jones, however, was interested in a description of the code.

He was lying quietly in his Clinitron bed, looking more pale than usual. His wife was seated beside him holding his hand. When I asked him about how he had been doing since the week before, he looked as though he wanted to cry. Instead he asked for a description of what happened, saying, "I understand that people came out of the woodwork." I agreed with him and explained that a great many people had been there.

> Colleen discovered that you weren't breathing and that your heart rate had slowed. She called the code. People ran, from anesthesia, the Emergency Room, Respiratory Therapy; nurses and doctors were there. Colleen was with you through it all. Sally came from another unit to help Colleen and to make sure that the [7H] nurses had enough help to take care of you. She got a nurse to stay with you, since staffing on evenings is decreased.

Mr. Jones listened. His wife told him that when she came to his room, shortly after the arrest, four nurses were standing over him. She told me that when she visited him a few days later, he pouted and said, "You haven't seen me for three days."

He could not recall that his wife had visited after his arrest and over the weekend. He asked me, "Why do you forget?" I explained that it is common to forget an event that is shocking, almost as if we have an innate, self-protecting memory loss. Mr. Jones had a difficult time accepting his loss of memory. He expressed his faith in God and his thanks at having a good life. When I said, "And you have her," both husband and wife smiled at this and at each other in a pleased, comfortable way.

Before Mr. Jones went home, the nurses cared for him and worried about him. He had one particularly upsetting episode of hematuria (gross blood in his urine) one evening. The nurses had been factually reporting his DNR status during most shift reports. Since his hemoglobin was 5.5, the DNR status was addressed again:

Morning Report:

He's a DNR—you know that. . . .

No, I didn't know that.

And you enforce that.

You didn't know that? [Amazed.]

That wasn't on report last night. I didn't hear that in the evening.

O.K. He . . . had no pain med during the night and he's O.K.

The nurses had no opportunity to let Mr. Jones die by abstaining from resuscitation efforts. Speculation about the quality of his life after Mr. Jones's resuscitation led them to the conclusion that it would be better for Mr. Jones to die at home, because his family supports were strong and loving.

A week later, after the 7H nurses taught Mrs. Jones some helpful nursing care skills, Mr. Jones went home to die. A patient who had been resuscitated once and "came back" despite his advancing cancer and low hemoglobin lived to die at home with his family.

DNR: A DILEMMA FOR THE FAMILY

Family members anguished over their involvement in DNR decisions. It was difficult for a husband, wife, son, or daughter to agree that he or she did not wish to have resuscitation efforts begun in the event of cardiac or respiratory arrests. The invasiveness of respiratory intubation and closed-chest massage intensified the drama of the life-and-death situation for family members, nursing staff, medical staff, and other involved hospital personnel.

While families did not wish to prolong the suffering of their loved ones, the thoughts of signing a paper that hindered life-saving activities left many locked in indecision. Often families seemed to avoid coming to visit so that they could simultaneously avoid confronting the decision and the signature that gave them responsibility for life and death. The following shift report illustrates a son's dilemma about his mother's DNR classification. By the nurses' account, the son loved his mother deeply.

Morning Report:

Lucille Petri. She's in with a large cerebral bleed. She has a history of diabetes and hypertension. It's my understanding that she's not compliant with therapy for both of these diseases. She's been in here two weeks. . . . Now I wrote DNR here because Dr. Karl came in this morning and wrote DNR. Now I find out that he has to categorize it. . . .

Who is Dr. Karl?

Her attending.

Plus he's gotta get the family to sign some papers. He just can't do that

[make the patient a DNR without family permission and signature].
He never got the signature.

Well the family is refusing to make her a DNR as of yesterday.

Yeah. They've been refusing. So . . . not that they've been refusing, but
he hasn't even visited her.

No, he visited . . . and he didn't want it [DNR].

Miriam described a negative situation for Mrs. Petri that happened at 5:15 A.M. Her blood pressure fell to 70, and her respiratory rate rose to 65. She was very diaphoretic. The resident told
Miriam that Mrs. Petri was to be a "slow code" if she arrested. "Everyone, that is, the doctors, were under the impression that Mrs.
Petri was not to be resuscitated," said Miriam. Colleen told Miriam
that she would resuscitate the patient: "Code her—I'm not takin'
that responsibility." The family wanted "everything done—if she
had to go on a respirator [ventilator], they wanted her on a respirator" (staff report).

Mrs. Petri lived on 7H in what the nurses labeled a bad luck room
for several days after this. Her son steadfastly refused to sign the
"do not resuscitate" permission. Relenting, he finally gave permission a day before her death. His daily visits confronted him with
the severity and irreversibility of his mother's illness.

In another situation, an elderly man with multiple myeloma
(neoplastic disease of bone marrow) was a 7H patient for many
weeks. When Miriam said during report that he was a DNR, Colleen said, "Mr. Feinstein is?" "No. Mr. Price," Miriam replied. "Oh,
I was gonna say I didn't think Mrs. Feinstein would dare make him
a DNR," said Colleen. Mrs. Feinstein was loving and attentive to
her husband. Her involvement in his care was intense. She did not
want to lose her husband of many years to his disease. Neither the
nurses nor the doctors had approached Mrs. Feinstein about a
DNR permission.

DNR: A DECISION BY THE PATIENT

Another patient's choice illustrates yet another aspect of the resuscitation problem. Betty Windrim had been coming to the hospital
for many years. She had been admitted to 7H about ten months
before and was back again. Tired of her chronic disease and ready

to die, Mrs. Windrim signed her own DNR permission in the doctors' progress notes.

Afternoon Report:

[7]49 Door: Just came up. It's Betty Windrim . . . sixty-eight years old. She came in on the 23d. On the 27th, she arrested. She extubated herself on the 30th. She's here with CHF, end stage, CAD [coronary artery disease], and HTN [hypertension]. She made herself a DNR. She is awake, alert and oriented, but won't do diddle for herself except feed herself. She was kind of malnourished, I think. She's got a right open 'cubital dressing. . . . She went into pulmonary edema over the weekend. Right now she's on a venti-mask for 50 percent [oxygen] which she takes off when she feels like it.

Mrs. Windrim was exhausted and ready to die. Her independent spirit was obvious. She informed the nurses that she was intolerant of hospital therapies, such as the irritation and confinement of the oxygen-supplying venti-mask, the annoyance of an endotracheal tube (which she removed), and life-extending resuscitation attempts.

Morning Report:

[7]49 Door: . . . She no longer has a fluid restriction. She made herself a DNR, number III.

She . . . it's all written and everything?

Yeah, she did. She has an INT in the left upper arm. She had some chest pain—at a quarter to six. I have one nitro for that. . . .

Afternoon Report:

. . . Yeah, she made herself a DNR . . . number III.

Did someone talk to her or did she. . . .

I don't know but she decided that. . . .

Why is she . . . is she that, is she bad off?

Yeah, congestive heart failure, coronary artery disease, hypertension. . . .

She's still getting Isordil every hour while she's awake. It's really not doing that much. They [doctors] talked about putting her on a nitroglycerine drip, but they can't do it while she's on the floor [7H], and they're not going to take her back into coronary care being a DNR.

Mrs. Windrim surely was planning to die. Barely able to feed herself, she occasionally requested the taste of orange ice, which the nurses got her. Talking was a great effort. She remained on bed rest for weeks until her death, too weak to get out of bed to a chair with the nurses' help. A cutdown incision in her arm healed slowly. She continued to submit to routine lab tests and special lab tests such as a red blood cell survival test.

Mrs. Windrim lived for two and one-half months after her DNR decision. Living every day was a chore. It was difficult to eat, breathe, and talk. She was considered "a sweet lady" by the nurses and suffered in silence except when she told the nurses about her chest pain. She died in early February at 5:30 A.M. Cecile, a new R.N., felt guilty because she was not with the patient when she stopped breathing and reported: "She coded at 5:30 A.M." No resuscitation attempts were initiated on the woman who had signed her own DNR permission.

Post-Mortem Care of DNR Patient

Betty Windrim was pronounced dead by the resident at 5:56 A.M. (Appendix 1). Miriam and the night supervisor did her post-mortem care together. They washed Mrs. Windrim and wrapped her in a plastic shroud, only to unwrap her because the resident told the nurses that the family was coming to see her. The nurses put clean sheets on the bed and cleaned the room.

By 8:15 A.M., Mrs. Windrim's family had come to 7H to see her. After they left 7H, Deidre, who had arrived for the day shift, went into room 749 to repeat the post-mortem care on Mrs. Windrim. Colleen and two nursing students were also in the room.

Mrs. Windrim's body was naked and lying flat in bed. Deidre and Colleen changed the shroud, since the first one was soiled from mucous and stool. They both washed Mrs. Windrim's skin. Deidre washed her face, arms, chest, and legs on the left. Colleen washed on the right, also washing the genital area. When asked if the family had come, Deidre said they had. Mrs. Windrim's eyes were fixed. She was blue-tinged around her mouth and nose and did not move. The reality of her death was confirmed by the ever-increasing coldness of her skin and her lack of respiratory movement.

Colleen washed the unhealed antecubital cutdown incision, which leaked serous fluid. She did this gently, as if Mrs. Windrim could feel her touch on a painful, never-to-heal incision. Deidre and Colleen turned the patient over toward Deidre onto her left side. She had lost sphincter control of bowel and bladder. This happens in death, as nurses know, so that frequently stool and urine have to be cleaned up by the nurses after death.

Colleen cleaned all traces of the bowel movement and urine from Betty's skin. It was obvious, however, that more stool would leak. Washing the patient gently with a wet towel, she said mildly and teasingly, "I'll bet you're doing that on purpose," referring to the incontinence following death. Colleen placed the shroud under the patient's back, and later turned her onto the shroud.

Colleen tied the toe tag on the patient's right great toe, crossed her legs at the ankle, and tied them together with the shroud pack tie. Deidre tied the arms together at the wrists, padding them in between with a soft abdominal (ABD) pad. She covered the patient's naked body with the plastic shroud, after propping her chin with a rolled towel. She wrapped the left side of the shroud over first, the right side over second, folded up the ends of the shroud at the feet, and tied another shroud cord at the ankles over the shroud. She then tied the shroud at the waist and, finally, flipped the shroud at the patient's head over her face and tied it with a cord at the neck.

Deidre finished the post-mortem care alone because Colleen left with a nursing student to check on another patient's "funny" breathing. Deidre taped the shroud to insure its closure. She said that she did not like to cover the patient's face. "I take a deep breath; it's almost as if they are still breathing." Deidre said that she was fanatical about cleaning the room before the family comes. She explained this by associating it with a "calm and a sense of peace" in the room.

Deidre sent the remaining nursing student out of the room to call the escort service to remove the patient's body. She covered the deceased patient in the shroud with a clean cloth sheet, bringing it up to the chin and leaving the head covered by the shroud but uncovered by the sheet.

Later, a male escort staff member nattily dressed in a blue blazer with gold buttons brought a litter with a special green sheet. He left the litter in the hall and soon returned with another escort person. Together they moved the body to the cold, stainless steel of the special litter and covered it with the green sheet. The body was taken to the morgue by the attendants. It would be refrigerated while awaiting the undertaker.

Mrs. Windrim's roommate sat in her bed in the corridor near the nurses' station from the time of the death until noon. She was in the middle of the 7H morning melee. She was moved back to the room after all remaining traces of Mrs. Windrim's occupation were cleaned by housekeeping service. The empty bed in 749 was ready for another patient.

Post-Mortem Care for a Slow Code Patient Whose Death Was Unexpected

Maria Fanelli was admitted to 7H in early winter. She came into the hospital through the Admissions Office and went next to the Admissions/Discharge Unit (ADU), where patients either wait for a bed on admission or wait for their families to pick them up and take them home on discharge. Mrs. Fanelli was to die on 7H in Room 752 Door.

Ann received a detailed report from Sharon about Mrs. Fanelli:

> [7]52 Door is a new admission—transfer—whatever you want to call it. She came from ADU. Maria Fanelli, seventy-three-year-old white female. She is in with urosepsis and diabetes. When she came in she was hyperglycemic and in a diabetic coma. Um . . . she was given insulin in the E.R. She was also given 10 units this morning in ADU. She'll respond to her name. She will open her eyes when you call her name. She did say a few words, but they were inappropriate to the questions that I asked her.

ANN: Oh, O.K.

SHARON: I told her where she was—she said she wasn't hungry.

ANN: Oh . . .

SHARON: She's on O_2, all right. They told me she was on O_2 at 5 L. upstairs [in ADU]. She transferred on O_2, however there is no O_2 written for her.

ANN: Oh, O.K. She did have an FBS?

SHARON: She did have an FBS. I don't know what it was. He called for it so it should come down on the lab slip.

ANN: Does she have a Foley?

SHARON: Yeah, she does have a Foley.

ANN: O.K.

SHARON: She's on I & O, S & A. I didn't get one on her. I forgot all about it. She is on aspiration precautions, O.K.

ANN: Um hm.

SHARON: She's on bed rest. She had been NPO [nothing by mouth]. Now he wants clear liquids to be started on . . . her. Apparently this is her normal state and she's been getting her nourish[ment]. . . . To me, she looks out of it.

ANN: I went into the other patient and looked at her and she doesn't look like she's ready to drink anything.

SHARON: When she came . . . her skin was warm, moist and clammy. It's dry now. She has an IV hanging. . . . They want her to have thigh high TEDS [thromboembolytic deterrent stockings]. . . . Her feet are real dry and scaly and flaky looking. It looks like caked powder between the toes.

ANN: Umm.

SHARON: Also has like benzoin around the heels and around the toes and she had a decubiti on her right foot . . . her right heel. But it's not broken. It looks like it was one that healed.

Six days after Mrs. Fanelli's admission to 7H, she "coded" during bath time of the morning shift. A graduate nurse called the code. The resuscitation team arrived, including Emergency Room nurses, an anesthesiologist, and a medical resident. The events moved slowly. An EKG machine ran continuously; EKG paper stretched from the machine at the foot of Mrs. Fanelli's bed to the wall by the door of the room. Mrs. Fanelli had an endotracheal tube inserted through her mouth into her airway by an anesthesiologist. The tube was connected to a ventilator. A respiratory therapist checked on her respiratory status. She lay in her bed in Trendelenburg position: head down, feet elevated. Her skin was mottled; blue and red areas contrasted with her pale skin. Her eyes were dull, and she seemed not to see her surroundings. Sharon stayed close to Mrs. Fanelli. She prepared drugs and observed any equipment requests of the doctors or the E.R. nurse. Mrs. Fanelli was receiving an intravenous Dopamine drip to stabilize her blood pressure. As her blood pressure fell, the drop rate was increased.

The senior medical resident checked on the code and left shortly to check on an available bed in the critical care unit for Mrs. Fanelli.

Behind a curtain in the next bed lay another patient, a woman who had previously suffered an allergic reaction to contrast material injected during a diagnostic test. Because of the test, she had had a respiratory arrest. The nurses thought that it was impossible to get this patient out of the room while her roommate was being resuscitated in the bed by the door and was surrounded by hospital staff and equipment. Chris and Sharon, both R.N.'s, worried about her but decided to talk to her later.

There was an almost carnival aspect to the slow code. At one point, in the middle of the resuscitation activities, the E.R. nurse calmly showed 7H's nurses how to use the doppler machine she had obtained from E.R. to get a femoral pulse. Despite the seriousness of the events of the resuscitation, a kind of patient, friendly mood prevailed that suggested that everyone involved was indulgent of disaster and getting used to it.

The resuscitation events continued at a slow pace. A conversation about Mrs. Fanelli's code was in progress in the utility room. Leslie was talking to another L.G.P.N. She said, "The patient was in A fib [atrial fibrillation] during the weekend. No one monitored her or did a digitalis level." That morning, Leslie had warned the resident, "The patient looks bad." She was pale, cool and diaphoretic. The resident had done nothing and incurred Leslie's disrespect.

The nurses in the utility room discussed the fact that during the previous week, on Thursday and Friday, Mrs. Fanelli's blood sugar had gone from 600 (very high) to 50 (very low). The patient had been "nonreactive." During the previous weekend, she had eaten and seemed better. This morning she had gone into respiratory arrest, and so Sharon had coded her.

The code efforts progressed in a slow, uneven way for over an hour and a half. The senior resident could not arrange to get Mrs. Fanelli into ICU. Beds were tight; there were no vacancies. Two X-ray technicians came in in the middle of the code and took a "stat" portable chest X-ray. Since Deidre and Kate were both off duty, the assistant nurse manager from the adjacent medical unit came to check and complained that the doctors were not giving "that much post code care."

Next a flurry of activity occurred in response to Mrs. Fanelli's EKG, which revealed complete heart block. The resident, a new doctor as of the previous July, had been checking the EKG tracing regularly, along with his senior resident. He was nervous. His deodorant had faded away, and he was visibly upset. He asked his senior resident, Nell, who had come back to the code, if the patient had a P.E. (pulmonary embolus) and was told, "Based on the initial respiratory problem, it is very likely."

Nell joked about the situation. Perhaps she was frustrated with her inability to move the patient to a critical care bed or with her failure to "save" the patient. The patient was stuck in her room on 7H. The room was crowded with people and equipment: two residents, three nurses, a roommate, two beds, two bedside cabinets, two overbed tables, a ventilator, an EKG machine, and a defibrillator outside the door in the corridor on the arrest cart along with the 7H drug box. Everyone spoke over the patient, waiting for the next blood pressure change, arterial blood gas result, and doctor's decision for the next medication. Every five to ten minutes, blood pressure and pulse were taken and recorded.

The doctors, especially Nell, seemed to be waiting for Mrs. Fanelli to die. Her pupils were fixed, dilated, and nonreactive to light, a universally ominous sign and generally accepted as harbinger of death. The E.R. nurse picked up most of the EKG paper from the floor and threw it into a plastic bag. A few minutes later, Mrs. Fanelli died. Her EKG was flat for several minutes.

The resuscitation team and the doctors left after recording notes on the patient's chart. Chris, Dotty, Jamie (a p.r.n. pool L.G.P.N.), Sharon, and Lynne, the neighboring unit's assistant nurse manager, were working on Mrs. Fanelli and her room.

Lynne got a suture removal kit to cut the sutures holding the subclavian catheter in the patient's skin. Jamie used a 5-cc. syringe to deflate the Foley balloon so that the urinary catheter could be removed. Jamie also obtained a towel and washcloth, then filled a basin with water and began to wash the patient's face after she touched her teeth to determine "if they were dentures or originals."

Jamie rapidly and efficiently washed chest and breasts, arms and legs "just like A.M. care." Next she washed the perineal area. There was a small amount of blood present. Dotty helped Jamie turn the patient over. Jamie washed the patient's back, now bluish-purple, and said, "Oh really" in a disgusted voice. There was a large amount of odoriferous stool present at the patient's anus. Dotty said to Jamie in reproach, "What do you expect, she's dead." Both Dotty and Jamie wore disposable gloves throughout the care, a usual practice for most 7H L.G.P.N.'s when giving a bath.

Mrs. Fanelli's eyes were open, their glistening moisture gone in her death. Her blueness, paleness, and lack of movement dominated the scene. Jamie asked for sheets, since all the nurses in the room wanted to help her. Sheets were brought from a chair in the corridor. With Mrs. Fanelli turned onto her left side toward Dotty, Jamie placed a clean sheet with the plastic shroud on top, under the patient. In order to help Dotty turn the body, Jamie rolled the plastic shroud up with the sheet. Jamie gestured for Dotty to turn the patient over toward her. Jamie put the cellulose pads in place at the anus.

Dotty helped and pulled the dirty sheets out and the clean bottom sheet and shroud through. Mrs. Fanelli was then turned flat in bed. Jamie put a clean gown on her, shielding her nakedness.

After stamping the toe tag, total body tag, and the personal belongings tag with Mrs. Fanelli's Addressograph plate at the nurses' station, Sharon reentered the room and tied the toe tag onto the patient's right great toe. Jamie was ready to tie the patient's arms together with the shroud pack cord at the wrists. Dotty stopped her. "Don't do that," she said. She wanted the family to have the opportunity to touch untied hands when they came to see Mrs. Fanelli. Both Jamie and Lynne said that they always tied the wrists together when they did post-mortem care. Jamie went along with Dotty, saying, "We'll do it however you want," in deference to her position as a 7H nurse. Jamie and Dotty tucked the shroud underneath the mattress as if it were a bottom sheet and pulled the top sheet over the patient up to her neck. Dotty combed Mrs. Fanelli's gray, shoulder-length hair.

Interspersed with the washing, tagging, and tying of post-mortem care were the nurses' rapid efforts to straighten the room for the family's arrival. They threw disposable trash away into the waste basket and saved the patient's powder and brush for the family.

Jamie went behind the curtain to sit with the roommate who had been trapped in the room throughout the long, slow code and post-mortem care. The roommate had confessed earlier that she "was a nervous wreck." She had a brace on her leg and had to use a wheel-chair whenever she left the room, but the 7H nurses had not wanted her to leave in the midst of the code and post-mortem care activities.

Mrs. Fanelli looked clean after death. Her sheets were spotless, and her side of room 752 looked neat, orderly, and clinical. No traces of the code or post-mortem materials were visible. She was obviously dead. The door to the room was left open, the curtain around her bed was partially closed. Anyone passing the door of the room could glimpse her from the hall.

Sharon left to go to Room 740, which was empty in preparation for the hospital's construction work. The nurses were using it tem-porarily for change-of-shift report. Sharon checked on the nurses' notes she had written about Mrs. Fanelli's respiratory arrest, resus-citation, and death. She was careful to change the starting time of the code from 8:30 A.M. to 9:00 A.M., crossing out the first time and writing "error" above it. Lynne advised her to do this since there was a discrepancy between the doctor's record of the starting time of the code and Sharon's, although Sharon's time was accurate.

Mrs. Fanelli's death was for Sharon, "the first patient that I was involved with" as a primary nurse when the patient died. When asked about her feelings about this experience, Sharon told me that she was "O.K., just tired" and did not mind that Dotty and Jamie did the washing part of the post-mortem care. Sharon did not know how to fill in the post-mortem stamp (Figure 6) information, so she left the room to learn how. She mentioned as she left that the new resident, Dr. Francis, did not seem to know what he was doing. Sharon checked on her other patients in District III after she left the room.

Around noon, a middle-aged man and woman, a son and daugh-ter-in-law, came to see Mrs. Fanelli. Dr. Francis spoke to them. Both seemed very upset. Sharon came out of another patient's room and

Time of Death: _____

Pronouncing Physician: _____

Family Notified: ☐ Yes   ☐ No   Time: _____

By Whom: _____

Post-Mortem Exam: ☐ Yes   ☐ No

Medical Examiner's Case: ☐ Yes   ☐ No   ☐ Unknown

Post-Mortem Care Provided by: _____
                                            Signature

Death Reported to: ☐ Admissions   ☐ Information Desk
                           ☐ Switchboard
                           ☐ Unit Management/Nursing Office

Disposition of Valuables: _____

Professional Nurse's Signature: _____

PLEASE CARRY THE COMPLETED CHART TO UNIT MANAGER/
NURSING OFFICE

Figure 6. Post-mortem stamp.

talked with them. She accompanied them into the room, pausing a few seconds, and left them alone with Mrs. Fanelli. After ten minutes they left the room and asked to see the resident. Mrs. Fanelli's daughter-in-law asked who would issue the death certificate. The 7H staff were unsure of this and could not answer. When the family left 7H, Sharon called Escort Service to remove Mrs. Fanelli's body. Ten minutes later two escort staff came with the special litter with the green cover on it and went into 752. One of them came out to tell Sharon that the patient was not wrapped. Since this was Sharon's first death and no other staff were available, I helped Sharon wrap the patient. She loosened the sides of the shroud that had been tucked under the mattress and tried to wrap the shroud around the body. She applied soft "abdominal" pads between the ankles and wrists as she tied them. I told Sharon that it was easier to slip the ties under the neck, waist, and ankles when the patient was turned onto her side before turning her onto the shroud. Since Jamie and Jackie had not done this, we had to turn Mrs. Fanelli side to side in order to get the ties in place. We covered the patient's body and folded up the end of the shroud at the neck and ankles. Sharon tied the shroud at the neck and waist; I tied it at the ankles.

The toe tag was in place, so I tied the waist tag to the tie that surrounded the shroud above the area of the patient's crossed hands.

Sharon summoned the escort staff to come into the room. One of them said, "Ladies, we don't need you anymore." Sharon said, "Are you sure?" "Yes," he responded. They lifted the green cover off the litter. They placed the patient on the cold, large stainless steel tray. Sharon shivered and said that this was terrible, as though Mrs. Fanelli could still feel the cold of the litter. Later in the utility room, discussion of Mrs. Fanelli's death stimulated discussion of other deaths.

Conversation about Mrs. Fanelli resumed after morning report the next day, as Marie and Camille, 7H's long-tenured nursing staff, discussed the code of the previous day. Marie expressed amazement, a noteworthy occurrence for this L.G.P.N. who never seemed surprised by anything. Camille mentioned how well Mrs. Fanelli had seemed to be doing over the weekend. Marie described how she had fussed with Mrs. Fanelli to get her to eat more food and to feed herself.

There were other repercussions from Mrs. Fanelli's death. The next day her roommate, who had been unable to get out of the room during the long resuscitation efforts, started to scream at her newly admitted, confused roommate:

Morning Report:

She's been screaming at her roommate last night, too. She was . . . everybody's getting carried away here.

I mean, really, really frightening. She was screaming for her to shut up and I explained that the lady's confused.

On four to twelve . . . [she] was screaming out and then she started shaking uncontrollably, and Pam went in and she had to sit her up and sit with her for a while and then kind of . . .

She was there all through that code yesterday.

Through what code?

Couldn't get her out.

Mrs. Fanelli's death and post-mortem care, only a few feet away, had forced this patient to confront the reality of death and perhaps to relive her own respiratory arrest.

Post-Mortem Care for a Slow Code Patient Whose Death Was Expected

Family members often had difficulty confronting death. In the case of Mary Kelly, a seventy-two-year-old with chronic obstructive lung disease and a severe seizure disorder, the family refused to grant "do not resuscitate" permission, despite requests by the doctors. Mrs. Kelly was admitted to 7H in a coma.

Mrs. Kelly lived on 7H for just over five days. The nursing staff was a minimal group because of the Christmas and New Year's holiday schedule. The nurses reported that there was "so much going on with her." She looked seriously, deathly ill during the time she spent in her "bad luck" room, 754. She received IV's through a right arm site through which aminophylline, Solu Medrol, ampicillin, and Tobra were infused at various times. Her IV orders were a problem, but the doctors and nurses finally regulated the fluids and medications she received.

Beth warned Loretta during report about the demands of Mrs. Kelly's care: "You have a full time job there tonight." Her tracheostomy tube was inflated with a cuff and connected to an MAI ventilator. She required frequent suctioning. She received Isocal tube feedings through a gastrotube. One evening she had frequent seizures, which necessitated intravenous phenobarbital infusions. Her eyes were open, and the nurses worried about corneal abrasions. They asked the doctors to order Natural Tears eye drops. 754 was a "busy, busy room."

During afternoon report, Loretta asked Beth about Mrs. Kelly's code status:

LORETTA: Is she a DNR?

BETH: No, she's a *full* code.

PAM: The family do not want to do this because they feel that they don't have the right.

BETH: The son came in today and asked if she was talking!

LORETTA: Talking to whom? [Laughs.]

PAM: I said, "I don't . . . I couldn't really say." You know, she just came up on the floor. [Laughs.] They [the family] don't want to make her a DNR because they feel it's not their responsibility to say who can live and who can't.

CECILE: Are they Catholics, or what?

PAM: Whatever religion they are, they're very strict.

After discussing the difficulty in auscultating Mrs. Kelly's irregular, apical heart rate, the nurses moved back to the discussion of the patient's DNR status. Their laughter had a ring of hysteria to it.

BETH: Do you know what Lester [a doctor] said? They're not going to do anything until the systolic falls below 60!

LORETTA: The systolic! [Laughs.] [Below a systolic blood pressure of 70, kidneys fail.]

BETH: And if she paces, you're to walk slowly to the phone and call Lester.

LORETTA: And he will call the code?

BETH: Well, it's not a code then. But then they'll . . .

LORETTA: Walk slowly down the hall. I'm running! I'm calling the code. I'm not calling the doctor.

PAM: When we knew Mrs. Jones [a patient who died recently after a prolonged illness] was going, we called him and he's in the room. [Laughs.] It's not funny; he just stands there looking. [Laughter.] "Can you feel a pulse?" "No, I can't feel one." It's not funny to say it but this is what they [doctors] do. "Can you feel the pulse?"

BETH: I heard you're supposed to walk to the code backwards. [Laughs.] Legally, there's no such thing, so if you don't feel comfortable . . .

PAM: I don't want to be held responsible . . .

LORETTA: And to think this lady's living! That's terrible.

Dotty expressed the nurses' reaction to coding an elderly patient: "When an eighty-five or ninety-year-old patient is coded, I think it's torture." The nurses transferred this belief to Mrs. Kelly's situation.

The District I nurses were confronted with Mrs. Kelly's slow dying. They commiserated over the fact that she lived. They were appalled that she was coded for another time over the weekend and "made it." They were concerned with the problems they had palpating her blood pressure. Knowing what her blood pressure was gave the nurses the temporary security of knowing whether she was "going" or not.

While Beth, the primary nurse, was happy that there were three recent successful codes on 7H, she regretted "that Mrs. Kelly made it." She knew that the other two patients were salvageable, whereas Mrs. Kelly's death was imminent and certain.

Marie, the L.G.P.N. on District I, bathed Mrs. Kelly for several days. She talked to her as she bathed one half of her body, then the other. Marie told Mrs. Kelly what part of her body she was washing and why she turned her onto her side. She shook her head, as if disapproving of the fact that Mrs. Kelly was still living. Her patient's skin was edematous and delicate, paper thin with bruises distributed on her arms where IV's and lab studies had required venipunctures. Mrs. Kelly had bedsores on her heels. Marie soon bathed her back, after turning her onto her left side. The patient was still kept on the "cooling" or hypothermia blanket to reduce fever when there were dangerous temperature elevations.

Marie finished washing, drying, and massaging her patient's back and buttocks. She turned Mrs. Kelly onto her back. Reluctantly she started removing dressings from the patient's right foot. An unpleasant, decaying odor permeated the room as she cut the old dressings off. She walked out of the room and said to me, "Did you smell it? I have a cold and I smelled it."

Marie placed as absorbent blue pad under Mrs. Kelly's foot. Her foot was "dead." That part of her was becoming gangrenous, as the tissue slowly died from poor circulation. Chris came in at Marie's request to see the patient's foot. She said, "It was just a blister the last day I saw it." Marie put on gloves as she prepared to redress the foot. Chris helped her as she put on Betadine dressings. Marie said, "The son should come and see this [foot]. We should uncover her so he can see her. Is this his mother? No? This isn't his mother [anymore]." Marie expressed her anger at the son's decision to employ all lifesaving measures necessary to prolong his mother's life, unnecessarily, to Marie's way of thinking. Throughout the A.M. care, Marie was very gentle with Mrs. Kelly. She talked to her. When the ventilator beeped to indicate accumulating secretions, Marie said in mild reproach, "Now, Mary, I suctioned you." After Marie adjusted the ventilator tubing, she left the room. Mrs. Kelly was dying slowly.

Later Marie "made eyes" to Chris as she saw a man approach Chris in the corridor. She eavesdropped and muttered, "He's from the hospice" (hospital crisis counseling service). Hospital crisis counselors saw themselves as objective, supportive, and skilled facilitators of communication between staff, dying patients, and their families. As Chris stood at the medication cart, she discussed Mrs. Kelly's situation with Michael, the hospice counselor. Chris painted a graphic picture of the situation. The patient's son, a Catholic, refused to sign the DNR form. He kept seeing signs of hope in his mother. Chris said, "The patient does worse all the time. There's nothing left of her. She's been coded several times. Her foot is turning black, and her abdomen is out to here," Chris gestured, indicating the degree of distension. "The family doesn't see it like we do."

Michael asked when Mr. Kelly had last visited; Chris told him, "Yesterday, around twelve noon." Michael noted that 7H nurses seemed pretty involved with Mrs. Kelly. "We don't want to have to code her again since there's nothing left of her," said Chris, who asked Michael to talk with the son again, maybe with a resident also present. The counselor reminded Chris that hospice and social services had been involved before. Chris beseeched them to intervene again. Michael promised that he would try but said that there was no fast answer. Michael explained that families needed support to make these difficult decisions.

Chris said that the son had left a present for Mrs. Kelly, saying, "This is a present from her granddaughter. She can open it when she wakes up." Marie laughed sarcastically, alluding to the son's false hope.

Mrs. Kelly lay in bed in a semi-reclining (semi-Fowler's) position. Her elevated arms were swollen with edema. An IV was running into one hand. Her tracheostomy tube was connected to the ventilator tubing; her nasogastric tube was connected to a pump regulating Isocal feeding by the drop into her stomach. Her mouth was open, her lips had skin lesions on them. Her eyes were closed. She did not respond at all to stimuli. Her bedside urinary drainage bag drained scant urine from a Foley catheter, an ominous indication. Her room had been "screened" (the Admissions Office had been notified by the nurses not to admit another patient to the bed beside Mrs. Kelly), and so she was the only patient in a semi-private room. There was a suction machine and other equipment, including a hypothermia machine, different bottles of solutions (water, saline, and Betadine), and a ventilator, in addition to the standard bedside cabinet, bed overbed table, and one large and one small chair.

Mrs. Kelly had lived through the previous weekend, following the successful third resuscitation attempt. She "coded and came back." Beth commented during morning report that she "literally has nine lives." Marie muttered in between Beth's report on tracheostomy suctioning, aminophylline drip, ventilator settings, and hypothermia blanket for temperature elevation that "they had brought her back from the dead."

BETH: She looks really bad.

DOCTOR: Maybe they [family] will come in to . . .

MARIE: They came in yesterday.

DOCTOR: They call every night.

Beth warned Tammy and Marie to have Mrs. Kelly's gastric feeding tube checked. She was afraid it had slipped out a little and worried about Mrs. Kelly's aspirating Isocal feedings into her lungs. Mrs. Kelly had not had IV's for twenty-four hours, since all veins in her arms "were gone." The doctors soon inserted a CVP line into a subclavian vein. Her urine output was extremely poor—60 cc. in eight hours. Greenish secretions were suctioned through her tracheostomy and around the tube. Her blood pressure was palpable, ranging from 70 to 80 mm. Hg. Her temperature fluctuated up and down from 35.6°C to 39.2°C. The nurses and the doctors did not want to "code" Mrs. Kelly again, but all signs indicated that they would face this "code–no code" dilemma again that day. But Mrs. Kelly clung to life.

The next day, Marie was taking care of Mrs. Kelly again. As Tammy and Marie made morning rounds on the patients in their district, they stopped at Mrs. Kelly's room last. Tammy took her blood pressure; Marie checked the ventilator settings. Mrs. Kelly looked worse. Her right leg was blue and mottled further up the leg. Her pupils were dilated and fixed. Her eyes were glazed and dull. She initiated reflex respiratory movements around her mouth which were not synchronous with the automatic ventilations of the respirator. Marie thought that maintaining her life in this state "was a crime. Her family should have to sit with her every day." A respiratory therapist and a resident also came in to check Mrs. Kelly on their rounds.

Mrs. Kelly was near death. Hospital personnel worked on her and around her. A resident removed her feeding tube and reinserted a new one that seemed to work better for Tammy and Marie. The respiratory therapist called for help from another therapist. They increased the tidal volume setting on the ventilator and that improved the ventilator's oxygen-air delivery through Mrs. Kelly's tracheostomy tube. Tammy adjusted the pump attached to the feeding tube, since its alarm had sounded.

A priest from a neighboring Roman Catholic church came to see Mrs. Kelly; he smiled and blessed her. When Chris told the priest about Mrs. Kelly's family and her recent successful resuscitation, he thought for a while and then answered that the ventilator was considered by the Catholic church to involve the use of extraordinary means to preserve life. If the family wanted the priest to come into the hospital, they just had to call the parish.

Later Tammy had a difficult time palpating Mrs. Kelly's blood pressure. Her fingernail beds were cyanotic; her hands were mottled up to her wrists. Her pulse was fluttering. Her blood pressure was 32 mm. Hg by palpation. Mrs. Kelly's apical heart rate was irregular and difficult to auscultate; it could have been 64 or 124.

Tammy did not want to call a code. Kate was in the room and suggested that Tammy call the senior resident. After talking to the doctor on the telephone, Tammy came back to the room and increased the IV flow to expand Mrs. Kelly's blood volume. Her next blood pressure was 50/32. Marie impatiently said to Tammy as she increased the IV, "What are you doing now?" Marie was implying, "Let her die."

A resident came to the floor to see Mrs. Kelly. When Kate asked him if he had seen her before, he said, "This could be the day" (that she dies). He called the attending physician and left his beeper number. Kate said, "We're crossing our fingers" (so she will die). The resident asked the attending physician over the telephone, "We don't want to start pressors on her, do we?" He was told, "No code."

Kate asked the resident, "Do we want her to be coded, so that there is a code note on the chart, so that the family will be happy, if they want to see the chart?" He said to Kate, "I know this puts you in the middle." Kate spoke to Tammy, "Have a cigarette before you call the code, if I were you." Kate, Colleen, and Tammy discussed how criminal it would be to code the patient. Marie later said that she "finally figured it out; the family hates her. A guilt complex can only go so far."

Tammy talked to Suzanne before going to lunch about a delayed code. Suzanne would "cover" District I for Tammy. "If she goes, call the code, but delay." The senior resident would come to the code and deal with the ICU resident who comes as part of the resuscitation team. The nurses obviously wanted the patient to die. Coding the patient was horrible to them, the worst action at this point. Her frail body "can't take any more."

The nurses went to lunch and came back to 7H, "covering" each other's patients as was their custom. At 3:20 P.M., Tammy found Mrs. Kelly pulseless. Tammy called Kate. After calling the senior resident, they decided to call the "code that wasn't a code." Jennifer, the medical clerk, called the operator. "Code Blue, 7H" was announced over the page system. Doctors and nurses from the hospital's resuscitation team came running. EKG leads were attached to Mrs. Kelly. The senior resident on Mrs. Kelly's medical team explained the "code that wasn't a code" to the ICU resident. Since the ventilator was not working efficiently, the respiratory therapist said, "I have to bag her." She disconnected the ventilator and connected an Ambu bag to hand inflate Mrs. Kelly's lungs. The tracheotomy tube leaked air around it. Respiratory secretions bubbled around her tracheostomy tube.

The resident could not find a femoral pulse in Mrs. Kelly's groin. Kate asked the ICU resident to identify the team member who would compress Mrs. Kelly's chest, that is, perform closed chest massage. Tammy then did closed chest message effectively but halfheartedly. Minimum actions included: EKG, sodium bicarbonate, epinephrine injections, airway-lung-ventilation, and chest compression. The Emergency Room nurse gave the obligatory sodium bicarbonate and epinephrine through the leaking CVP line. The patient was not receiving the full amount of these drugs. All leads of the EKG were flat, indicating no heart activity. After five minutes, the ICU resident pronounced Mrs. Kelly dead. All in the room were pleased and smiled in an embarrassed, bittersweet fashion. They had little respect for themselves for going through the motions of resuscitation. They thought their participation in the patient's death pathetic.

The written log of the resuscitation read as though Mrs. Kelly had lived for the duration of the team's effort, despite the fact that the ambu bag ventilated her lungs and all of her cardiac activity had ceased. When her death was officially pronounced by the resident and the time recorded, all present were relieved. Mrs. Kelly's slow code had ended in her death. The resuscitation team left with the cart containing the cardiac defibrillator.

Marie was still angry at the family. She expressed her opinion that the family should see the secretions, the bruises and the harsh realities of Mrs. Kelly's suffering that the nurses had to face.

Mrs. Kelly had been unintentionally bruised from therapeutic interventions: venipunctures for blood studies and IV "sticks." Her hands, feet, and legs had become increasingly mottled during the recent days. Foul mucous secretions leaked around her tracheostomy tube, spattering the respiratory therapist and Tammy during the code. Her eyes were glazed with the look of death.

Kate started to do Mrs. Kelly's post-mortem care. She deflated the air in the cuffed tracheostomy tube. She removed the tracheostomy tube and threw it in the trash. Cutting the skin suture, Kate removed the CVP line tubing. Kate gently washed Mrs. Kelly's face, neck, and CVP site and closed her eyelids. Kate and Tammy put a clean gown on Mrs. Kelly. Marie deflated and removed the urinary catheter. When Marie and Kate turned Mrs. Kelly onto her left side, they observed that she had lost bowel control. Kate cleaned her and placed the cellulose pad from the shroud kit at her anus. Marie complained about changing the sheets as she placed the plastic shroud under Mrs. Kelly's back, and absorbent blue pads underneath Mrs. Kelly's head.

Kate and Marie turned Mrs. Kelly back onto the shroud. Marie crossed her ankles and tied them, after placing an ABD pad in between to prevent trauma. Marie and Kathy threw out, with great speed and efficiency, all supplies that were in Mrs. Kelly's room that had been opened. Other unopened supplies were distributed by Kathy to other patients in District I. Marie instructed Kathy about what to do in this post-mortem care situation. Marie crossed Mrs. Kelly's wrists and tied them, also placing an ABD pad between them.

Post-mortem care was shared. Kate washed, Marie tied and wrapped, Tammy and Kathy threw out opened equipment. Rachel, a nursing assistant, came into the room and offered to help. She returned with large trash bags to remove all of the discarded equipment, including the CVP line and the tracheostomy tube. Kate called the priest from the neighboring parish, in the event that Mrs. Kelly's family needed him or wanted him to come. She had already received the Sacrament of the Sick when she was in ICU.

Mrs. Kelly's body was held on 7H for her family to view. The room was cleared of equipment and of all traces of suffering except what evidence of suffering was left on Mrs. Kelly's body. Much of this evidence however, was hidden by the clean patient gown and sheets. The resident called the family, who said they would come to the hospital, but later they were unable to come.

When it was change of shift time, Wanda finished wrapping Mrs. Kelly in the plastic shroud and tied her at the neck, waist, and ankles. Her toe tag had been tied in place by Marie. The 7H nurses then released Mrs. Kelly's body to the escort staff, who took her to the morgue to await the undertaker. Mrs. Kelly's son later came to 7H to get the brown paper bag containing Christmas cards and the granddaughter's Christmas present that Mary Kelly had never opened.

Post-Mortem Care: Historical Antecedents and Current Procedure

Two nursing journals published in the United States before 1900 provide evidence that American nurses have long been giving post-mortem or after-death care. Articles found in old issues of *The Nightingale* and *The Trained Nurse* (later called *The Trained Nurse and Hospital Review*) contain discussions of care of dying patients and details of post-mortem care.

Many of the procedures described in these journals are similar to those currently practiced by 7H nurses. The repetition of a succession of practices during post-mortem care and the fact that these practices have been going on for at least a century confirms the ritual nature of after-death care.

In an article entitled "Laying Out the Dead," published in 1889 in *The Trained Nurse,* a nurse gives detailed instructions about how to perform post-mortem care. She also indicates that nursing students from her training school were insured "a training in this part of the nurse's work" when calls came to the hospital for someone to "lay out" the remains of a woman. A carriage picked up the nursing student or nurse, who left the hospital and performed that service for the dead. Laying out was to be done in the following manner:

> Straighten the body. If there are false teeth put them in at once. . . . If the person had been bathed frequently during the illness, it may not be necessary to give a full bath. See however that the body is *clean*, the teeth, hands and nails requiring special attention, besides a local bath, since owing to muscle relaxation the bladder and rectum usually empty at death. Hold the hands firmly together by means of a small book, roller bandage or anything, that will fit closely between the lower jaw and collar bone. . . . Dress any discharging wounds. . . . The body is turned on the side for the first and only time, to sponge back, remove soiled clothing, put on clean clothes and adjust the band and napkin. . . . Tie the knees together with a broad bandage, when the body may be placed upon the cooling board by the undertaker's assistants . . . cover all with a sheet and restore things to order. (Vol. 3, No. 5, P. 170)

It was particularly important that trained nurses begin to straighten and clean the body and insert dentures before rigor mortis set in. The undertakers would have an easier time and be more successful in preparing the body for viewing. Less washing of body parts was required if a man died, but the nurses were to give special attention to the condition of teeth, eyes, hands, face, and feet. The article stresses cleanliness of the body and removal of all evidence of urinary, fecal, and respiratory drainage.

In *The Nightingale,* a weekly nursing periodical, a story appeared in the issue for July 12, 1890, entitled, "The Night Nurse." The anonymous author details the duties of a night nurse in a scenario that included the death of a beautiful Spanish immigrant. The night nurse was "watching for the end."

> The nurse has unconsciously strained her own muscles in sympathy with the last struggle. When it is over she trembles and feels faint, but habit

is strong and this young woman never has fainted and never had thought much of herself. . . . She touches the pallid surface and she carefully performs the last offices for the dead. A large sheet of beautifully fine linen had been found among the patient's effects. The body having been prepared the nurse literally rolls it in the linen sheet; . . . the nurse had arranged the hair in a regal coronet; . . . the "dead men," as they are called, dispose the body upon the bier. They do it gently as they cover the face with the sheet. (Vol. 5, No. 5, P. 217).

Another article in *The Nightingale* details the care of the dying patient. Post-mortem care is referred to as "the most painful part of the hospital nurse's work" (p. 235).

In "After Death," published in 1890 in *The Trained Nurse,* the author, Julia Tudor, admonishes nurses that washing the dead body is "far more easy if the work is done at once." Tudor also emphasizes cleaning face, hands and "lower regions. . . . See that the eyes are shut." She describes the washing and wrapping procedure in detail along with the tidying of the patient's room.

> Burn at once anything in the room that has been used and would be of no value, tooth brush, flannel, etc. . . . Dust the room and make everything tidy and pretty. (Vol. 5, No. 5, P. 226).

Almost one hundred years later, nurses still clean the room of the patient and bathe the patient after death.

Nurses at the end of the nineteenth century were also sensitive to the possibility that their dying patients might still be able to hear. A hospital nurse, writing in *The Trained Nurse* in 1890, describes nursing the dying and suggests that the sense of hearing may be the last sense to go.

> Sight and speech *may* go before hearing, so, I think, we cannot be too careful not to say anything that is not intended for the patient to hear. (Vol. 5, No. 1, P. 19).

For a long time, nurses have paid attention to this idea as they care for dying patients. They still talk to patients, as Marie did, as though they can hear. They are usually careful about what is said in the unconscious patient's room.

While the 7H nurses performed post-mortem care, none consulted the *Hospital's Policy and Procedure Manual* to determine the hospital expectations of the nursing staff. "Post-Mortem Notification, Documentation and Care" takes up five pages in the manual and details nurses' and doctors' responsibilities when patients die (Appendix 1). The details of the nurses' responsibility comprises the greater part of this procedure. On 7H, however, the nursing tradition of giving post-mortem care was passed along to the neophyte only by action and word, not by consultation with the published procedure. For example, only by action and word does the neophyte on 7H learn the tradition of not crossing the arms of a Jewish patient. Nowhere in the hospital's procedure on post-mortem care can this information be located.

Post-Mortem Care: First Experiences and Other Memorable Experiences

Mentioning post-mortem care stimulated vivid recollections for 7H nurses. They reminisced about the first death experience or about deaths that for a special reason stood out from others. It was evident that these memories were stored just below the surface of the nurses' awareness. Each nurse carried these stories of former patients within her, seldom sharing her thoughts with another. Therefore, it was necessary to ask another question: What are nurses' subjective recollections of post-mortem care of dead patients? This section includes some of these recollections.

Gloria, staff development instructor for 7H, recounted her experience with an infant's death. When Gloria worked the twelve-to-eight shift, she had periods of free time between in-service programs. She typically offered her services to whatever units needed her.

Once Gloria answered a request for help and went to the pediatric unit. A baby had just died. "I did post-mortem care on the baby. The nurses on the floor couldn't do it."

It was a strange story. The baby was left with a baby-sitter. The baby fell and was found on the living room floor by the baby-sitter, who did CPR. The baby revived but was brain dead. She was four months old and was on the ventilator on Peds for two to three days. She was taken off the ventilator and died. I got her ready for her parents [by giving post-mortem care]. I took the baby to the treatment room. I put the baby in a buggy. The longer we waited [for the parents] the angrier we got. We didn't know that night, but the parents were seen by counselors. They had been away on a trip when the accident happened. We waited the whole night. You'll think this is crazy, but I checked the baby periodically to make sure she was O.K. Finally, I wrapped the baby [in a shroud] and sent her to the morgue. We tried not to judge the parents, but it was hard. There was not a bruise on the baby—she was beautiful. She looked well cared for and well nourished. I guess we wanted to be angry at someone because of the death.

Gloria checked the baby in death as a nurse would check an infant in life. The beauty and the look of life that the baby displayed conflicted with the reality of her death. The nurses' anger at the parents was strong, yet misdirected. They needed to express their anguish however, at the unnecessary death of a lovely child. It was evident in Gloria's descriptions that she vividly remembered this death and post-mortem care.

After Deidre shared the post-mortem procedure with me, she was stirred by another recollection of dying and death:

There was a scary story. There was a patient who was real mean; nothing ever pleased this man. He was mean to his wife and mean to his children and mean all of his life. He was discharged from the floor to home. He had severe COPD [chronic obstructive pulmonary disease].

He was gone a week and the ambulance brought him back. He was really short of breath. Naturally we tried to get a "line" [IV] in. He kept yelling at the doctor and me, "Goddamn you, don't stick me." He was determined to be a "no code." He was dying then. When he died, there was something about his facial configuration. His chin came up to meet his nose. I said to myself, "If there's a God or a devil, he was going to the devil." It looked like a vendetta; he looked so scared as if he saw something.

After this, Deidre, Kate, and I talked about life and reincarnation and about belief in God. Deidre spoke of her belief in kindness to people and joked about her belief in an afterlife. We returned to the man's death; I asked Deidre if anyone saw the man's face when she did. His wife and son did. "His son ran out of the room." It was as if he had seen something horrible—his eyes got as wide as saucers.

Deidre described her anger at a group of nurses who were doing post-mortem care together. Once when she was the night supervisor, she came to a floor when there was a death. "I couldn't find the R.N.'s. They were all in the room doing post-mortem care. I was angry, because I wanted them to care for the living. Later I realized that they must have needed to do it together." Deidre's realization was a reflection of her maturity and thoughtfulness.

Pam recalled a time when, as a new graduate nurse, with little experience with dying and post-mortem care, she did not want to complete post-mortem care on a patient. "A tiny lady just blew up [before her death], bigger than me. When she died, she was bleeding from everywhere. She had esophageal varices. I just couldn't finish it. Wanda had to finish it. It wasn't my first post-mortem care, either."

Pam's recollection seemed full of fear. Her inability to explain why the patient "blew up" and the horror of a patient "bleeding from everywhere" were intensely upsetting. Her superstition seemed to fill in where knowledge ended.

Kate joked about post-mortem care, saying, "Post-mortem care is always fun." Then she added, "There was the patient that I killed." Kate described a patient who had been shot in the spine. One day, since he was paralyzed, Kate performed range-of-motion exercises on his legs. He began to complain of pain in one leg. Next his breathing became labored. Kate sought the opinion of another nurse, "who knew about as much as me, only out of school one year."

Kate's patient "threw a pulmonary embolus and coded." During his post-mortem care, Kate remembered feeling overwhelmingly guilty. She thought that she had caused the death with the exercises. She had been giving nursing care that had an intended therapeutic effect, but instead it had had a negative result. She knew that she did not cause the death, but the guilt still remained with her seven years later.

Sarah described the death of a patient to whom she was emotionally attached. Before she became a nursing student, she worked for a short time as a nursing assistant and was caring for a female patient. Her patient died.

> I went into the room with the nurse and I said, "We can't wrap this lady, her arm just moved. You'll have to get someone else to do it." When there are patients I have really gotten attached to, such as Mr. Bowman, I couldn't go in and do his post-mortem care. I wanted someone else to do it. Over the years, you just mellow out about it. I guess you get used to it.

While Sarah said she had grown used to it, she apparently had not, since she was unable to do Mr. Bowman's post-mortem care. Sarah described what was important to her when she did post-mortem care:

> The way you handle the body, not just handling like a dead piece of meat. Closing their eyes, fixing their jaw, leaving jewelry on the family wants on, generally cleaning them so that when the undertaker gets them they are not full of BM.
>
> The last thing [part of the body] wrapped is the head, especially since the family might view the patient. Sometimes the family wants to spend time with the deceased. The deceased can stay on the floor two to three hours. Then you have to take them to the morgue. I would hate to see my father in the morgue. The bed [on the unit] is a more natural state.
>
> I don't close the doors. I even let the patients who know the patient look in.

Sarah's approach to her patient's death reflected a temporary kinship with the patient and his family. The greater the emotional attachment, the harder the death was for her to deal with. She liked to carry out family wishes by leaving jewelry on if they preferred. She wanted the patient to be clean when the undertaker received the body. Her feelings emphasize the high value that nurses place on the cleanliness of patients and also suggest that nurses might fear criticism if a patient is soiled.

Nancy recalled her thoughts about several patients' deaths and in particular her first experience with the death of a patient:

> The first time I did post-mortem care, I was working at another hospital. During shift report, they told me that my patient was probably dying at that time. Sure enough, after I left report, I found out that she died. I didn't know what to do. It was my first time. Then a Mr. Green, a nursing assistant, told me that there was nothing to it; he would show me. He put everything he needed on a cart, went into the room, and showed me how to do it. He hummed all the way through it, when he removed the IV's and the Foley. He had it all done in eight minutes, humming all the way through it. He said, "If you don't like to do some things, you don't have to spend a lot of time doing it." I guess that the way you do it first, it really affects how you do it. That's the way I've always done it.

Nancy did not perform post-mortem care in a businesslike manner, although she did do it fast. When Nancy prepared a body, she preferred that the body be on the shroud, with the edges of the shroud rolled up close to the body. She did this because she did not want the family to see the shroud. Nancy covered the face last, because she imagined that she could still see the face through the shroud.

> I tie up the neck real fast and leave the room. I don't like to look back for fear I'll see they're breathing. . . . Another thing, I won't do post-mortem care on a patient who has been dead awhile. A patient died at 2:30 in the afternoon. We got out of report at 4:50 and he still didn't have post-mortem care done. I told Kate that I wouldn't do it. There's something about touching a body that is cold, like there is not life there anymore. I just won't do it when the body has been on the floor [unit] for a while.

Nancy described peaceful and not-so-peaceful deaths.

> There was this patient they had on 7H who had emphysema. This lady was transferred to ICU, intubated, and connected to a respirator. While in ICU, she developed a systemic fungal infection. Later she came back to 7H. She always looked uncomfortable on the respirator. Her face changed [after death]. She looked happy. Her daughters came in to see her before we did post-mortem care. They had a peaceful, sedative conversation with her. They told her that she didn't have to suffer anymore. *Then* they cried. This death was really different. It was almost as if she was listening to them. There were four daughters. They lived near here. This happened three years ago. . . .
>
> There was a Jewish man who you could think was ornery, but he wasn't really. He was on 7H, left for a rehabilitation hospital, and came back to 7H. The family came every day to check on him. They were in the room when he passed away. They watched him take his last breath. They ran to get us and asked if he was dead. The one sister broke into a wail. It must have been Yiddish. She cried out his name. They held him and talked to him. Then they left. You could see and feel her [his sister's] loss and sorrow. It wasn't exactly American, their mourning.
>
> There was another old man I took care of, a Jewish man. We had developed a good relationship. His son visited him the night he died. We knew that the father wasn't doing well, but we couldn't tell when he would die. I noticed that the son had a hard time leaving the floor. He walked up and down and sat at the end of the hall by the elevators. I guess that he finally figured it was all right to leave. The father called me in and asked me to hold his hand and I held his hand for about ten minutes. He said, "Thank you," and then he died, right then. I sup-posed he didn't want to die while his son was there. He was his only child.

Nancy continued to pour out her memories of death. A young woman was admitted to 7H. She was four years older than Nancy and the wife of a policeman. Although she stood by him while he studied and earned promotions in the police department, he began to neglect her and the children. She began to shoot speed. The doctors said that, at 32 years old, she had heart function equivalent to that of an eighty-year-old woman. One evening the nurses were afraid she was going to code. She did, that night, and was transferred to ICU. Nancy went to see her.

> Her eyes were wide open and she looked out of it, like she was dead already. I didn't go back to see her one day and I was off another. I went back to ICU and was looking for her. The medical clerk told me that she passed. I went back to 7H, hit the frame of the door and cried. The head nurse told me that she understood. I was upset because she was close to my age. I was bitter against her husband. It seemed unfair. It could have been someone I knew, who was close to me.

Nancy seemed to say that the more she could identify with a patient, the more upset she was with the death.

Nancy also shared her memories of the deaths of three other patients.

> 743 Door or Window. It was a black lady in her mid-fifties. She had lung cancer and was in and out with radiation treatments. It was a bizarre Fourth of July weekend. Two people were coding in E.R. One man jumped out of a building across from 7H. This lady had increased problems breathing. The respiratory therapist was here. The doctors were here. She was on aminophylline. She vomited bile. Her eyes were wide as if she was suffocating. She *was*. She was panic stricken and there was nothing that we could do about it. Her visitors were here. Her postmortem care was unremarkable. Her face still looked scared, as if it was frozen there. It didn't fall into a peaceful expression, like some do. I wouldn't . . . I didn't close it [the shroud] because she suffocated. The rest of her body was living while her lungs were dying.
>
> Another black lady, about forty-four years old with four kids. One came to see her. Her husband saw her twice and she was in for a month at least. Her kids were always calling from home. She had uterine and breast cancer. They coded her because the family wasn't in to get a "no code" status. Eventually they stopped. We cleaned her up to get her presentable. The family would visit. Another L.G.P.N. said, "All these people and she's dying alone." She evoked a lot of feeling from us. Black and young with a family. We felt hostile about the family. When we

washed her off, we talked to her. We could understand. It was a long-suffering round.

There was a twenty-eight-year-old black female. Thrombocytopenic purpura. She was married. It was the first marriage for her, the second for him. His first wife died. While they were phlebotomizing her, she had uncontrolled bleeding. They couldn't stop it. She was aware of what was happening. Her husband was there and we had to get him out of the room. He went to the lounge area and paced between the phones and the hall, looking down the hall. She coded and they coded her for forty minutes. When the doctors told him, he screamed. Here was his wife who he wanted to live with and have children. He screamed as if he would tear his heart out and give it to her to make her live. He hugged her and kissed her. When I did post-mortem care on her, I cried. She was a young woman. Later when Rachel came in, not knowing about her death, I stopped her. She wailed and threw herself over the bed and cried. My heart ached for her.

Nancy's recollections of death all revealed the suffering of the patients and their families as well as the sadness of the 7H nurses as they reacted to these deaths.

Nancy wanted to learn more about helping her friends and their families and her patients as they were dying. She reported that she had listened carefully to the hospice nurse and had tried to emulate her clinical skills. As a result, Nancy was able to help a friend who had suffered the death of someone she had loved. Nancy was glad she learned more skills about the handling of death from the hospice nurse.

Wanda, an L.G.P.N., like Nancy, who worked during the evening shift, described her perspectives on post-mortem care. She said that she did not like to cover the face, and she joked with the other nurses: "Don't cover my face, I won't be able to breathe." To her, there was "nothing" to doing post-mortem care. She had been doing it for seventeen years and did not mind it, except that she covered the face last.

One goal of post-mortem care is to get the patient presentable for the family. The nurses must find out whether the family will come to see the dead relative. Wanda was matter-of-fact and explained that she did not mind if the deceased patient remained on the unit in the bed for awhile, since the nurses have the shroud underneath the patient and the patient is clean. "Maybe the family wants to touch the patient's hand. . . . That's why I partially wrap the body. I just have the sheet [shroud] underneath him."

After the death of a long-time 7H patient, Rachel recalled her first death. She had just finished nurses' aides' school. She knew that she never wanted to touch a dead person. One evening she was taking an obese patient's blood pressure and pulse and could not get these vital signs. She asked Camille to take them for her. Camille "took one look at the patient, closed the curtain around the bed and said, 'I guess not, she's dead.'"

Rachel was upset. Camille was unsympathetic and told Rachel, "No one is going to wrap your dead patients for you." Camille made Rachel help her.

> She was so fat we needed two sheets [shrouds] to wrap her. I just touched the patient like this [indicating just with her fingertips]. . . . Next about a month later, I was with a young nurse's aide who didn't want to touch a dead person. Well that night I did three [post-mortem cares]. I got over my fear and I made her stand there and watch me.

Rachel had handed down the tradition of post-mortem care to other nurse's aides, just as staff nurses taught other, uninitiated, nurses of the unit.

When Dotty spoke about her first death, she described caring for a patient who had a decubitus that was so large "it went down to her bone." After Dotty cleansed and dressed the patient's decubitus, she turned the patient over from her side to her back. The woman groaned. "I thought I killed the lady." Dotty laughed as she recalled her experience. Her anxiety made her laugh.

Often the nurses' recollections were stimulated by a death "on the floor" or by a question about post-mortem care. One morning, Miriam finished doing closed-chest massage on a patient. She showed her reddened wrists, sore from compressing the patient's sternum, to three other nurses. CPR had taken its toll.

Following report, Miriam walked into the utility room and began to describe the resuscitation. Her description highlighted both how nurses handle bodily excreta and how she tries to protect the family from witnessing this evidence of suffering:

> MIRIAM: They tried to . . . they intubated her and they got into the left side [left bronchus] but they weren't getting a really good air flow. The minute they stuck that tube in and I hit a compression [performing

CPR]—I mean—feces flying out at—I mean it was all over the floor. I mean, look at me—I'm still—covered.

z.r.w.: What was the diagnosis?

MIRIAM: She's CA of the lung with bone mets [metastasis] and she also had an [intestinal] obstruction. That's why she had the Cantor [tube] in. . . . She was—well basically she was up to her ears, 'cause they were trying to clean out. So it was like every time you turned around there was feces coming out of either the mouth or the rectum.

z.r.w.: What did the family do when they came?

CECILE: The family hasn't been here yet.

z.r.w.: So she's still here?

MIRIAM: Yeah. She—they pronounced her at like a couple of minutes . . . 5:56 [A.M.]. And initially they wrapped at a quarter after and then they said they're coming in so we unwrapped her, put the sheets back on the bed, and cleaned up the room.

z.r.w.: When you clean up the room, one of the things I've noticed is you absolutely make it look perfectly organized, neat. It's almost like removing all traces of suffering . . . or unpleasant things that the family would even have to see.

MIRIAM: Yeah. I think it's hard enough for them to accept death and they wanna try and remember them—you know, their last picture of what they see of her is going to be their most memorable. We try to make them as pleasant, you know, as pleasant as possible. I mean you don't want to see blood and gore and everything else 'cause you'll only have nightmares. It's hard. I'll tell you—like today it wasn't so bad but my first time I couldn't go in the room by myself. Usually we do it in twos, threes, because it gives you such an eerie feeling—like Mrs. Brown—she let out a breath afterwards; she went "Ah." It was like . . . the first time you hear that whether it was sometimes it was an arm flings loose when your muscles let—it's like, "Whoa, what's going on here?" . . . You really get psyched out. It's an eerie feeling initially. . . . I think a lot of it is mental, too. You feel a lot of guilt. It's your way of saying, sort of, goodbye—your final whatever for her . . . your nurturing type of instinct. I found myself talking to her today. When she put the strap on her chin, I thought that just doesn't look like Lillian—she looks better—more natural with her mouth open.

It's hard. It really is. I mean, my first code I remember. I had the whole floor. It was the first day back from a few days off. And I always make it a point if I'm down at the end of the hall or going to be in a room more than a few minutes, to let someone . . . know where I'm going to be. I was down in 51 and one of the girls came down and says "43 [is a code], we got one in 43." . . . Nobody had done anything other than turn the bed on to raise it up. . . . The CPR board wasn't there, nothing. I looked at the lady, ran out and got everything, 'cause everybody disappeared on me. I was like the only one up here. Got the board—finally somebody came in and helped me put the board under her arms and I was doing compressions. I couldn't remember her name, her diagnosis, nothing. I had no idea . . . I had been in here [the room] maybe twenty minutes before [the code] but . . . I just didn't remember looking at this lady to see how she was breathing. I felt guilty as hell. And the doctor said, hey, she couldn't have been dead more than ten or fifteen minutes maximum 'cause she was too warm—her color was too. . . .

A particular supervisor, whose name I will not mention, came back, didn't . . . bother to ask if it was your first code or anything. During the code she's trying to rearrange the stuff on the crash cart and they threw her out of the room. [Laughter.] Then she's looking for her scissors on the bed and one of the nurses threw her out. After the code, she comes back an hour later, doesn't ask me . . . are you O.K. or anything. She could see I was upset. Her first words to me are, "Did you give the lady forced air cage ventilation?" I'm like, "What?" I said I didn't even find the lady. I walked in in the middle of the thing, you know. I said, "No. . . ." "Well, you should do them for her" [the supervisor said]. Well, how long can I code? I mean, very infrequently that you see people do mouth to mouth. . . .

z.r.w.: I mean, I've done it, but . . .

miriam: So have I. I mean the first. . . . 'Cause the cancer patient—I'll never forget it—her dentures bit me—I got bitten on the lower lip from her dentures—she didn't make it. The second one . . . we happened to find him. We're sitting at the desk and we heard a [deep, short, inhaled breath demonstrated by Miriam] like that. And we had a patient who used to wake up with nightmares. So I sent one of the girls down the hall. I started checking out the rest of the rooms. I walked into 53 Door—we had just admitted a guy there—he said, "Oh, my roommate called out in his sleep." I went over and he was blue. Didn't even check for pulses. I mean, he was gone. Called for the code. I was on my third set of compressions before anybody got down here. I was screaming, but we got him back. A young guy, forty-five years old or so. And he was supposed to be discharged the next morning. He was a cardiac patient. They wanted to do surgery; he refused. He ended up dying about two weeks later. He ended up having five or six more arrests. . . . But he was clean and everything, but he . . . something you could smell clear out in the hall. . . . The girl [L.G.P.N.] came in to help me . . . brought the board in but didn't bring in the bag and I said, "Get on the mouth." And she looked at me like I was going to report her if she didn't get on the mouth. [Laugh.] . . . See, that's why I did it.

[Another patient coded.] There was no way I was gonna put my mouth to this man. . . . He had a nasal tube in him, but his mouth had something green in it. . . . I was like, no way, five [of us] saying we're not putting our mouth to this man. [Laugh.] Yeah, well somebody finally got the bag for us, but you know. In that time somebody was on the chest in the meantime.

z.r.w.: Um. No use.

miriam: It wasn't. What good was it [CPR] doing [without ventilation of lungs]? I mean Chuck [M.D.] went right for the chest—the heck with the mouth. He was the first one in there. He was in there. He went right for the chest, and Sally was in there and she grabbed the board. And he finally got the mask on.

That time lapse is enough to do it. I recommended to Respiratory to have those bags prehooked.

Miriam explained that she gave mouth-to-mouth resuscitation to a patient for the first time, so that she would be able to do it to save another, more salvageable, patient. Her repugnance about putting her mouth on that of the near-death patient described above was understandable. His respiratory secretions were visible. He probably would also have vomited, since many patients do during resuscitation. Miriam explained her guilt about one of the patients' deaths described above. She forgot whether she had checked his breathing when she was in his room before the code. She alluded to a doctor's tendency to avoid the nurses' "dirty work," mouth-to-mouth resuscitation. The use of an ambu bag and a mask was imperative for respiratory ventilation and resuscitation. It also served another purpose. The hospital's nursing and medical staff were able to avoid mouth-to-mouth contact with secretions and excreta of the patient who was in cardiorespiratory arrest.

Resuscitation as Context; Post-Mortem Care as Ritual

The nursing and medical staff who worked with the 7H patients admitted that daily facing the diseases, illnesses, and deaths of their patients reminded them of their personal mortality. When a patient died quietly, the 7H nurses were pleased. For example, when a ninety-year-old woman died Sharon said during shift report, "The patient went quietly." Beth smiled. She had eluded the resuscitation drama. When a patient was dying or died on 7H, many of the nursing staff were stimulated to discuss death. They predicted the deaths of other patients on the unit and recalled their past experiences through these death stories.

Many of the 7H nursing staff who told stories of dying patients and post-mortem care at length seemed to seize the opportunity to recapture an intensity of experience that was apparently not sufficiently shared at the time of the experience but stored just below the surface of their awareness.

The 7H nurses clearly appreciated the opportunity to discuss past and present deaths and first post-mortem care experiences. The importance to a nurse of her first experience with giving post-mortem care to a patient was dramatized by the fact that the nurses were all always willing to describe these memories when the subject of death was introduced by a general question or was stimulated by the death of a 7H patient. Nurses seem to remember many details of their first post-mortem care experience. Their ability to "handle" death as a health care provider is tested during this experience. They compare their performance to some internalized standards acquired through the passing on of traditions.

The 7H nurses required emotional support from other nurses when their patients died. Some never got it. One young nurse, Miriam, never forgot a supervisor's emphasis on the techniques of resuscitation rather than on Miriam's reaction to the crisis of a first death and resuscitation attempt. While Miriam did not overtly ask for support, she needed it. Instead she had to listen to criticism, and she judged her supervisor to be insensitive.

The 7H nurses were never comfortable with dying, death, and the possibility of a code. Their nervous laughter during report and their "do not resuscitate/resuscitate" comments highlighted their reaction to the uncertainty of the occurrence. They questioned their abilities to recognize imminent death in time for effective resuscitation and emphasized their need for proficiency in the skills of CPR. They felt insecure because they occupied a gray zone while waiting for a doctor to ask for family agreement to a "do not resuscitate" decision, for a family to make this decision, and, finally, for a doctor, a nurse, and a family member or patient to make the official chart notation and signature that made the inaction of "do not resuscitate" seem more legal. They felt morally compromised when they enacted a "slow code."

These nurses were angry at their "being stuck" in the middle of the "do not resuscitate" dilemma. It was clear that they ultimately bore the responsibility for the decision to resuscitate or not to resuscitate when the harbingers of death presented themselves. They feared litigation if they did not resuscitate a patient. Yet they knew that CPR is an intervention to be performed for sudden, unexpected cardiopulmonary arrest.

The nurses thought that it was torture to resuscitate patients they considered deathbound. Perhaps their reactions can be explained by the continuous, shift-by-shift confrontation with slow dying that nurses witness first hand. This identification of resuscitation with torture may explain the anger that 7H nurses bore toward families who could not bring themselves to sign DNR permissions for dying patients but often did not regularly visit the patient. They saw some resuscitation efforts as futile and were angry at their own participation in this futility.

The neophyte nurses of 7H learned some of the distinctions among the resuscitation or code categories from discussions with the unit's more seasoned nurses. There were four choices of action when cardiopulmonary arrest and death were evident: no code, almost no code, slow code, and full code. From the nurses' point of view, a no-code status translated at death to a peaceful parting for the patient. While an EKG often was taken to document the end technologically, the absence of emergency ambience surrounding the death made it stand out for the nurses. They smiled approvingly when an elderly patient died peacefully, without the fanfare of the code.

In the "no-code" situation, the nurse, doctor, family member, and sometimes the patient were involved in the decision about the death event. The family member or the patient and the nurse and doctor witnessed the placement of a note in the doctor's progress record that documented the decision to avoid resuscitation in the event of cardiac or pulmonary arrest. The patient was classified as a DNR, Category III.

An "almost no code" situation meant that the doctor had the family member's verbal permission not to resuscitate the patient but no witnessed statement had been entered into the patient's chart as a progress note. When an almost-no-code patient experienced a cardiopulmonary arrest, 7H nurses usually "called the code" and resuscitation efforts began.

A "slow code," meant that, although the staff judged the patient as "no hope," the family had refused to give the permission to nurses and doctors not to resuscitate the patient. The nurses "called the code." Resuscitation efforts were delayed and slow paced resuscitation efforts were eventually started. Resuscitation seemed largely motivated by a desire to go along with the family's wishes and to avoid lawsuits.

The slow code choice held the greatest ambiguity and conflict for the 7H nurses and the doctors of the dying patient's team. The decision to call the code rested squarely on the nurses. They had the choice of waiting for a time after the blood pressure "bottomed out" to call the code. Their waiting insured a faster death and a less effective code. During the slow code the nurses and doctors wished for a fast death, gave the minimum cardiac compressions and ventilations, and waited for the flat EKG. The futility of the slow code was evident.

The "full-code" situation was for the unanticipated, suddenly approaching death of a patient for whom the staff had hope, either in a situation in which it had not occurred to the staff to ask for DNR permission, or in a situation in which the patient or family had refused to give the nurses and doctors permission not to resuscitate the patient. The full code was fraught with tension. Resuscitation efforts were vigorous. The vigor and speed with which resuscitation efforts progressed seemed to intensify the drama of the situation. Even for a slowly dying patient, a "regular code" was aimed at saving life. On an implicit level, all resuscitation efforts seemed aimed at future patients deemed more hopeful or more salvageable by nurses and doctors. All codes seemed to be "practice" runs for the totally unexpected death.

It was evident that 7H nurses valued being technically competent to handle the code, including the chest compressions and respiratory ventilations necessary to support a dying patient's life. They wanted to be efficient dispensers of the code medications. Their values about care surrounding death, however, extended beyond technical expertise. They wished that their patients would not suffer as they died. If a patient's death was preventable, they hoped that their clinical ability to detect the cardiopulmonary arrest and to care for the patient during the code would be sufficient to help.

The classification of a patient as a DNR, Category III resulted in the nurses' viewing the patient differently. Fluids and food in the form of IV's and gastric tube feedings were always provided for the DNR patient, along with bathing and position changes. Hospital equipment, such as the Clinitron bed, however, was allocated to the more salvageable patient or the patient who did not have the DNR label.

7H nurses were clearly attached to some of their patients. The longer they knew the patient, the greater was their approval or disapproval of the family's degree of attentiveness, visiting style, or DNR decision; the closer the patient was to the nurse's age, the more the nurse identified with the patient's death. When patients became more like kin, some nurses were unable to do post-mortem care for them. At these times, they relied on the other nurses to do the post-mortem care for them.

The less experienced 7H nurses used resuscitation and post-mortem care as a sort of proving ground of their ability to "handle" death, that is, to be brave and courageous in the face of death. G.N.'s awaited the resuscitation experience in order to test their clinical ability in maintaining life. More experienced nurses checked inexperienced nurses to see how they managed resuscitation care, the influx of hospital personnel, and the post resuscitation aftermath of death or survival. During the code, another nurse might ask the G.N. if she needed help. This nurse would also assume the care of the patients in the resuscitating nurse's district. No matter which nurse was involved in resuscitating one of 7H's patients, all however, gave post-mortem care to people, their patients, not merely to dead bodies.

The ability of a new nurse to deal with post-mortem care was self-assessed and was also evaluated by the more seasoned nursing staff. The new nurse was frequently helped through post-mortem care by more nursing staff than was available during the resuscitation effort preceding the death. The post-mortem care work was shared. Tasks were assigned and efficiently and rapidly taken care of. The nurses' group approach to post-mortem care helped each nurse get through the confrontation with her patients' and her own mortality. More experienced nurses relied on words and actions to pass on the practices of the post-mortem tradition to the less experienced nurses. Directions and demonstrations were given as nurses dealt with the washing and positioning of the patient's body after death.

The younger nurses felt a need to "practice" post-mortem care so that they would be able to successfully resuscitate patients and help families and patients through the crises of dying and death. As nurses gave a patient post-mortem care, they did it with the implicit intent of washing away the traces of suffering so that the family would not have to witness the harsher realities of death.

Certain physical signs made the distinction between life and death obvious to the nurses: the cessation of vital functions, the immobility of the patient, and skin color and body temperature changes all confirmed death. However, whatever warmth was left in the body reminded the nurses of life. Some acknowledged life by referring to a spirit presence: "The person is dead but the spirit is still here." The transition between life and death was blurred; immediately before death was pronounced, nurses and doctors paused, usually waiting for a flat EKG to confirm death. This pause was a poignant waiting for the end of human life.

After the death of the patient, the nurses washed the patient as they would wash someone in life during morning care. They had help during the bathing. Another nurse would hold the dead patient over while the back and buttocks were cleaned and dried and the plastic shroud was rolled against the patient's back. The 7H nurses admitted having a great deal of difficulty with covering the patient's face with the plastic shroud. Some also disliked tying the hands at the wrists and covering the hands and trunk with the shroud prior to the family's arrival to view the body. Both the face and the hands had defining, uniquely human characteristics and a special meaning, which the nurses related to individual recognition of the person and the way we greet people and say good-bye. Eyes were closed to emphasize the fact of death. Non-seeing open eyes were disturbing. Both face and hands were left exposed. 7H nurses felt that they must be, until family members had witnessed death in their loved one and said good-bye. The imagined possibility that the patient might breathe again was linked to the nurses' aversion to covering the face with a plastic shroud.

The nurses also seemed protective of the patient's body. They liked to think of themselves as treating the patient's body as they would treat one of their family. One nurse admitted that she wanted those in attendance in death to be respectful of the body. Escort personnel and nurses would be stopped if they treated the body as "a piece of meat." She preferred lifting the body from the bed to the morgue litter with a sheet rather than dragging the body over. Part of this protectiveness may relate to the nurses' uneasiness that life was not "long gone." At times the line between death and life was not clearly demarcated.

The 7H nurses had some superstitions about death. For example, when patients died with upsetting expressions on their faces, nurses' thoughts about good and evil were stimulated. They agreed with the notion that "death comes in threes," waiting for the third death if two had occurred. They also talked about unlucky patient rooms. These rooms were identified during change-of-shift report and earned their reputations by association with patients who died in the room or who "went bad," and eventually died in the ICU or CCU.

Although matter of fact about their contact with fecal and urinary excreta, the nurses were also repulsed by the fecal and urinary incontinence associated with death and the mouth-to-mouth resuscitation that was expected of them. Such contacts with excreta and secretions documented the fact that nurses do a special kind of dirty work. It also separated the nurses' dirty work from the doctor's dirty work. Nurses' dirty work concerns more intimate types of bodily contact than does that of doctors.

The nurses have to be able to deal with excreta and secretions at the same time they face questions of mortality and the spiritual aspects of life and death. 7H nurses also showed fear of death and knew the dramatic changes in the physical appearances of their patients that death brought.

It was important to the nurses that the dead patients were clean when they left their care for the morgue and the undertaker. They washed the patients' bodies and cleaned the rooms with a fervor that was partially explained by a need to wash away all traces of suffering.

Newer nurses, more than the more seasoned staff, exemplified the value orientation that nurses must be brave and courageous in the face of another's death. Not only were they interested in the technical skills associated with resuscitation and post-mortem care but they also wanted to handle death well, despite the fears they had. They wanted to develop interpersonal skills so that dying patients and their families would find strength in them. The seasoned nurses possessed these skills.

Some of the seasoned nurses took pride in their ability to predict when a patient would "go bad." If a doctor failed to listen and the patient "went bad" and died, the nurse selectively used that story as support of her intuitive clinical knowledge. When the nurses failed to predict death, they regretted their failure. Deaths of patients reminded both seasoned and new nurses of their own mortality and the deaths of their own family members.

The 7H nurses made judgments about the manner in which family members attended dying patients and about the manner in which patients died. If family members failed to visit and failed to give DNR permission for what the nurses considered a useless, intrusive violation of the patient, the nurses became angry. They expressed this anger to each other. They pitied the patient who was abandoned by his or her family, even though they knew at some level that the relatives may have had their own difficulties facing the death. This could have included fear of being backed into a DNR decision.

The nurses became angry when they could do little to ease the suffering of their dying patients. Their anger seemed directed at their own inability to mediate pain and anguish.

After a patient died, for the nurses, the body's inanimateness and coldness only partially confirmed death. Their recollections of death events contained examples of alarming after-death movements of an arm or leg, or a sudden exhalation. The fact that it took the body some time to cool reminded the nurses of the life recently present. Several nurses discussed their views that the spirit hovers around the body and that therefore they feel that they must protect the body from being treated roughly. Gentleness of touch was evident during post-mortem care, during which nurses sometimes spoke to their dead patients.

Peaceful deaths were valued by the nurses. These were deaths unimpeded by the resuscitation technology of the defibrillator, monitor, ventilator, and electrocardiograph. Patients who "passed" quietly pleased their nurses. If a patient died alone, however, his death unwitnessed by a busy nurse, the nurse felt guilty and worried. Nurses ruminated on what they could have done differently in order to have been there for the dying patient.

Using the definition of DeCraemer, Vansina, and Fox (1976), the post-mortem care that nurses perform for their dead patients is a nursing ritual. Seldom, if ever, witnessed by other hospital personnel and patients' families, its character is not widely known. Post-mortem care as a therapeutic nursing ritual is comprised of patterned symbolic actions that represent the values and norms of 7H nurses. Therapeutic rituals improve the condition of patients. Post-mortem care holds latent meaning for nurses as they care for patients after death, continuing therapeutic nursing interventions. The symbolic meaning of the post-mortem ritual rests in the nurses' need to remove the manifestations of suffering, to purify the patient's body and the hospital room of the soil and profanity of death, and to gradually relinquish their tenure of responsibility for the patient, given up only as the escort personnel transports the dead patient to the morgue. Explicitly, post-mortem care helps nurses make their dead patients presentable for family viewing.

Post-mortem care is part of nursing's long tradition with the laying-on-of-hands. Even after patients die, nurses care for them, touching them with gentleness.

III

The Nursing Ritual of Medication Administration

Giving medications is a high priority nursing function. Nurses regard medication administration as a serious trust, shared with doctors. This trust is embedded in the nurses' therapeutic goal to do good and to avoid harm. Medication administration represents the reciprocal relationship between patient trust and nursing responsibility. The customs of nurses giving medications link the scientific aspects of medication administration to the magic of giving drugs.

Nurses classify medications according to their therapeutic effects: stabilizing medications, curing medications, preventive or prophylactic medications, and placebo medications. Stabilizing medications are given to maintain bodily functions. Curing medications are given to remove the signs and symptoms of disease. Preventive or prophylactic medications are given to stop the onset of disease and keep the patient from becoming ill. Placebo medications are given to placate patients, and because the drugs do no harm and might do some good.

The nurses on 7H witnessed that medications worked and knew implicitly that scientific rationale did not always explain their effectiveness. The therapeutic benefits of medications convinced nurses, doctors, patients, and family members of their almost magical, unexplained powers. The statement "The medication is working" conveyed this belief in the efficacy of prescribed drugs.

Medications were effective, despite their obvious side and toxic effects.

One of the ritual aspects of medication administration is the "three-time check" that the 7H nurses relied on to insure that the correct medication was given to the right patient. The three-time check is outlined in the *Hospital Policy and Procedure Manual*. This practice has persisted for years in the nursing literature specific to medication administration. 7H nurses neither consulted the abundant medication procedures in the manual, nor verbally stated the three-time check as they prepared medications. Instead, they silently checked the medication Kardex, in which the ordered medications had been transcribed, removed the medication from the patient's drawer in the medication cart for the district, read the label on the medication itself, and again checked the patient's Kardex.

The nurses persisted in using supplies, such as the small, fluted paper soufflé cup (Figure 7), in a manner that seemed inefficient. The soufflé cups were often stuffed to overflowing with unit-dose medications, still in their identifying package. Some nurses said that the drugs were left in their packaging so that the nurses could review the drugs and their side effects with the patient. The practice of using a small paper cup, however, was ritualistic. Like the three-time check, the soufflé cup was used to protect the nurses from making a medication error.

Medication administration was a clearly identifiable, visible nursing function. Its standing as a public function was emphasized by the fact that doctors, nurses, medical clerks, and pharmacists shared in the work involved in the ordering, preparation, and giving of drugs. Many hospital forms, including patient chart and Kardex forms, were involved in recording the business of medication administration.

At the same time that medication administration was public it was also somewhat parochial. New G.N.'s were gradually initiated into the special knowledge needed for medication administration. Moreover, the most secret, abbreviated, and archaic language and recording style used by nurses and doctors when medications were involved kept medications to a restricted domain. Explicitly, the

Figure 7. Soufflé cup.

special language was used to reduce the time needed for discussing medications and for charting medications. Implicitly, the language served another purpose, that of maintaining an aura of secrecy about the work of ordering and giving medications. The language contains such words as "pouring" and "holding" along with Latin abbreviations.

Military influences on nursing and hospitals remained in the medication language and procedure of 7H. Military time was used to mark the times of medication administration during every hospital day. Medications arrived on 7H transported by an escort staff member. This "pharmacy drop" was symbolically reminiscent of war supplies left in a combat zone. Furthermore, medications fought disease.

When nurses made medication errors, they revealed the seriousness and moral concern with which they viewed medication administration. They openly yet hesitatingly admitted their own and each other's errors and feelings of guilt in the arenas of staff meetings, change of shift report, and incident reports. These admissions of guilt served a latent function. Through public confession, the nurses were able to share the guilt, blame, and punishment in a corporate or group way.

The nurses often blamed medication errors on their failure to follow hospital procedure or the failure of other hospital personnel such as pharmacists or doctors to correctly carry out their responsibilities for medication administration. Regardless of where the blame lay, to the nurses on 7H, medication errors meant, on a latent level, failure of responsibility and loss of patient trust; it meant inadvertently doing harm to those who needed their help.

The 7H nurses placed medication errors into two categories: errors of commission and errors of omission. The most serious error of commission was to intentionally give a wrong medication to a patient. The next most serious error of commission was to unintentionally give a wrong medication to a patient. Errors of commission varied in degree of seriousness according to the effects of these errors on patients.

Errors of omission were both intentional and unintentional. The degree of seriousness of these errors depended on the importance of the drug to the patient's recovery. Not giving a patient an ordered drug could have severe effects on his or her recovery. Not receiving an antacid was not as serious as not receiving a postoperative antibiotic.

The data on medication error emphasized the symbolic association of medication administration with nursing responsibility and revealed the seriousness and the moral responsibility with which nurses regard their drug-giving function. Medication administration is tied to nurses' implicit intention of doing good and avoiding harm for their patients.

Medication Administration

A NURSE'S SPECIAL KNOWLEDGE

Medication administration was a nursing function that required special knowledge for those involved. 7H nurses took their responsibility for medication administration seriously and resented intrusion into what they perceived as their domain.

The nurses resented having patients identify and request medications that they thought they should receive while in the hospital. They could not accept the idea that the patient knew best about medications. They resented, for example, a patient who stayed in the hospital for two months and decided that he should get Dilantin, a seizure-preventing drug. He persistently requested the Dilantin from the nurses and doctors. Although the doctors were lukewarm about his request, they finally prescribed the Dilantin. During change-of-shift report, the day shift primary nurse, smiling sarcastically said, "Mr. Sparks was thrilled at getting his Dilantin." The nurses disagreed with the patient's request and the doctors' decision. They felt that they knew better about this medication than did the patient and his doctors.

The nurses learned a little about medication administration during their basic nursing education prior to working on 7H as G.N.'s. They learned much more of the intricacies of medication administration after coming to 7H.

G.N. INITIATION

The G.N.'s slowly increased their knowledge of medication and their skills in the administration of medications. They found that nursing 7H patients and administering medication on 7H was not similar to their experience in their nursing education programs. 7H was a harsher, more demanding, more complex environment than school. The many permutations of medication administration reminded all 7H nurses, new graduates and seasoned nurses alike, that they would never be certain of their knowledge or absolutely secure in their skill. There were always unfamiliar drugs and patients who responded to drugs in idiosyncratic ways. Both experienced and inexperienced nurses consulted the P.D.R. and the pharmacy when they lacked knowledge of a drug's action.

The G.N.'s were supported in their quest for experience with medications by Gloria, the staff development instructor, and by 7H's seasoned nurses, Deidre, Kate, Sarah, Beth, Tammy, and Miriam. All of the experienced R.N.'s answered the G.N.'s many questions about specific medications, the patients who received them, and how to deal with the doctors who ordered them.

Gloria spent several days teaching and evaluating each G.N.'s medication administration performance. She was direct and gentle with the new nurses. She discussed written examination results with them and reminded them to work at becoming more secure in their developing skills. She admitted to Chris, a G.N., "I'm compulsive. I get nervous and sometimes get other people nervous. Tell me if I am getting you nervous." Gloria worried about the seriousness of her responsibility.

When Gloria finished the orientation or "initiation" period with the new graduates, she made herself available to them by telephone. The G.N.'s relied heavily, however, on Kate, Deidre, and their R.N. preceptors, including Beth and Sarah, and Tammy and

Miriam, to help them through the difficult times with dispensing medications.

Frequently the G.N.s worried about IV's. Their inexperience with IV's and medication additives was obvious in the questions they asked and illustrated by an incident that occurred when Colleen, a new graduate, was the sole R.N. on the night shift. A doctor changed an IV heparin (an anticoagulant) dosage late in the evening shift. When Colleen discovered this on the night shift, she had difficulty calculating the dosage per cc. so that she could order the IV with heparin on the pharmacy slip. She sought the help of an experienced R.N. The 7H nurses had many problems monitoring IV's and managing medications added to IV's. The G.N's had to learn how to time flow rates, how to safely flush IV's, how to add drugs, and how to handle other aspects of these infusions. They showed their delight when doctors discontinued IV orders. On evenings and nights, when there were fewer nurses on duty, IV's kept nurses busy.

Electronic IVAC pumps helped the new nurses to monitor the ordered drop flow rate of IV's. These pumps beeped to signal a problem. This sound was difficult for the nurses to ignore. They checked on the patient's IV as soon as possible and began working on a solution to whatever problem they found. Often the solution was identified after consultation with an experienced R.N.

G.N.'s resented the amount of time that medication administration consumed. They valued the ability to pour medications with speed and precision during scheduled times, to maintain correct milliliter per hour flow of intravenous fluids, and to time and regulate the periodic infusions of IV medications.

Often a G.N. had a difficult time balancing the administration of medications with other nursing responsibilities. Meredith, a G.N., exhibited this as she worked during the evening shift. Since she had problems setting priorities and getting organized, particularly about medication administration, she was moved back to the day shift and was "shadowed" by Sarah, an experienced R.N., who said, "She was putting people on the bed pan while she was passing meds three hours on evenings, and ignoring chest pain." Sarah preceptored Meredith and helped her work out her problems with medication administration and priority-setting.

Often during shift report, a G.N.'s lack of knowledge and confidence about medications was aired especially when unusual medications were ordered by doctors for patients.

> G.N. Oh, he also had . . . he was ordered this medication—the chole. . . .
> How do you say that?
>
> R.N. Colchicine. Colchicine. And it [the order] says to stop it if he has
> diarrhea or until pain relief.

The medication was so unfamiliar that the new nurse did not know how to pronounce it.

Along with the difficulties the G.N.'s had with their knowledge of the actions and side effects of medications, there were patient problems that troubled the G.N.'s as they tried to administer drugs skillfully. When Pam, a G.N., mentioned a problem to the other nurses, they decided, after discussion, to put the patient on aspiration precautions because she had difficulty swallowing, "especially big pills." They would carefully help the patient eat her meals and swallow her medications.

Another incident revealed how insecure the inexperienced nurses felt about dispensing medications to patients with problems that interfered with taking medications. Colleen was caring for Charlotte Evans, who had polymyositis and a mediastinal tumor. The patient's gag reflex was still absent after she had a diagnostic test. Colleen was unsure about whether to give the patient medications that had been postponed because of the diagnostic test. She knew that Mrs. Evan's gag reflex had not returned. She asked the resident if she should try to give the patient her late medications. Following the resident's suggestion, she attempted it, but with some hesitancy. Her patient "nearly choked to death."

During change-of-shift report, the experienced R.N.'s took time in between patient reports to teach the G.N.'s some of the details of medication administration. In the following example, Sarah explained the timing of an antibiotic medication to Ann:

> ANN: And when does he get this ampicillin? Is that q. 8 [every eight
> hours] or two additional doses after he comes back?
>
> SARAH: After he comes back, so if you give it to him 12:30 [P.M.], so it's
> eight hours after that and eight hours after that.

ANN: And then repeat one dose after twelve hours after that?

SARAH: Yeah, so if he gets this . . .

ANN: Yeah, we can figure it . . .

SARAH: Yeah, do it on the cards, so if he gets his last dose at 9:00 in the evening tomorrow, so 12 hours after that would be 9:00 in the morning. . . . So he gets the whole thing. . . . So you just have to . . . when he's due that, take his index card and write out the times. You can look at it like this, just write out a card with the next two q. 8 hours doses.

The responsibility of teaching medication administration to the new nurses was taken very seriously. During report the seasoned nurses quizzed the G.N.'s about their medication knowledge. This initiation period was most intensive during the first five months of the new nurses' tenure on 7H. However, the seasoned R.N.'s frequently "pitched in" to help relieve the new nurses of some of their work load and make possible an easier adjustment to medication administration and other nursing duties.

MONITORING CONTROLLED DRUGS

Medication administration was a visible and highly documented part of nursing care. Throughout each twenty-four-hour day, on each eight-hour shift, of the hospital, nurses were observed giving medications at scheduled and unscheduled times. At routine times the medication cart (Figure 8) was rolled into the corridor, and nurses moved the cart from one patient room to another. After giving a patient's medications, the nurse recorded her initials beside the time and beneath the date of administration on the medication Kardex. In this way they "signed out" the medication, acknowledging their responsibility. Their full signature was located on another section of the medication Kardex for verification (Appendix 2).

The importance and seriousness of medication administration when compared with other nursing functions was emphasized by the amount of paper work associated with this duty. The hospital records that contained information on medications were many. They included: the doctor's order sheet, the medication Kardex for

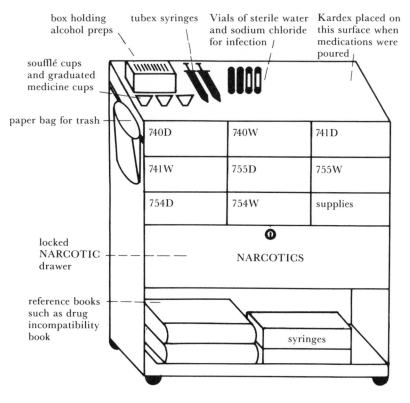

Figure 8. Medication cart.

each patient, the order slips that the night nurse completed; incident reports that were completed when medication errors occurred, the intake and output record where common IV medication additives were listed, the additive sticker that was taped on the IV bags, and the narcotics flow sheet.

The most visible and frequently used of these forms were the medication Kardex and the doctor's order sheet. By using these forms, each professional group daily acted out and acknowledged their responsibility. The nurses checked the doctor's order sheet to determine if the medical clerk transcribed orders correctly onto the Kardex. The nurses signed this record along with the doctor and the clerk. When the clerks were not working (between 9:30 P.M. and 8:30 A.M.), the R.N. transcribed the doctor's orders onto the medication Kardex.

Doctors checked the nurses' medication Kardex to determine whether ordered medications were given and to get a clear summary of the drugs patients were currently taking. Even patients' self-administered medications, such as eye drops and ointments, were noted by the nurses on the Kardex.

The medication Kardex was made of light-weight cardboard inserted into a metal frame and consisted of two folding cards. Included on the routine drug Kardex cards was the following information: the patient's Addressograph stamp, the title "Medication Kardex," and a routine record of medication administration. The record of medication administration included: order date, renewal date, discontinuation date, medication name, dose, route of administration, time given, site, nurse's initials, nurse's signature and status (R.N., L.G.P.N.), and patient's medical diagnosis, name, and room number. The second Kardex card also included the patient's Addressograph stamp. This card was entitled, "P.R.N., Stat and Sliding Scale, Pre-Operative and Scheduled One Dose Medication Administration Record." It included allergies, a large section for p.r.n. (as needed) medications and pre-operative and scheduled one-dose medications, and a diagram of injection sites, with two front and two side views of a patient for the location of subcutaneous and intramuscular injection sites. The second card also included space to record the specifics of the medications given.

The time spent recording narcotics and other controlled drugs was another indication of the seriousness of medication administration. 7H nurses signed for the receipt of these drugs, counted them, and "signed out" as they poured and recorded the administration of these legally controlled, government-monitored, potentially addicting substances. Every day at 7:30 A.M., 3:30 P.M. and 11:30 P.M., a nurse going off duty on each shift was obligated to publicly count and compare the count with that of another nurse coming on duty. They counted the number of controlled drugs used during the shift and the number of drugs remaining in the narcotic drawer of the medication cart. Sometimes, because of patient care demands, the nurse going off duty did not count with a nurse coming on. Two day shift nurses might count controlled drugs at 7:30 A.M. when Miriam, the night nurse, was giving shift report or finishing some aspect of nursing care.

R.N.'s or L.G.P.N.'s completed these eight-hour nursing audits for injectable and oral preparations of controlled drugs. They checked the numbers recorded at the end of the previous shift with the numbers remaining at the start of the next shift. Since the nurse who had given the controlled drugs during her shift was mandated to record the time and the patient's name and room number, to check the specific drug given, and to sign that she gave the medication, it was usually easy to document the drugs used on that previous shift. Occasionally a nurse would forget to chart this information on the twenty-four-hour controlled substance record, but it was easy to find the necessary information. There were two other places for recording these controlled medications: the medication Kardex and a charge slip that was filled out and carbon copied as each nurse gave a dose of a controlled drug to a patient.

If a nurse had to "waste" or dispose of part of an injectable or oral controlled medication, she was obliged to have another nurse as witness. For example, Meredith prepared an injectable narcotic for a patient. The prescribed dosage was less than what was packaged in the premixed tubex syringe. Meredith squirted a few milliliters of the medication into the trash bag taped to the side of the medication cart. A night nurse, also a G.N., witnessed this and signed on the Pharmacy Service form along with Meredith.

Controlled drugs were brought to 7H by a pharmacist who waited as an R.N. counted the drugs and recorded them on the twenty-four-hour controlled substance record. The new supply of medications was placed in the narcotic drawer, which was then relocked.

7H had only one narcotic drawer, located in the medication cart for Districts I and II. The rest of the nursing units in the hospital had one drawer in each of their two medication carts. One of the R.N.'s carried the narcotic drawer keys on her person, around her waist, around her neck, or in her pocket. The keys, according to the policy and procedure manual, were to be visible at all times: "Wear keys around the waist so that they are visibly on your person while on the unit" (Appendix 3, section V., M.). The narcotic keys were never supposed to leave the unit. When a nurse accidentally took them home, the clinical director was notified and the nurse was called at home. She returned the keys as soon as possible.

When a patient asked a nurse for a narcotic pain medication, required a preoperative medication, or had a routine order for a controlled drug, the responsible nurse searched for the narcotic keys. "Who has the keys?" was the often repeated question.

When the keys were located, the nurse checked the Kardex, unlocked the drawer in the medication cart, removed the medication, such as Percocet, and placed it in a soufflé cup, relocked the drawer, signed the tablets out on the 24 hour oral controlled substance record, and completed the Pharmacy Service slip along with its carbon copy. She rechecked the Kardex and carried the medication to the patient's room, where she gave it to the patient, with water in this case. After the patient took the medication, the nurse left the room and recorded the time, date, site, and her initials on the medication Kardex.

The nurses were aware that controlled substances disappeared occasionally from 7H and other units of the hospital. They quietly discussed these disappearances when news of them traveled along the grapevine. Either Deidre or Kate would investigate a controlled substance problem and stay with it until it was resolved. Once, Librium disappeared from the narcotic drawer. Colleen knew that it had been received during the previous day shift. She reported the missing drugs to Deidre. Deidre investigated the incident thoroughly, but the drugs never reappeared nor were they accounted for.

When the narcotic count was "off" or inaccurate, the nurses who were counting and recording announced this aloud, making public a potentially serious situation. Since the counting and recording were typically done during change-of-shift report, it was possible to ask the previous shift's nurses what happened to the drugs that were not recorded. One morning, Kate and Chris found the narcotic count off an "outrageous" amount for one drug. Kate called the pharmacy and discovered that there had been a pharmacy and nursing recording error. Another time a narcotic count that was off was "cleared up." A patient who was dying with lung cancer received three doses of the drug during the night shift. His nurse forgot to chart them as given. Once this was detected, she recorded the drugs on the usual forms.

When medications were not given, the responsible nurse signaled her responsibility by making notations on the medication Kardex. She drew a circle on the Kardex across from the time and under the date when a patient refused to take a medication or when a medication was out of supply, that is, unavailable in the patient's medication drawer.

Seldom was a medication that had been "poured" by one nurse given to a patient by another nurse. When this was done, each of the nurses involved, the nurse who "poured" the medication and the nurse who dispensed the medication, checked that the medication was recorded in the Kardex. When a nurse forgot to sign out a medication, she was reminded by other nurses and hastily corrected this on the medication Kardex. Again, the nurse's initials represented an acknowledgment of responsibility for administering the medication.

PROCEDURE

While the *Hospital Policy and Procedure Manual* contained many pages devoted to the administration of medications, 7H nurses seldom referred to it. The details of medication administration were often passed from experienced nurse to inexperienced nurse by verbal exhange or by demonstration. For example, when a Z-track, intramuscular injection of Imferon was ordered, the nurses discussed the technique of injection in detail. Although they discussed the procedure, they did not consult the *Policy and Procedure Manual*. Nurses on the evening and night shifts consulted the manual most often, probably because fewer personnel were available to answer questions.

The *Hospital Policy and Procedure Manual* contains a large subsection entitled "I.V. and Medication Administration." Topics included are: "General Administration of Medication" (Figure 10); "Preparation and Administration of Oral, Parenteral and Rectal Medicines"; "Administration of Post-Op Narcotics"; "Anti-Lymphocytic

Globulin Preparation, Distribution and Administration"; "The Role of the I.V. Nurse"; "Hyperalimentation"; "Intralipid Therapy"; "Use of Reseal Injection Cap"; "Blood Transfusions"; "IVAC Infusion Pump"; "IVAC Infusion Controller"; "Use of Dial-A-Flow"; "Final Filter"; "I.V. Care—Peripheral Site, Changing I.V. Tubing—Peripheral and Deep Vein"; "Application of Armboards"; "General I.V. Management"; "Discontinuing Peripheral I.V. Catheter"; "Care of Central Venous and Cutdown Injection Site"; "Mixing I.V. Solutions on the Nursing Unit"; "Pre-Operative Medications for Ophthalmology Patients"; and "Chemotherapeutic Drug Administration on the Oncology Unit."

These published procedures served as guides to action, even though they were consulted infrequently. Nevertheless there is a system of checks outlined in the *Policy and Procedure Manual,* under "General Administration of Medication," section V., D.:

Select the correct drug and read the label three times:
1. when selecting the drug.
2. when comparing the label with the data on the Kardex.
3. before returning the drug to the patient's drawer.

This system of checks has persisted for nearly a century. A similar three-part system of checks was described in a pre-1900 American nursing journal. The purpose of the three time check, then, as now, was also to help the nurse avoid error and maintain accuracy by the following approach:

When you are about to measure a dose of medicine, look for your bottle, read the label, and then reach for it. As you raise the measuring glass to a level with your eye, look at the label again. Measure the medicine, and as you return the bottle to its place, again read the label. Here are three chances to correct a possible error; always take advantage of them. (Groff 1896, 638)

Even though 7H nurses seldom consulted the *Policy and Procedure Manual,* they nevertheless knew and used the system of checks as a behavioral code. They acknowledged their use of this system when describing their customs of medication administration, but they used it silently, as an almost magical protection against medication error.

ROUTINES

As soon as change-of-shift report ended, the primary nurses made rounds on all of the patients in their districts. Medications were well integrated into the fabric of these nursing activities. For example, nurses discovered that patients needed pain medications during rounds. Most medications were given at regular times, although p.r.n. and one-dose medications were given at irregular times. The regular times identified for medications included: b.i.d. (twice a day); t.i.d. (three times a day); q.i.d. (four times a day); q. 1 h. (every hour); q. 2 h.; q. 4 h.; q. 6 h.; q. 12 h. The "twos" (2 P.M. medications) were "out" much faster than the "tens" (10 A.M. medications). There were generally fewer medications to give in the afternoon than in the morning.

The afternoon pace began to accelerate after 1:45 P.M. when all of the staff had finished their lunch breaks. The work to be completed by the nurses of the day shift included carrying out treatments, taking afternoon temperatures (and other vital signs), checking IV's, moving patients back to bed, and dispensing 2 P.M. medications. Most of the time-consuming work of the day shift, such as bathing patients, was completed before 2 P.M.

During the evening shift, the staff divided 7H into three geographical districts. Ann reported that, "Most of my time on 4–12 is spent on the pouring of medications, as well as taking off [doctors'] orders." Ann moaned frequently during report if there were many IV's to monitor during the evening shift. The 6:00 P.M. (1800) medications were poured from 5:15 P.M. to about 6:15 P.M. at the same time that patients ate or were being fed dinner. The 10:00 P.M. (2200) medications were poured from 9:30 P.M. to about 10:10 P.M. Midnight or 2400 medications were started at 11:00 P.M. because night change-of-shift report almost always started promptly at midnight. Pam, Ann, and Nancy each usually gave medications to one district apiece.

With a smaller staff on the evening and night shifts, administering medications and monitoring IV's exhausted much of the nurses' time. The heaviest times for medications on nights were 2:00 A.M. and 6:00 A.M. IV's were watched and replaced when "low." The R.N. gave most of the medications during this shift. The two L.G.P.N.'s gave p.r.n. medications and ordered medications for one district each, using the medication Kardex. The R.N. ordered the medications for two districts.

The night nurses' duties included ordering medications for each patient for the next twenty-four hours, reporting to the night supervisor about 7H patients, keeping IV's running on schedule, taking vital signs, washing and changing bed linen for incontinent patients, taking off doctors' orders, and checking intake and output records. Despite the other duties required of 7H nurses as they cared for their patients, they always gave medications. Nurses frequently interrupted other duties to get the narcotic keys so that a patient in pain would receive some relief from an ordered p.r.n. analgesic.

There were days when the nurses on each shift were unable to maintain the scheduled times for medication administration. Patients may have been absent from rooms, perhaps to have a diagnostic test; medications may not have been "back" from the pharmacy; and p.r.n., preoperative, and prediagnostic test medications may have been abundant. The nurses liked to be finally "done these meds." It seemed as if they were never finished. On the busy weekends, medication administration may have been one of the only ways the R.N. saw all of the patients during the shift, except for the quick morning rounds after shift report.

In addition to time spent actually dispensing medications, considerable time was spent sorting the order/charge slips and checking and storing the medications that arrived in the zippered green bag of the pharmacy "drop." Routinely, one nurse would sort the yellow slips, check them against the medications received, and note which of the ordered medications had not arrived. The nurses next distributed the medications to the appropriate patient drawer in one of the medication carts. This pharmacy "drop" system was created to reduce the time spent by nurses in ordering and checking on drugs. Besides the routine ordering of drugs during the night shift, it was necessary to order drugs from the pharmacy when medication orders changed or when newly admitted patients needed to start their medication therapy. Nurses anxiously awaited these drugs from the pharmacy.

The 7H nurses stocked the medication cart with straws, juices, syringes, soufflé cups, plastic medicine glasses, a small trash bag, and reminder notes on 3 × 5 cards before beginning the rounds to give medications to the patients of each district. Nurses also periodically ran to the medication refrigerator in the nourishment area of the nurses' station to obtain refrigerated medications or IV's.

The details that nurses had to consider concerning medication administration were many. Nurses used various devices to help them recall the detail of a one dose or "single dose" medication (red stickers on the Kardex) and the fact that a patient was not in his or her room during routine medication times (reminder notes on 3 × 5 cards on the medication cart). Identibands on patients' wrists were supposed to be checked to insure that the right patient received the right drug. The most annoying interruption of the medication routine occurred when newly ordered drugs did not come from the pharmacy when expected.

During change-of-shift report, 7H nurses starred the patients' names on the primary nurse worksheet so that special or single dose medications such as preoperative medications were not forgotten. Nurses also verbally reminded each other during report and slipped a note in the Kardex as an additional reminder. So many details were associated with the nurse's role in administering medications that the nurses always seemed rushed during the busiest time of their shift.

All nurses are taught in their nursing education programs and reminded in the *Hospital Policy and Procedure Manual* never to leave medications unattended at the patient's bedside or with the patient. The nurse must see the medication swallowed. The real pressures of clinical practice, however, sometimes forced nurses to disregard this teaching. All 7H nurses who were observed administering medications occasionally left medicines either at the bedside when the patient was out of the room, or with the patient before the nurse saw the patient swallow it.

In one such situation, Beth entered room 743 with IV and oral medications. She quickly changed the IV tubing and the IV bag and dated the tubing. After the patient turned from his side to his back, Beth poured water for his medications and left him swallowing his oral medications as she went out of the room. The patient did not see that there was a tiny, sublingual (under the tongue) tablet left in the soufflé cup. Beth's haste modified a time-honored safety routine and inadvertently jeopardized a patient's welfare.

THE ART OF MEDICATION ADMINISTRATION

The art of medication administration was revealed at the patient's bedside. Nurses adjusted sluggish IV's; patiently coaxed weak, nauseated, and querulous patients to take their medications; and almost painlessly gave injections to patients. At times it was difficult for the nurse to get a weak patient to swallow an oral medication. For example, Beth prepared a medication for Ellen Paul. She crushed the medications at the medication cart with a mortar and pestle. She went into Mrs. Paul's room and put the medications into a tablespoon of cream of wheat cereal. The patient did not want to take the medicine. She resisted gently but with the tenacity of an ill, long-suffering woman who could die at any time. "There'll be pills in there," Beth said to me. "I'm hiding them in the cereal; she had such a hard time swallowing. I'm doing one at a time." "I'll give you some orange juice so you can wash them down," Beth said to Mrs. Paul. "Oh my God, I'm too sick," she replied. Beth fed Mrs. Paul the cereal mixed with crushed medication one spoonful at a time. She helped the patient drink some juice. Slowly, Mrs. Paul managed to take her medications and eat a little breakfast.

Kate bargained with Irving Mann, a confused seventy-nine year old, considered to be a difficult patient. Kate poured Mr. Mann's tablets into a soufflé cup. She left the medicine cart in the hall and entered the patient's room. Mr. Mann repeatedly muttered to himself that he needed an "enemy" (enema). As Kate told him to take his pills and put the soufflé cup to his lips, he pushed her hand away. Kate managed to tip the pills into his mouth. He removed the pills from his mouth and threw them to the floor. At this point Kate said, "Irving, take your pills and we'll call the doctor" (about the enema he wanted). Later, he swallowed his newly poured morning medications. His nurse was finally successful on the second attempt.

The above examples and the following indicate that the routines of medication administration were integrated with other nursing duties. One day Kate stood in the hall beside the medicine cart (Figure 8) pouring medications for an elderly patient with congestive heart failure and dysphagia (difficulty swallowing). She explained to me that she would "hold" his Diabinese, since he was going for a "broncho" (bronchoscopy) today. She poured Lasix (a diuretic), digoxin (improves cardiac contraction), and Pronestyl (an antiarrhythmic), which were packaged in unit doses (one dose of the drug was enclosed in a labeled package). The medications in a patient's drawer of the medication cart were separated into plastic envelopes. After checking the medication Kardex and putting the oral "meds" on the top of the medication cart, Kate put the medications still in their package into a paper soufflé cup. She then went into room 740, where she found a pulmonary fellow (a medical resident) aspirating a blood gas specimen from the patient's artery. The patient was in pain since an arterial puncture was needed for the blood specimen. Kate told the patient that she had pills for him, and that she would give him his "meds" when the doctor was finished. The patient seemed upset at this. Kate took the blood gas specimen out of the room and returned to help the patient sit up.

The patient had obvious problems swallowing. Kate got him water and encouraged him as he slowly swallowed one tablet at a time. The largest tablet was saved until last. Kate poured more water. Finally the patient successfully swallowed the tablet. Kate began to "set him up" for his morning care. She obtained a comb, wash cloth, towel, patient gown, mouthwash, toothbrush, and lotion out of his bedside cabinet. Next she put water in a yellow plastic wash basin and encouraged him to bathe.

In the next patient room was an alcoholic patient who had been recently admitted with "ketoacidosis," a complication of diabetes mellitus. Mabel was giving the patient a bath because Kate was occupied with medications. Mabel asked Kate if she could get the patient out of bed to change the linens since he had wet his bed. Kate said yes, even though he had a bed rest order. Kate poured three tablets for the patient at the medication cart. She first read the Kardex, said aloud the names of the three drugs, opened the patient's drawer in the cart, and removed the prepackaged medications. She put the medication in a soufflé cup and recorded the "meds" she was going to administer on the patient's Kardex. She placed her initials next to the time under that day's date (Appendix 2). She poured water for the patient to drink with his medications. (Water pitchers and styrofoam cups were kept at each patient's bedside.) Kate poured the tablets from the soufflé cup into the patient's hand, after she asked him if he was ready to take his medications. She told him that he was taking Decadron, Dilantin, and a multivitamin. The patient swallowed the Dilantin but dropped the other two pills in his lap. He told Kate that he "lost two." Kate carefully looked into the folds of his patient gown, found the pills, and watched as the patient took them. Kate then interrupted her medication duties to answer a telephone call.

Kate returned to prepare medications for another patient, again checked the Kardex, and poured three tablets onto a soufflé cup. She signed her initials on the medication Kardex to indicate that the medications had been given. She walked into the patient's room and conferred with the patient's wife. She placed the soufflé cup on the bedside table and then helped the other patient assigned to the room walk from the bathroom to the chair. This patient was so unsteady on his feet that he almost missed sitting on the chair. Kate helped him avert a fall.

Kate moved back to the first patient to administer his medications. His wife helped with the task. Kate did not interfere or limit the wife's participation. She poured the medications directly into the patient's mouth from the soufflé cup after helping him into a more comfortable position. He seemed confused and had trouble following her directions. He swallowed two of the medications. His wife helped by holding a cup of water with a straw. Kate held the soufflé cup again to his lips as he swallowed the other medication. After this success, both the patient and his wife seemed pleased.

Commonly 7H nurses administered medications while attending to other patient needs. The following description provides an example of the interruptions that the nurses encountered while giving medications. Deidre prepared to give 10 A.M. medications to one of her patients. She interrupted her "pouring" duties for one patient by responding to an electrical alarm ringing on an IVAC pump. She then listened to the first patient's apical heart rate and gave her some digoxin. Ann came into the room and asked Deidre how to remove air from a CVP line connected to the IVAC pump. Deidre first gave the patient the medications she had prepared. She then left the room, poured medications for the patient with the IVAC pump problem, and joining Ann, took the medications into his room. Deidre "purged" (cleared of air) the IV line and reset the IVAC pump. She gave the patient his medications.

On her return to the medication cart, Deidre met a resident doctor who gave her a verbal order for a change of dosage on a thiamine (vitamin B_1) order. The doctor said that he "got the wrong information from the pharmacy." Deidre repeated the verbal order to the doctor. He later changed the medication order on the patient's chart. Deidre prepared another patient's medications: a tablet, a subcutaneous injection, and an elixir. After asking the patient about his preference, she poured the elixir into enough orange juice to suit the patient's taste. Next she gave him an orally inhaled medication and the other medications. Deidre moved on, pouring the 10 A.M. medications for the other patients in the district, and completed the administration of 10 A.M. medications.

THE LANGUAGE OF MEDICATION ADMINISTRATION

Nurses use old terms when speaking about the work of medication administration. These terms are holdovers from times before scientific advances and technology changed medication manufacture and therapeutic effectiveness.

"Pouring" medications refers to many aspects of medication administration. When 7H nurses said they "poured" medications, they used the word to include the checking of the medication Kardex to determine the specific medication, the route of administration (oral, subcutaneous, sublingual, inhaled, topical, rectal, vaginal, ear, eye, transdermal, via gastric tube), the time and frequency of dosage, the patient's name and room number, and whether the medication was routine, p.r.n., or one dose only. They also used pouring to refer to the selection of the medication from the drawer in the medication cart, checking of the Kardex so that the drug would be given, the final transportation of the medication to the patient, and helping the patient take it orally or by another route of administration ordered by the doctor. Pouring also seemed to include the last step of recording the medication the patient received, as the nurse initialed the medication Kardex.

When describing events or facts specific to the administration of the pouring of medications, 7H nurses most often abbreviated the word medication to "med." For example, when discussing a patient with coronary artery disease, Sarah matter-of-factly stated during afternoon report, "He's refusing his meds." This type of contracted or abbreviated language pervaded the verbal and written exchanges of the nurses. Nurses often shortened words and employed abbreviations to use time efficiently and to avoid unnecessary talk at the patient's bedside.

The word "hold" was used as a shorthand way for the nurses to say that the medications would not be administered at this time (for example, "I'm holding the Diabinese, since he's going for a broncho [bronchoscopy] today").

When the patients were "off the unit" for diagnostic tests, medications were given to the patient late and the nurses staggered the remaining doses of the medication therapy throughout the day. This meant pushing the scheduled time of medication administration to a later time while maintaining a therapeutic interval between doses as required by the doctor's order and procedure. For example, a patient had a chest X-ray and bone scan taken on the day shift. During report, the primary nurse for his district reported that his medications were staggered: "You have to stagger his meds. I gave him his two o'clocks late. The Persantine [vasodilator], the Ecotrin [enteric-coated aspirin], and the Inderal [antihypertensive and cardiac drug]. . . . The three of them get staggered. The others he can get at the regular time." Some nurses used the terms "split-schedule" and "staggered" interchangeably.

Abbreviations used to identify the frequency of the medication administration such as b.i.d., o.s. (left eye), stat (immediately), and p.r.n. came directly from Latin. These abbreviations saved time in communicating about medications. The abbreviations were used in doctor's orders and in the transcriptions of these orders onto the medication Kardex.

The names of the medications themselves, whether trade names or generic names, sounded exotic to the uninitiated. Patients, nursing students, and G.N.'s mispronounced drug names such as Nifedipine, mercaptopurine, and Metamucil. Some drugs are referred to by trade names and some drugs by generic names.

Another aspect of the language used for medications was the use of military time for specifying scheduled times when medications were administered. In the following discussion during change of shift report, the nurses planned the times of administration of Theodur, a bronchodilator.

> You know what? I just noticed this. This . . . it should be . . . it says b.i.d. It should be [given] at 22.
>
> No.
>
> B.i.d. is 10 [A.M.] and 18 [6 P.M.] . . .
>
> O.K. Theodur has an eight-hour effect. . . . But it can be 10 [A.M.] and 18 [6 P.M.]. But we usually give it [at] 10 and 22, so he had enough to carry him over to the morning.
>
> Right.
>
> Give him the [medication] 22.

The special language used by nurses helped to keep the business of medication administration somewhat secret, by preserving an aura of difference between those who were responsible and knowledgeable about medications and those who were not.

A HIGHLY VALUED NURSING FUNCTION

The nurses on 7H seemed to value their role in medication administration above other responsibilities. They were noticeably upset as they considered the remote possibility that pharmacy technicians might pour their medications at some future time. They doubted that the technicians would be aware of the patient's status, that they would recognize or ask for medication order changes in response to changes in patients' conditions, or that they had enough knowledge to give medications.

What meaning medication administration did have for 7H nurses was revealed in the following discussion. Beth called the administration of medications one of my many responsibilities. It is needed to give the medications, to teach the patient about the medications, and to give the right medications. Sometimes I think of it as a chore. It is part of helping the patient, part of caring for the patient; being gentle, firm, and unobtrusive.

Medications are part of how the patient gets better. My caring for the patient alone won't get him better. My judgment is vital, since the doctor is not there and doesn't see the interrelationships with the symptoms of the patient. . . . It's important. Because it's a chore, I can't make it routine. It's always dynamic. If I'm stuck in a [patient's] room, I don't get to see all the patients. When I give medications, I get to see all of the patients. I felt "out of it" when my G.N.'s were pouring meds. When I do them, I'm conscientious.

Beth spoke about her sense of urgency when she gave medications. She admitted getting angry at patients who refused medications. She balanced this anger with an admission that since patients were participating in their care more, they were often knowledgeable in their comments and correct in their refusal to take medications. She emphasized the special role of nurses' administering medications and the socialization of doctors and nurses.

In nursing, we give meds when ordered. We recognize the inappropriate, too much, too little. At least for the first six months of a new doctor's residency, we have to be careful. We have to be interpreters of the various doctors. We have to translate what they say.

Beth acknowledged problems nurses have with IV medication administration and that nurses must rely on "all sorts of tricks" to get oral and injectable medications into patients. Beth admitted that she skimped on other aspects of care when giving medications during the weekends that she worked: "Control is maintained by giving meds, seeing patients. The care gets done. I'll get to my care later." Beth acknowledged that she and the other nurses bathed patients after medications were given.

The importance of the administration of medications in relation to other nursing functions was also illustrated at mealtime, when nurses gave regularly assigned medications before they fed patients who needed help with eating. The nurses worried about the patients who were waiting to eat. They knew that helping people to eat was an important nursing duty but that it was more important to give patients their medications on time. In fact, giving medications was a higher priority than feeding patients.

In comparison to the rest of nursing care, Tammy ranked medications a high eight on a ten-point scale: "I try to do my teaching [about medications] along with other teaching. Meds predominate." The G.N.'s ranked medication duties higher than bathing patients and change-of-shift report, both nursing priorities. Perhaps the interdisciplinary and public nature of medication administration added to its importance.

Sarah emphasized that knowledge of the use of medications in relation to a disease process is important. So also is the fact that patients need to be informed about their medications. "There is a lot of patient teaching with meds. Like taking the pulse and cardiac meds. If it is high or low, the patient should notify someone. The teaching part of meds is more the domain of the R.N."

Explicitly, medication administration was important to 7H R.N.'s. While they agreed openly that medication administration, including ordering, sorting, and dispensing, was very time consuming and at times dominated their care, they did not want to abandon this function to another group. Sarah emphasized this point, saying that as medications were dispensed, "The patient will sometimes tell the R.N. about something they will not tell the physician."

Implicitly, medication administration represented the seriousness and responsibility with which the nurses regarded their patient care duties. Medications were dangerous; errors could result in catastrophic effects for patients. Nurses were accountable for their mistakes. Side effects of drugs could also be harmful.

Drugs and their attendant nursing functions served as a visible focal point that emphasized, on a symbolic level, not only the seriousness of the nurses' duties in relation to the dispensing of drugs, but the nursing care of patients in general. Nurses desired more experience with medications and expected accuracy when medications were given. These factors emphasized the responsibility that nurses assumed and expected as they dispensed medications to their patients. Sarah spoke for all nurses when she commented about the seriousness of medication administration from the nurse's point of view: "You cannot cut corners on meds. It could hurt the patient."

R.N., M.D., L.G.P.N., AND MEDICAL CLERK ROLE RESPONSIBILITIES

Medications, according to one G.N., were a "hospital and doctor priority, . . . the highest ranked" care function. Medications were recorded specifically, with greater detail than bed baths and other nursing care. This G.N. stated that, "you get 'static' if you don't give meds." Medication administration may have been more highly valued than other nursing priorities because this function represented a shared domain of responsibility with the doctors.

Physicians who cared for 7H patients ordered the medications and recorded their prescriptions on the doctor's order sheet in the patient's charts. Either the medical clerk or the R.N. transcribed the order to the medication Kardex. When the clerk transcribed the order, the R.N. was responsible for checking the accuracy of the transcription.

Doctors determined what drugs to order, wrote the orders, and sporadically checked that patients were receiving what was "written for." Their system of checks emerged during rounds as more senior doctors checked on junior house officers and as they countersigned their orders.

The R.N.'s helped the new residents and medical students learn their functions in relation to medications, as in the following example. Kate was standing at the desk of the nurses' station, telling a junior medical student how to write IV orders with medications added. She told him how to write the order, using correct notation, so that the order would be clearer to the nurse who would prepare the IV. When Kate explained the art of medication order writing to the medical student, the senior resident standing nearby did not interrupt.

Kate admitted later that she had never thought about the fact that experienced nurses teach new doctors to write medication orders. Repeatedly, Deidre, Kate, Sarah, Tammy, and Beth were also seen doing this teaching.

At times, nurses tried to convince the doctors to order medications. Fearing the violence of DT's (delirium tremens), one nurse asked a doctor to order Valium for an alcoholic patient. During a discussion of the problem, the nurse stated, "So he [the doctor] said they do not want him on Librium. They just feel he shouldn't be on it." Another nurse asked, "Did they order leather restraints up here?" One nurse said that they had, as the first nurse continued, "Then he says to me, 'Give him IM [intramuscular] Valium if he gets out of hand.' So how are we going to get close enough to him to give him that?" The nurses disagreed with the doctor's handling of the potential DT situation. While they found the patient a "nice guy," they worried about being physically injured if he went into DT's. The doctors had their reasons for avoiding a Librium order, but it was the nurses who would first detect and immediately deal with the "DT'ing patient." They were afraid. In another situation, the doctors agreed with the nurses' suggestions.

The 7H nurses were not permitted by hospital policy to administer medications in concentrated, undiluted form by IV "push." These theoretically more dangerous medications were relegated to the domains of the critical care nurses' domain or the doctors, including the inexperienced medical students. The "less dangerous" medications belonged to the domain of the "floor" or unit nurse.

The 7H nurses assumed the responsibility for calling the doctor when these IV "push" medications were scheduled to be given. They worried about inexperienced medical students giving powerful drugs IV "push." On one occasion, Beth followed two senior medical students who eagerly went to a patient's room to administer, for the first time, IV digoxin that Beth had drawn up into a syringe for them. As was typical of the nurses, Beth had assumed the responsibility for calling the doctor when the time had come for the drug to be given. She also was very concerned about whether the medical students would give the medication safely. A resident had allowed the medical students to administer the drug unsupervised. This trusting attitude on the part of the resident contrasted sharply with the cautious concern that nurses held in relation to teaching neophyte nurses the intricacies of medication administration.

Nurses and doctors shared the responsibility for observing the effects of medications on their patients. Both professionals evaluated serum chemistry values carefully. For example, when a "K level" (serum potassium level) fell or rose beyond normal limits, the nurses called the doctor who then ordered appropriate medications.

7H nurses thought that they had special knowledge about their patients that the doctors did not have, but they did not believe that the doctors valued that knowledge. According to Tammy, "The doctors do not believe us. They do not think we know. We are with the patient[s] and have a sense about when they have pain and when they do not."

The nurses had limited independence in adjusting oral medication orders. When a patient had difficulty swallowing a tablet or capsule of a medication, or when the crushed medication did not easily go down a gastrotube, the nurses changed from the tablet form to a suspension. The nurse informed the doctor of the change. Nurses never changed from oral to parenteral preparations of drugs. When they thought that this was warranted, because of a patient's vomiting, for example, they called the doctor for a change in order.

The nurses exercised limited judgment in adjusting dosage of medications. When prescribing narcotics for cancer patients, the doctor might order morphine SO_4 2 mg.—10 mg. q. 4 h. p.r.n. pain. Often the nurses would choose the lowest dosage of the narcotic and move it up as the patient's pain increased or as the selected dose failed to reduce the patient's pain.

The R.N.'s saw the business of medications as their responsibility. They did not resist this responsibility, even though they complained about "heavy" shifts when medications and intravenous solutions kept them busy. The R.N.'s looked up the medications in the P.D.R. more frequently than did the L.G.P.N.'s and were seen repeatedly teaching patients about their medications as they dispensed them at routine times and when patients were being discharged from the unit.

R.N.'s shared the dispensing of medications with L.G.P.N.'s. At times the L.G.P.N.'s who worked on the day shift gave medication to their patients. During the evening shift the permanent L.G.P.N. staff also gave medications without prodding from the R.N.'s. The night shift L.G.P.N.'s reluctantly dispensed medications, most often giving p.r.n. pain medications. The R.N.'s, however, bore the overall responsibility for medication administration during each shift.

The R.N.'s checked that doctors' orders were transcribed from the order sheet. R.N.'s signed doctors' verbal orders (given in person by the doctor or over the telephone). The R.N. signed the verbal order and either administered the medication immediately or asked another nurse to do so. L.G.P.N.'s and the unit's medical clerks did not have the responsibility of checking the accuracy of doctors' transcribed medication orders, either written or verbal. The R.N.'s countersigned the doctors' orders as did any medical clerk who transcribed them to the Kardex. It was the R.N.'s, not the L.G.P.N.'s or medical clerks, who directly shared the responsibility of medication administration with the doctors.

Medication Error

VIOLATION OF A PATIENT'S TRUST

The ritual importance of medication administration was derived from its symbolic importance in relation to nurses' responsibility and the trust of patients. Medication error dramatized the seriousness of medication administration. Patient harm resulting from medication error was equated symbolically with failed responsibility and violated trust.

Mistakes happened on 7H as they do when humans are involved in any activity. R.N.'s, G.N.'s, and L.G.P.N.'s made medication errors. G.N.'s, the neophytes of the 7H nursing staff, made medication errors more often than the other nursing staff.

The 7H nurses worried about the effects of medication error mistakes. They knew that serious medication errors could result in harm to their patients. Seasoned R.N.'s still recalled serious medication errors years later. Describing her most serious medication error, Sarah stated that she had been working on the cardiac stepdown unit. After realizing that she gave a patient eight medications intended for another patient, she became very upset. She called the doctor to report the errors, cried, and wrote an incident report to document the error. Later, after going home, she called the unit during the evening shift to ask whether the patient was all right. The vividness of her recollection was evident. She confessed her guilt and repeated the story of her most serious medication error twice. She blamed the error on the fact that she had started to give medications to the patients in the last or highest numbered room in the unit instead of the lowest numbered room. She had violated the nursing routine of giving medications from the lowest numbered room in the unit to the highest. Although the patient was unharmed, Sarah still felt guilty about her medication error years later.

TYPES OF ERRORS

7H nurses described medication errors in degrees of seriousness. Less serious errors were verbally acknowledged by the nurses. Other, more serious medication errors, were "written up" on incident reports.

Beth stated that the most serious medication error, an error of commission, was intentionally giving the wrong medication to a patient. No medication errors of intentional commission occurred during the course of this study.

The next most serious medication error of commission, described by Sarah, as inadvertently "giving the 'med' that was not ordered," was classified as an unintentional error of commission. Unintentional errors of commission included giving a drug that was not ordered to the patient, giving a drug to a patient known to be allergic to the medication, giving an excessive dose of a medication, giving an "underdosage" or too little of an ordered medication, giving prescribed drugs too late or too early, and giving a medication by the incorrect route administration—all unintentionally. An example of the latter error of unintentional commission was infusing an intravenous solution with an added medication through a biliary tube, not through the intravenous tubing. Of these errors of unintentional commission, the least serious was giving a patient a medication too early or too late.

Errors of omission also fell into a hierarchy of seriousness. One very serious error of unintentional omission involved a postoperative patient who failed to receive his intravenous antibiotic for several days. The next most serious error of unintentional omission involved a patient's failure to receive the correct narcotic to reduce his pain from metastatic cancer. This error of omission was not considered very serious, since the patient did have pain relief from the wrong narcotic. Another serious error of unintentional omission involved a diabetic patient not receiving Tolinase, an oral hypoglycemic agent. The last two errors troubled 7H nurses, but not as much as the error involving the postoperative patient's omitted antibiotic.

The least serious medication error of unintentional omission cited by 7H nurses was failure to give a patient Colace, a stool softener. This was less of a problem, from the nurses' perspective, than not getting an oral hypoglycemic drug. An example of a medication error of intentional omission occurred when a doctor ordered an ointment in a percentage of strength unavailable at the hospital. The patient did not receive the ointment for his hands because the nurses would not apply the ointment of a different strength than that ordered by her doctor.

PUBLIC ACKNOWLEDGMENT OF ERROR: RITUAL CONFESSION

Medication errors were acknowledged in unit staff meetings and change-of-shift reports, on doctors' progress sheets, and in incident reports. These methods of acknowledgment informed nurses, doctors, and sometimes patients and family members about errors. The hospital staff were then able to act to prevent or minimize the effects of the error so that serious harm to the patient was avoided.

In general, incident reports were written to document the following unit events: medication and IV errors, a patient's falling out of bed, a patient's escaping from the unit and leaving the hospital, a patient's getting temporarily lost in the hospital, a patient's staying for an excessively long time in the X-ray Department, a patient's losing personal property, and anything else that seemed out of the ordinary.

Nurses taped the incident reports detailing medication errors onto the wall of the 7H nurses' station. There they awaited completion of doctors' and nurses' descriptions of the medication errors made and signatures of the nurses who discovered the error and the doctors responsible for the patient. All who entered the nurses' station were able to read the report and share the knowledge of the medication error. In addition, the patient's attending physician was notified of the error, signed the incident report, and described it in the patient's chart on the progress notes.

Sarah explained how she identified a medication error and emphasized her concern about such incidents:

> We all have to be on the ball. If I am giving out meds, I question whether someone forgot to give a medication. I checked on a med that was in the cart. It was not on the Kardex. Lasix was in the drawer. I filled out an incident report. The patient did not get it for three days. It could hurt the patient. We have to find ways to cut down [on errors].

Sarah discovered this error by finding a medication in the patient's drawer of the medication cart that was not written on the medication Kardex. She evaluated the seriousness of the error. Sarah also gave her opinion about when nurses should and should not write incident reports for medication errors:

> Not giving Colace you do not make out an incident report. Write them when you give the patient the wrong antibiotic. If you D/C [discontinue] an antibiotic or give too much of a med, or when the patient does not receive a med, you should write an incident report. A leaking IV with heparin—incident report. Too much IV in a short amount of time—incident report.

Individual nurses acted independently as they determined whether or not to write incident reports after evaluating the gravity of an error.

Medication errors that were acknowledged during change-of-shift report received public treatment similar to that of an incident report. Admonishments were included with the report. For example, Kate said, "Show Arlene [a p.r.n. pool nurse] the difference between half normal saline solution and normal saline solution. She hung normal saline solution. She hung 0.9."

Sometimes nurses were puzzled when they discovered medication errors. Sharon once was: "I don't know what the story is. . . . That's what he [the doctor] told me so apparently she was given Coumadin [an anticoagulant] and she shouldn't have been or something." In this instance, the nurses going off the day shift were unable to identify either the nurse responsible or the source of the error.

Often the nursing staff became aware of a newly discovered error by word of mouth. When medication errors were discussed during the nurses' staff meetings, Deidre and Kate exhorted the nurses to be careful and reminded them of the perils of these errors. During one staff meeting, Deidre acknowledged that medication errors will occur and suggested methods of reducing errors.

> We all make mistakes, when orders are transcribed incorrectly, as medication errors. Recently two [transcriptions] were incorrect. Take your time taking off orders. Two checks and there are still problems. Five days a patient got Tagamet [peptic ulcer medication] when he shouldn't have. Also consolidate your meds. Send discontinued meds to the pharmacy. Don't hoard [medications left over when a patient has gone home or when medications in the drawer of the medicine cart and used for another patient].

Through incident reports, change-of-shift reports, and staff meetings, medication errors became the shared property of the 7H nursing staff. The guilt spread beyond the specific nurse who was directly responsible for the error to those nurses who failed to detect the error rapidly. The open acknowledgment of error and guilt seemed to diffuse the blame among the nurses. All of the nurses, whether directly or indirectly involved, participated both in the guilt and in the confession of guilt.

Disciplinary action was always considered when a nurse made a medication error. Deidre was cautious about initiating the disciplinary process, but she believed it was necessary, as in the following situation.

Four months after the G.N.'s started their employment on 7H, an R.N. made her second "med error" in a short time. Deidre admitted that she was concerned. It seemed to her that the errors were out of control. In this instance, the nurse missed transcribing an antibiotic medication from the doctors' order sheet to the medication Kardex. The patient received no antibiotic for three days. Deidre considered disciplinary action, yet wished to avoid devastating a nursing unit with already low morale.

Deidre described the hospital disciplinary process. Disciplinary action was taken when there was any violation of policy identified in the employee handbook. Events warranting disciplinary action included medication error, unprofessional conduct, excessive lateness, excessive illness, and unavailability for "on call."

The steps in the process included talking about the problem with the involved nurse, completing a "yellow slip" counseling session with the nurse manager, a "green slip" or warning suspension from work duties, and finally, discharge from the Nursing Service Department. Deidre admitted that generally the disciplinary process, "works like the law, although not necessarily in that order, depending on the gravity of the problem." In the case of the missing antibiotic, Deidre used the "green slip" method to discipline the R.N. who made the error.

A SERIOUS ERROR

An elderly man was admitted preoperatively for transurethral prostatectomy surgery. Since there were no surgical beds available "in the house," he was admitted to 7H. Postoperatively he was returned to his 7H room, since there were still no surgical beds available.

Unintentionally, an R.N. failed to transcribe some of the patient's postoperative medication orders from the doctor's order sheet to the medication Kardex. For three days this omission went unnoticed. Suddenly the postoperative patient who had been "doing well" had a temperature elevation. His life was threatened by septic shock, most likely caused by a combination of errors. He did not receive several doses of his ordered postoperative medications, most importantly antibiotics. Also, a resident had reinserted an indwelling urinary catheter, pushing pathogens into the bloodstream. These errors most likely resulted in septic shock.

The nurses did not realize that the patient had missed his antibiotics until they discovered his temperature increase, septic shock, and cardiopulmonary arrest. The magnitude of the nurses' error was great. All involved with the patient feared for his life as he was moved to the critical care unit. They knew that their omissions were connected to a life-threatening illness.

This was not the only medication error that had occurred since the G.N.'s and new residents had come to the hospital and to 7H. There had been a spate of medication errors on 7H which had originated with nursing, pharmacy, and medicine. Angry and agitated, Deidre discussed the errors at length with all of the nurses involved in the error. The R.N. who made the error and the R.N.'s who missed the errors were directly and indirectly blamed in these discussions. In addition, Deidre reviewed the errors and methods to reduce medication errors in staff meeting.

Deidre was very upset about the serious situation. During a three-week period she analyzed the medication errors involving the missed antibiotics. The R.N. who made the error was disciplined through a warning suspension, documented in her employee file. However, more severe punishment did not take place. Kristen, the nursing clinical director of the medical units, advised Deidre not to single the R.N. out for disciplinary action, since three other nurses were involved. These nurses failed to "catch" or detect the errors. Deidre admitted that she "hated to discipline the young graduates [nurses], since it would have been devastating" to them. The blame and responsibility was shared by a small group of nurses. One nurse actually was directly responsible for transcribing the doctor's order to the medication Kardex. But the three nurses who were responsible for the patient on successive days during successive shifts shared the burden. Perhaps this solution was necessary.

While the patient was in the critical care unit, his condition improved. At one point he seemed well enough that transfer to 7H from the critical care unit was considered.

Deidre viewed this transfer back to 7H as a "second chance," a chance for 7H nurses to rectify or make good the errors. Just before the patient was to be transferred back to 7H, Deidre's hopes were abandoned. "The patient 'coded' and died," Deidre said. The responsible R.N., Deidre, and the other 7H nurses were not soon to forget this patient and these errors. The blame for the error and the fallibility of the hospital staff were blatantly revealed in this unfortunate incident of medication error. The doctors and nurses did not directly discuss each other's blame in this incident.

METHODS OF REDUCING ERROR: ROUTINES AND RITUALISTIC PRACTICES

Deidre knew that medication errors occurred during the process of transcription from the doctor's order sheet to the medication

Kardex. She instituted a system of checks in order to "catch" or eliminate medication errors.

Miriam checked all of the 7H patients' doctors' order sheets nightly against their medication Kardexes in order to detect transcription, omission, and dosage errors. The day shift nurse checked on the night nurse's accuracy by examining newly "rewritten" medication Kardexes when Miriam transcribed medication orders from a fully used medication Kardex to a new Kardex.

In her worry over the excesses of medication errors, Deidre was determined to reduce and eliminate errors: "Everybody's to check charts. Everybody's to check orders to see that they're taken off. And that means your associates [most often L.G.P.N.'s], too. Check charts and absolutely in no circumstances do you go home without these charts checked. I'm gonna put a note by there to check rooms. . . . No matter how busy we are, no matter what's going on, the orders are checked."

Deidre admonished the nurses during morning report to relate the medications ordered to the patient's diagnosis. "Check the diagnosis with what we're doing. We're looking at the medication, medication Kardex, and look at what the diagnosis is." She reminded the nurses to think about what they knew to be common medications linked to common medical diagnoses.

There were additional hospitalwide checks which helped nurses avoid medication errors. Identilines, tapes that included the patient's name, room number, and bed (D for door or W for window) were taped in place in a slot over patients' beds. Identibands, placed on patients' wrists, could be checked to determine facts about the patient, including name and hospital number. Nurses admitted that they used the identiline as they looked over the patient's bed, when bringing medication to the patient. However, the name band was checked only when the nurses did not know the patient. "I'm more thorough when on a district I'm not used to," one R.N. admitted.

Noteworthy because of its persistence, the system of triple checks, as mentioned in the *Hospital Policy and Procedure Manual* and carried out by nurses for years, was also intended to avoid errors. Checking the medication Kardex, the medication package, and the Kardex again were the three steps of this time-honored, ritualistic practice.

The nurses frequently checked the doctors' orders and the transcriptions of these orders onto the medication Kardex. Deidre had exhorted them to do this since medication errors resulted from orders that had been overlooked.

Even the simple custom of starting the pouring of medications for the patients in the lower numbered rooms and then in sequence until completion of the higher numbered rooms of a district or the whole unit seemed a necessity. It was a way of eliminating error. The Kardex organization paralleled this room-arranged sequence. The first patient Kardex to be seen as the nurse opened the Kardex of a district was that of the lowest numbered patient room.

Still, errors occurred despite the fact that nurses knew these checks, often carried them out, and supported them as worth using to avoid error. Errors happened not only because of violations of procedure and tradition, but also because the many details and demands of the floor nurses' existence on 7H made the ideal not always practical or possible.

The 7H nurses used more informal methods of avoiding medication errors. Facts about medications were sprinkled through change-of-shift report. Most often, the fact that a patient received a medication was mentioned. "He got his Tobra today," or, "He's still getting Ancef." When a medication was discontinued, this was mentioned during report: "They discontinued his Maalox today." Nurses on the oncoming shift checked if a patient who usually received a medication got it during that shift: "Did he get his nitro today?"

When an unusually large dose of medication was ordered, the nurse acknowledged this during change-of-shift report: "Her [urinary] output is tremendous. There's less edema now in both legs. They increased the Lasix to 120 t.i.d." The other nurses whistled. "Jesus, I pity her kidneys." In addition, dosage changes of a medication were mentioned. For example, Kate said, "They cut back on her Lasix. I started the order. The Lasix is now cut back to 8 A.M. and 1500. Decreased to 10 mg."

The nurses often requested that problem medication orders become clarified by the nurses coming onto the next shift. A day shift nurse, unable to contact the doctor about a confusing medication order, would pass the responsibility on to the evening shift nurse.

Deidre used change-of-shift report to follow the events associated with specific medication errors. For example, one morning she questioned Ann and Miriam:

> DEIDRE: One gram [of Ancef], q. 6 hours. And it was one started right away. And you just never got the rest of it.
>
> ANN: Oh.
>
> DEIDRE: Now this amazes me. Everybody knew he was septic. His Ancef was sitting in the refrigerator. Two days in a row, pharmacy sent the Ancef up. Which is another strange thing because from what's on the Kardex, how was this [Ancef] reordered?
>
> MIRIAM: Well, wasn't it? I checked; I went back and checked the Kardexes. It's not on any of them.

SOURCES OF ERROR

The unfinished business and the many details of medication administration lent an atmosphere of confusion as the nurses tried to sort and resort facts before they felt confident enough to proceed with the actual "pouring of" the medications. Systems problems confounded them. Patients were "off the unit," doctors "did not answer their pages," the pharmacy "had to be yelled at," some patients refused medications, and the nurses, doctors, medical clerks, and pharmacists made mistakes.

Frequently the pharmacy was the butt of complaints. "She gets a Nitrodur today when it comes up through the pharmacy. I've yet to see it," a nurse sarcastically commented. Deidre admitted that she had "yelled at" the pharmacist when the nurses were not notified by the pharmacy that a drug was unavailable in the hospital.

There were a few incidents when ordered medications were simply missing. An R.N. complained about not receiving the 10:00 A.M. "pharmacy drop" of medications ordered by Miriam during the night shift. The green bag of medications had disappeared.

At times the IV laboratory and the pharmacy were jointly responsible for error. Both departments failed to notify the nurses of medication problems. Occasionally the pharmacy did not have certain medications in stock. The slow relaying of this information back to 7H resulted in delays for patients supposedly hospitalized in order to benefit from ordered drugs. The nurses informed the doctors of these problems and eventually new medication orders were written.

The nurses occasionally forgot to send medication slips for newly ordered drugs to the pharmacy, and so medications did not arrive. Nurses forgot to use the reminder system, including the single dose medication red sticker warning and the nurse-instituted 3 × 5 reminder card to jog their memories to give medications. It was difficult to avoid rapid infusions of intravenous fluids containing medications when a patient's position in bed and an occasional adjustment by a patient disturbed the regulated flow. Nurses hung incorrect IV's at times, most likely because of rapid reading of the IV label or forgetting the ordered solution.

Doctors were also guilty of blame where medication errors were concerned. In one situation, a middle-aged man was admitted for pain control related to metastatic prostatic cancer. A young resident wrote an order for liquid morphine elixir in an incorrect dosage. During the evening shift the patient received methadone elixir instead of the ordered morphine elixir. The pharmacy compounded the problem and the error. Later the error was corrected, but only after a nurse contributed to the complexity of the incident.

The nurses acknowledged the error during shift report: ·

> Well, there was a whole big confusion. There's a big incident report out there.

> What for?

> Because pharmacy sent up methadone hospice [mixture]. It was signed out on the narcotic sheet as methadone instead of morphine last night. So we sent back the methadone and got the morphine up here. I don't know where the confusion happened between here and downstairs. Why they [pharmacists] didn't look at the original order or what. But whether pharmacy made the original error, Pam gave it anyhow without reading—rechecking the bottle label.

This medication error involved a doctor, the pharmacy, and a nurse.

Medication errors were blamed on the different departments in the hospital that bore the most obvious responsibility for the error. However, many hospital departments shared in the error. While a medication error was coded as "Pharmacy" or "Nursing" by the quality assurance nurse, the guilt for the error seemed to diffuse among the nursing staff rather than among other hospital personnel.

Other medication errors were related to the inexperience of the new nurses and doctors, to their preoccupation with patient care demands, and to the fact that hospital personnel make mistakes randomly as other humans do.

Medication Administration: A Nursing Ritual

On a symbolic level, the patterned act of medication administration represented the responsibility toward their patients that 7H nurses accepted and assumed. Medication administration was a therapeutic nursing ritual. Nurses gave medications to improve their patient's health. The trust that patients implicitly granted to 7H nurses in relation to medications was evident.

In order to avoid error and harm, 7H nurses practiced many routines, customs, and procedures. When error occurred, 7H nurses confessed this error in three public areas: change-of-shift report, staff meetings, and incident reports. The blame and guilt for the medication error was diffused among the group of nurses.

Of the many rules associated with medication administration, the persistent three-time check was a ritualistic practice: "I triple check: the Kardex; the medication; and the Kardex again." The nurses' persistent use of the small paper soufflé cup, despite its having outlived its function, was also a ritualistic practice.

One 7H nurse seemed to be superstitious about the correct sequence of dispensing medications. When she "went backwards" or first gave the medications to the patients in the highest numbered rooms on a unit, instead of first giving drugs to those in the lowest numbered rooms, she made what she considered a horrible medication error. Giving medications in the right order, lowest patient room number to highest patient room number, seemed to work magically to eliminate errors. Giving them in the wrong order seemed to magically invite medication error for the nurse.

Patients, nurses, and doctors were convinced of the therapeutic benefits of most medications. Some drugs had obvious, immediate, and measurable effects. Occasionally patients complained, along with nurses and doctors, that a drug did not work as expected. Nevertheless, hospital personnel and patients expected most drugs to work and indeed seemed to invest almost magical powers in the capabilities of medications.

A G.N. volunteered that patients looked at medications "magically or religiously." Patients became particularly upset if they did not receive their medications at the exact time due. The timing of medications was important for hospital staff as well as patients. In fact, excessively late or early times of drug dispensing were considered medication errors.

The nurses on 7H believed in the therapeutic power of medications, for both potent and less potent drugs. They attested to the effectiveness of drugs during change-of-shift report and during verbal exchanges throughout their shift. Implicitly, they viewed the efficacy of medications in a magical or unexplainable way and often did not consider the possibility that other care-giving actions or self-healing could have been responsible for improvement in a patient's condition. Drugs dramatically relieved patients' symptoms.

One important reason patients were hospitalized on 7H was to receive disease-appropriate medications following diagnosis by doctors. The motivations of patients who refused to take the medications that nurses offered were questioned. The nurses asked patients why they stayed in the hospital if they refused to take prescribed medications.

During the hospitalization experience, patients, nurses, doctors, and pharmacists were the chief actors involved in the dispensing of drugs. It was the nurses, however, who finally and most often gave drugs to patients in the hope of "doing good" and helping. In the end the nurses bore the chief responsibility for medication administration. And when errors were made, the nurses needed to confess them, since doing good and avoiding harm is a highly held nursing value.

IV
Nursing Rituals in Medical Aseptic Practices

Medical aseptic practices are the hygienic routines that nurses go through as they care for patients and perform some of the more profane aspects of their work. For 7H nurses, hospital work involved frequently bathing patients and handling their excreta, secretions, and infected bodily products.

Part of the 7H nurses' identity was associated with keeping their patients clean. Bathing patients with skill and efficiency and with the intention of comforting was part of each nurse's agenda. Nurses bathed their patients quietly and privately, while respecting their needs to maintain dignity. Implicitly the bath served a symbolic function of washing away the traces of disease during the repeated bathings of each daily cycle.

The nurses handled private body parts with respect as they bathed patients. The many washings helped nurses remove the soil of bodily products. Simultaneously, the clean and the dirty were kept separate by the nurses. Failing to keep a patient clean was considered a violation of a nursing norm. When emergencies such as codes or patient requests delayed bathing activities, nurses apologized.

Failing to bathe a patient was considered a violation of the wishes of a patient and his family. At an implicit level, not bathing patients was associated with disorder. The scheduled washings of patients during each eight-hour nursing shift helped nurses maintain order and certainty in an environment that could easily become disordered.

The ritual aspects of bathing were emphasized when the 7H nurses ignored the nurse manager's attempt to institute a new policy of bathing patients every other day during the day shift. The importance of bathing patients and keeping them clean transferred from shift to shift as an expectation. Ritual, not scientific rationale, was the basis of some of the bathings.

The purpose of the bed bath was traditionally and explicitly seen by nurses as protecting the patient's skin, the first line of defense against disease. New nursing students who came to 7H early in their hospital experience learned to give "complete care," including the bath, to their patients. Seasoned nurses demonstrated and explained the variations of the bath to the G.N.'s, passing on alternative and skilled modifications of the bath that were required by a patient's conditions and hygenic needs.

Neophyte nurses as well as seasoned nurses were in close, personal contact with their patients. Giving the bath required that nurses handle infected materials, excreta, such as urine, perspiration, and stool, and secretions, such as mucus, blood, and wound drainage. The nurses responded to their contacts with profane materials with humor, tolerance, complaint, and magical thinking; with the protective medical aseptic practices of bathing, handwashing, and wearing gloves; and with the pathogen-specific precautions of isolation procedures.

The less experienced nurses consulted more experienced nurses instead of the *Infection Control Manual* when they were in doubt about the handling of infected patients. Here was another instance where the nurses seemed to prefer word of mouth and demonstration to published hospital procedures and policies.

Nurses, more than any other hospital personnel, cared directly for infected patients and handled their bodily products. Nurses frequently expressed their fears about herpes zoster, AIDS (acquired immune deficiency syndrome), lice, and other communicable disorders in the privacy of the utility room. The nurse manager and assistant nurse manager realized that they were responsible should staff refuse to care for infected patients. The nurse manager held the standard before the staff that all patients, even those who were infected, deserved care that respected the dignity of the human being. Responsibility for patients was supraordinate to nurses' fears.

Even the most seasoned nurses, who seldom expressed fear about caring for infected patients, admitted that they were afraid of taking communicable diseases home to their families. In the past nurses have died after caring for infected patients. Today nurses continue to contract infectious diseases from their patients and some die as a result.

When the nurses suspected their patients' bodily products to be infected, they warned each other during shift report of their suspicions. Their efforts to keep clean and dirty separate through medical aseptic practices helped them to feel more confident about reducing the spread of communicable diseases and to maintain order on the unit.

Bathing

THE BED BATH

Medical asepsis includes practices that reduce the number and spread of pathogenic microorganisms. Also called clean techniques, medical aseptic practices help nurses deal with the contaminations of the hospital environment, including frequent and direct contact with patients' bodily excretions and secretions that may carry pathogenic organisms.

The ability to give a bed bath was a highly valued and early mark of achievement for the new nursing student. "Giving complete care" during the day shift included a "complete" bath for the patient, oral hygiene, hair care, and a change of bed linens. Nursing students and seasoned nurses alike marked the work load of their day by complaining or boasting that they had so many "completes" on their shift. "Cleaning up" or "washing up" was done during each of the three nursing shifts. Nurses of each shift were responsible for hygienic care of patients in their districts.

Morning care, which included the bed baths, started on 7H with the conclusion of morning change of shift report. Nurses who were waiting for their district's shift report to begin stocked the "patient units" or patient rooms with the washcloths and other necessities for morning care.

Supplies for the bath and oral hygiene were distributed to each patient upon admission to one of the rooms of 7H. These supplies included a rectangular plastic basin for bath water, plastic emesis (kidney-shaped) basin, soap dish, soap, water pitcher, disposable cups, hospital lotion, and hand wipes. These supplies were used by the nurses for the personal care of patients during bathing.

Following shift report, the nurses moved from the utility room to their districts and made rounds on their patients. The nurses did not merely check on the patients. They encouraged them to begin A.M. care. When necessary, they "set-up" the patients by filling the bath basin with hot water from the bathroom and by making bath equipment, toiletries, and linens available in a convenient place, usually on the overbed table but sometimes on the bedside cabinet and chair.

Bathing patients was not always an easy task. Patients often had IV's running into one or both of their arms. The nurses had to remove the patient gown, threading IV bags and tubing through the sleeve, before beginning the bath and replace the gown after the bath. Since IV's were a routine therapy, the nurses were accustomed to moving around IV's as they bathed patients. Some patients had contractures of their extremities, that is, their arms or legs were bent stiffly and held close to the body. Other patients were in pain. The nurses moved them carefully and bathed them gently.

The nurses also extended their concern with cleanliness to the patient's room. Patients' rooms often became cluttered and dirty. When Deidre found such a problem, she approached housekeeping personnel to clean the room. Beth would permit the patient to have clutter up to a point. "I never think of control. . . . I see more of a balance" between "getting accomplished what I want" and "what the patient wants."

The bath often competed for time with other nursing activities. But for 7H nurses bathing patients was an absolute. The whole tone of an eight-hour shift could be disturbed if linens were unavailable to finish bathing patients and changing beds. Nurses on the day shift insisted that able patients "get washed up now." Their insistence was hard to ignore. Even the most bath-resistant patients usually complied.

THE LANGUAGE OF BATHING

An "insider's," peculiar language was used by the nurses to describe the activities of bathing patients. "Setting the patient up" involved obtaining basin and other supplies to begin the morning bath. The language was condensed, full of detailed meaning to the initiated.

Patients were classified as either "self," "partial" or "complete" baths. Patients in the category of "self" baths were able to bathe themselves. Generally they were ambulatory, able to walk around their rooms, to the bathrooms in their rooms, and into the hall. "Partial" bath patients needed some help from the staff with part of their baths. They could usually wash their faces, hands and arms, chests, axillae and "private parts," or genitals and anal regions. Nurses caring for partial bath patients completed their A.M. care by washing their feet, legs, and back. The nurses helped patients with oral hygiene when necessary by cleaning their dentures, brushing their teeth, or assisting them to rinse out their mouths with mouthwash.

Patients classified as requiring "complete" baths required maximum assistance from the nurses with bathing and other aspects of morning care. These patients were unable to "do" for themselves. They were limited by their disease process or treatment.

Patients who were capable but who refused to bathe themselves were often bathed by nurses. When nurses were able to convince able patients to bathe themselves, they were pleased. Nurses believed that "doing for yourself" had therapeutic effects.

THE COMPLETE BATH

One morning Kate was the primary nurse of a district. She walked into Joe McGuire's room. She was worried about this patient, because she had discovered during report that his abdomen was distended. After listening to his abdomen with a stethoscope and palpating it, she asked him if he had pain and whether he had "passed his water" (urinated). Mr. McGuire said that he had, but that he could not find his urinal. Kate discovered it under the bed, empty.

She found that his bed sheets were wet. Obviously, he had been incontinent of urine. She said, "That's good, because I was worried about you," indicating that she was relieved his kidneys and bladder were functioning. Her patient replied, "The days are long but the nights are twice as long." He had been in the hospital three weeks. When Kate told him that she wanted to bathe him, he replied, "I think they bathed me ten times in one day." Kate replied, "Were you wetting yourself? Was it your bowels?" He answered, "I think they just like to wash me."

As Kate talked to her patient, she systematically collected a plastic basin, soap, a soap holder, lotion, and a disposable washcloth and towel from his bedside cabinet. Kate started to wash his face with water from the basin, talking to him about what she was doing. When she finished his face, she washed his left arm, right arm, his chest, and his abdomen with soap and hot water, rinsed them with water, and dried them with a towel. She then asked, "When was the last time you moved your bowels, Joe?" as she stood by the right side of the bed washing and drying him. He did not answer.

Kate next asked, "Joe, do you sweat a lot? Let me see your armpit. Joe, you have a good grip." Her patient nodded, not answering but looking quite comfortable. Kate next uncovered him, washing his genitals with soap and water. After rinsing him and drying him, she covered his genital area with a sheet. After this she changed the water in the basin and threw out the disposable washcloth, using a fresh washcloth to wash his right leg and left leg. She turned Mr. McGuire onto his left side with his help. The side rail was up, so he could hold onto it. She washed his back and dried it. She washed his buttocks, then his perineal area last. When she noticed an area of reddened skin over his sacrum, she told him about it, and told him that he must turn from side to side while in bed. After drying him, she massaged his reddened skin, using lotion.

Kate helped Mr. McGuire to get out of bed and sit in a geri chair. Suddenly he became dizzy. Kate called his name, noting that he did not respond to her for a few seconds. Kate persisted in calling him. She took his blood pressure. It was 82/58. One minute later she found it to be 100/70. Then it was 210/110 and finally 160/90. She rapidly got Joe back to bed with the help of Gloria, the staff development instructor. She expressed concern about his abdomen. Did it "look bigger" (more distended)? She checked on her patient throughout the day shift. Kate assigned herself to Mr. McGuire's care because she was worried about his condition, specifically about his distended abdomen, the sudden drop in blood pressure, and his failure to respond for a few seconds after sitting upright in the chair. It was clear that Kate was not annoyed at her patient's urinary incontinence but instead was relieved to have this evidence of kidney and bladder function. She used the time spent bathing Mr. McGuire to make assessments about his medical condition.

Mr. McGuire did not resist the bath, although he complained about how often he had been washed previously. Patients sometimes refused to be bathed because they were in a state of confusion. In most instances, however, the nurses managed to bathe them when they became more receptive, or as in the case of Sam Brown, an elderly, confused man, less combative. Kate said to Mr. Brown, "Let's get washed up." He asserted, "I'm clean." When Mr. Brown pushed Kate's hand away, refusing to go along with the bath, she placed a clean sheet on his bedside chair and helped him out of his bed into the chair. Kate could not let him lie in a bed with sheets soiled by stool. Although she didn't argue with him, she had to act on her nursing imperative to get him cleaner that he was. She worried about his skin breaking down from the irritation of his excreta. Later that shift, an L.G.P.N. was able to bathe Mr. Brown. He was in a "better mood."

During another day shift, Dotty, bathed Lorraine Best, a comatose, elderly black woman who suffered the devastating effects of an intracranial hemorrhage. Mrs. Best's depressed deep tendon reflexes, dilated pupils, decreased response to pain, poor lung and heart sounds, and Cheyne-Stokes respiratory pattern suggested to 7H nurses that death was imminent. Dotty discovered that Mrs. Best's family had given their approval for a gastrostomy tube insertion (a doctor would surgically insert a tube into Mrs. Best's stomach so that she could receive nutrition). The nurses had been having difficulties feeding Mrs. Best through a nasogastric feeding tube. Mrs. Best had a small amount of bleeding from her vaginal or urethral area. This bleeding was a source of concern to Dotty and a medical student assigned to Mrs. Best.

Dotty assembled bath equipment and explained to me that she did not talk much when giving "the bath." She said, "Lorraine, I'm going to wash you and get you all clean." Dotty removed the patient gown, exposing Mrs. Best's breasts. Her pubic area was covered with a sheet. The plastic wash basin was filled with warm water and Alpha Keri bath oil, which gave off a sweet odor. Since Mrs. Best was on her side, Dotty deliberately turned her onto her back so that she could begin the bed bath in the customary way. Standing on the right side of the bed, Dotty washed Mrs. Best's face first. She was interrupted by the medical student and helped him place Mrs. Best's leg in a lithotomy (gynecologic) position so that he could inspect Mrs. Best's perineum to determine the source of the bleeding.

Dotty and the medical student discussed the bleeding. The medical student thought that the blood came from the urinary tract. He was not certain; it could have been vaginal.

As the medical student left the patient's room, Dotty resumed Mrs. Best's bed bath. She washed and dried Mrs. Best's arms, axillae, and hands and moved next to her chest and breasts. She observed skin lesions at Mrs. Best's neck and acknowledged this aloud. Dotty bathed her patient's left leg and foot before washing her right leg and foot. She performed range of motion exercises on Mrs. Best's legs. When Dotty washed Mrs. Best's perineal and pubic area, she soaped her washcloth more vigorously than when she washed the other body parts. She carefully washed the patient's genitalia and rinsed twice to remove the soap residue before drying. She had cleaned some blood and stool from the genital area. She was careful to clean around the patient's Foley catheter.

Turning her patient onto her side with the help of a turning sheet, Dotty noticed the odor of stool. She removed the stool, washed Mrs. Best's back, buttocks, and anal area, and threw out the disposable washcloth. She used another disposable washcloth to finish cleaning the skin. Dotty said, matter of factly, "This is the first bowel movement I've seen her have." Putting on a disposable glove, Dotty inserted a Tylenol suppository (anti-fever drug) into Mrs. Best's rectum to lower her temperature.

Despite the fact that Mrs. Best's eyes were open, she was not responding. Her respirations continued in an irregular pattern. Dotty applied Keri lotion to Mrs. Best's arms and legs, while she was positioned on her side. She then put a clean patient gown on Mrs. Best's left side and began to change the bed linens, saying, "I'm going to make your bed, hon." "Linen is a problem here," Dotty said to me as an aside. She placed two sheets under the mattress. It covered the eggcrate foam pad that was on top of the regular mattress to relieve skin pressure. She placed two blue pads (incontinent pads) over the bottom sheet and folded a standard-sized sheet to be a turning sheet. Dotty admitted that she preferred using folded standard sheets for turning rather than the smaller draw sheets. These sheets were wide and helped the nurses to turn heavy patients more easily.

Dotty explained that she liked to place the blue pads on top of the large turning sheet and then place a draw sheet over the pads. She said, "The bottom sheet for turning, the top for soiling." Dotty could remove the blue pad and replace it with another, if the patient was incontinent. Dotty rolled these sheets neatly against the patient, put the right side rails up, moved to the left side of the bed, and turned the patient over the rolled sheets and blue pads. Tucking the bottom sheet under the mattress and mitering the corner at the head of the bed, Dotty skillfully straightened the bottom sheet, the large turning sheet, and the draw sheet by pulling and tucking. As I helped Dotty pull Mrs. Best up in the bed using the turning sheet, a doctor came into the room and inquired whether the patient had been in a comatose, or nonresponsive state. Dotty answered affirmatively. He pinched the patient's skin (to elicit a pain response) and said, "Well, we're practicing benign neglect."

Dotty placed a towel under Mrs. Best's chin and used glycerine swabs to clean her gums, tongue, and teeth, and thus completed Mrs. Best's morning care. Dotty straightened the equipment on the window sill, which included 4 × 4 gauze squares, suction catheters, flashlight, a room deodorizer tablet, and plastic bottles of hydrogen peroxide and sterile water. Dotty left Mrs. Best's room to care for another patient. Despite the interruptions, the patterned actions of the bath had persisted.

Often, the morning bath for a male patient included shaving the face and neck if the patient was unable to do this for himself. I observed Tammy shave one of her elderly patients, Meyer Schwartz, "who had this habit of spitting," according to Tammy. She described him by saying, "He's fine, except for the spitting." Tammy got a prep set (for preoperative skin shave) and filled the wash basin with water. She said, "Here we go," and started to gently shave the patient. "I hope I don't nick you," she said. She used skin lotion and the soap foam from the prep set to soften his beard. She patiently shaved Mr. Schwartz as he quietly lay in bed with his arms folded. As she finished his shave and washed his face, Tammy said, "Now you'll get washed." Mr. Schwartz moaned a little as she carefully washed his face, neck, arms, hands, and chest. She was particular in using an orange stick to clean his fingernails, which had blood on and underneath them. Tammy quietly directed Mr. Schwartz, "Give me your arm. You can relax your arm. You can put it down, Meyer." Tammy used more friction when washing Mr. Schwartz's hands than when washing the other parts of his body. She was solicitous about his becoming cold. Observing that a cleaning woman had come into the room, Tammy washed Mr. Schwartz's genitals without uncovering him, by raising the sheet over him. She carefully washed him and rinsed his genitalia, since a urine odor pervaded the room.

Tammy changed the water in the basin and finished bathing Mr. Schwartz's legs, feet, back, and buttocks. Helping him out of bed onto a bedside commode, she next answered a question from the doctors on rounds: "Meyer is fine except for spitting." The fact that he failed to use disposable tissues and had sputum indiscriminately spread on his geri chair and patient gown upset Tammy. She straightened his unit, cleaned the overbed table, and changed the soiled linens. Before moving Mr. Schwartz from the commode to the geri chair, Tammy cleaned his gums and teeth with pink toothpaste. She helped him into the geri chair after removing the mucus from it with soap, water, and paper towels.

Tammy considered Mr. Schwartz "an easy one" to bathe. "I like to get him out of the way," she said. She knew that Mr. Schwartz's condition was fairly stable and set her priorities so that she had time for other patients needing more of her skills.

Next Tammy prepared to bathe another of her patients. Once again the patterns of the bath would be repeated.

THE BATH DURING THE EVENING AND NIGHT SHIFTS

During the evening shift, 7H nurses had a scheduled time to bathe their patients. They were obligated to keep their patients clean before the scheduled time to begin P.M. care, 8:00 P.M., arrived. The nurses worked the bathing of patients around medications, IV's, and other duties.

When the time for P.M. care arrived, nurses moved quickly from room to room, washing patients' faces, hands, and backs and straightening or changing sheets.

One evening, Beth and Loretta entered a patient's room together. The middle-aged patient, Mary Phillips, look emaciated. She had breast cancer with extensive bony metastasis and was terminally ill. She was awake, with her eyes open, but was not responding to questions. She moaned softly throughout her P.M. care.

Beth discovered what she knew was the patient's third episode of diarrhea, since she had cleaned her twice previously on this shift. Beth, the more experienced nurse, gave Loretta directions in a gentle way. "I put a towel in a pillowcase; it helps to absorb." Beth planned to insert the towel and pillowcase between Mrs. Phillips's legs after she was cleaned. The stool was brownish yellow and watery. While the odor of stool was evident, it was not overpowering or very offensive to the nurses in the room. Beth put water in the basin, complaining that it was not getting hot fast enough. Loretta turned the cancer patient over onto her side. She was on a Clinitron bed to relieve pressure and avoid bed sores; she "floated" in it.

In a gentle tone, Beth said, "We're going to turn you over, Mary." Beth told Loretta to use the disposable washcloths that she had brought into the room along with the linens. She repeated her intention to turn the patient over again. Loretta put on disposable gloves and began to clean the diarrheal stool from the patient's back, buttocks, and perineum and from between her legs, using several disposable washcloths, throwing the soiled ones into the trash can one by one. Beth continued to give Loretta specific directions about how to move the patient gently in order to wash her legs. Beth was initiating Loretta into the more skilled practices required when bathing difficult patients. Beth and Loretta turned Mrs. Phillips to her other side. Again, she moaned softly.

Beth asked Loretta for toothettes for the mouth care. (These were small pink foam sticks and were stored in the bedside cabinet.) Beth used glycerine and lemon swabs instead, however, because they were more readily available. Loretta continued to wash Mrs. Phillips's buttocks, perineum, and legs, this time as she lay on her right side. "Isn't it hard that we have to do this, Mary?" Beth asked. Mrs. Phillips did not respond. Loretta massaged her skin with lotion, and Beth changed the diarrhea-soaked sheets, leaving clean sheets in their place. Beth carefully had placed the towel-enclosed pillowcase between Mrs. Phillips's legs, so that the constant diarrheal stool would be absorbed and the soiling of the skin restricted to a smaller area. Loretta drained the water and cleaned the plastic wash basin in the bathroom. She replaced the basin in the bedside cabinet.

Beth turned off the overhead lights and placed the soiled linen in the hamper in the hall. The room was dimly lit. Mrs. Phillips's roommate quietly watched TV. Mary Phillips was clean for now, having been moved and washed as gently as Loretta and Beth could manage.

Adaptations in bathing patients were necessary for patient comfort and protection from complications. Patients with special needs such as continuous diarrhea or severe pain required nursing skill of a higher level. Skill in bathing patients increased with a nurse's experience.

During the night shift, the bathing of incontinent patients continued. On all shifts, bathing an incontinent patient meant bathing his back, buttocks, and other parts soiled by the stool, urine, or other discharge. Linens were changed and the patients were repositioned on their sides or backs. The L.G.P.N.'s moved a cart with supplies from room to room so that they did not have to make repeated trips to the places where this equipment was stored. Although the night R.N. also bathed incontinent patients, it seemed that the L.G.P.N.'s chief responsibility during the night shift was keeping incontinent patients clean. They sometimes had to be urged to perform other jobs. Keeping patients clean or "changing" them was seen by these two nurses as the unavoidable, "bottom line" of their work on that shift.

According to hospital policy, rounds were to be made every hour during the night shift by the R.N. and the L.G.P.N.'s. They used a flashlight in the patients' rooms to check on their breathing and incontinence. It was not always possible for the L.G.P.N.'s or the R.N.'s to "round" every hour, since other duties interfered.

The night shift was also structured by a hygenic routine. The scheduled time to check patients to determine if they needed to be bathed was 5:30 A.M. Both of the L.G.P.N.'s made rounds, washed and changed incontinent patients, and took vital signs (temperature, pulse, respirations, and blood pressure) on all patients.

Patients who were awake at 5:30 A.M., those scheduled for early surgery or a diagnostic test, and incontinent patients were bathed by the night nurses. Miriam would report at change of shift, "His bed and bath's done" or "His A.M. care's done," to signal to the day shift nurses not to repeat the work. After report, the day shift nurses started their A.M. care, continuing the twenty-four-hour pattern of hygenic care.

MODIFICATIONS OF THE BATH

On the day shift during the weekend, staffing of the unit was poor. The nurses adapted to the staffing shortages by bathing only certain parts of the body of patients who required complete baths. Marie commented, "They need the bath every day. If you don't wash all over, certain parts of you need it every day. The sign of the cross, every day: face, armpits, groin." Marie recalled that one of her head nurses used to say, "Only do the sign of the cross," on the weekend.

When patients' needs required a different approach to the bath, 7H nurses rapidly put their bedside skills to use to help the patient. One elderly woman, for example, required a complete bath. She had a recto-vaginal fistula (an abnormal track connecting her rectum and vagina). Because of the fistula, rectal contents flowed through the fistula to her vagina and drained out of her body to her skin. Her perineal skin was very excoriated, raw from the irritating effects of the stool. Beth had called the enterostomal therapist who suggested special skin care in addition to the Mycolog-Karaya powder that had been ordered. The Karaya powder, a vegetable preparation and a time-tested skin application for excoriation, was to be applied to clean, moist, excoriated skin. The sore skin was to be first flushed with a sterile water and Betadine solution, then patted dry with a soft abdominal pad. Beth explained this modification of the bath, emphasizing that regular bathing would hurt the patient's skin, and adding that the "leftover Karaya powder, by now gummy from the moisture, should be left on the skin."

Another elderly patient who required a different approach to bathing had an unstable fracture of the cervical spine and lay in a regular bed. Although her neck was stabilized by a cervical collar, the nurses feared the danger of neck flexion. Her spinal cord could be severed by the bone fragments. Beth and Cecile bathed her together, but they worried about her severing her spinal cord by the movement of bone fragments from her spine.

The nurses took turns bathing and drying alternate parts of the patient's anterior body. Beth washed one side, Cecile the other. They were aware that the patient had been incontinent of stool and that she had to be bathed and her sheets had to be changed. Otherwise, her skin would break down and decubitus ulcers would develop. Beth and Cecile carefully turned the patient to her side, taking special care to keep her neck rigidly extended in a cervical collar. They bathed her back, changed her sheets, and turned her flat in bed again.

The nurses knew that eventually patients had to be bathed by nurses, no matter how potentially serious the bathing activities could be for the patient.

BATHING PATIENTS—THE DOMAIN OF THE NURSE

Bathing patients and keeping them free from odor and excreta belonged to the domain of the nurses. The following example illustrates how the nurses viewed this responsibility. When a doctor wrote an order, "a nice note," for the nurse to "check q. [4] for loose stools and cleanse," the nurses resented the doctor's effrontery. One nurse sarcastically commented, "We're gonna leave the man sit [in diarrhea]!" The nurses were saying, "We know how to keep patients clean. That's our domain."

Kate described the value of the bath:

The bath means take a look at their skin. They are not playing in mud. The only thing, the family gets upset with no bath. The mother has blush on with her perfume, she had great nursing care. I think that everyone on admission should have a bath. It's perfect for assessment. I think that skin assessment is really important. A first bath is important on admission for the patient to be clean. Lots of times, they're cleaner if washed by a nurse.

Sarah added her view:

You have to use your judgment. Her back and peri [perineal] area are necessary. When people come into the hospital, if they haven't bathed and have crud between their toes, you bathe them. People who are paying for nursing care [through the daily hospital rate] sometimes want a bath. Well, I think they deserve it. When people have preoperative showers, I don't know what it does for their skin, in terms of the surgery. A preoperative bath gives you the chance to talk to a patient. They're frightened. I don't know how much it [preoperative bath or shower] decreases the bacteria on their skin.

When nurses bathed comatose patients, they were certain that these patients were aware. Dotty reflected this view when describing her day shift bathing of a comatose patient.

I still think that she's here. She's a human being. I think that she can see us and hear us talking. I don't like it when the doctors treat them [patients] like a number, a diagnosis.

Baths helped nurses show concern for their patients, according to Colleen. "Respect is shown. If a patient is smelly and dirty, they would be embarrassed if they had visitors." Nurses worried aloud about the effects of incontinence on their patient's skin.

Beth spoke about the necessity of the bath. She thought that giving a bath to patients was evidence that the nurse cared. "Not giving a bath might mean that you don't care enough."

At one point, Beth's view of bathing patients each morning included a litany of descriptors: a way of caring for someone, like a mother cares for a child; loving care, in between toes and behind ears; a loving attitude while you did it, even if rushed; cared for in the sense of being loved; a great deal to do with how they see the rest of the day; a good time for assessment; a quiet, somewhat uninterrupted time when they let off steam or just relax after not sleeping; a back rub or lotion on the skin makes them feel good;

therapeutic touch; feeling as good as can be. Beth worked many of her views about the bath into her response. She pointed out that if the nurse neglects other details when caring for a patient, these are forgotten, "because of the care" involved during the morning bath.

Miriam stated that a bath means "skin care, hygiene, controlling bacteria, and their own [patients'] self-esteem. It doesn't help if they're laying around dirty and smelly." She added, "To nurses, clean means visibly palatable. The patient looks clean and they're not smelly. The way you bathe a person is personalized, in terms of your own personal hygiene." She thought that a nurse would clean other people the way she cleans herself.

Miriam related her amusement about a paper she once heard a nurse present entitled, "Nurses Who Wear Dirty Shoes Give Poor Nursing Care." She felt that the rule did reflect some nurses' care accurately. She reminisced about one of her nursing instructors in school who had "a fit" when her students wore dirty shoes or shoe-laces, to the point that she would put incredible pressure on the deviant student to comply. A clean nurse kept patients clean.

Dying, being resuscitated, or experiencing severe pain were patient situations that temporarily altered the inevitability of nurses' bathing patients. If patients lived, survived a resuscitation, or had less pain, nurses rapidly cleaned them if they were soiled.

Nurses thought fifteen minutes the outside limit of acceptability for leaving an incontinent patient uncleaned. Longer than that was unacceptable. If a patient slipped by the nurses' hygienic vigilance, the nurses considered this unusual, even disgraceful. For example, Gloria described an incident when a patient went to the Operating Room "dirty." The intensity of Gloria's condemnation underscored nursing's value of cleanliness for patients.

Gloria's daughter, also an R.N. at this hospital, told Gloria about a patient who was admitted to 7H on a Monday, and went to surgery on Wednesday for a cystoscopy (the bladder is visualized through the transurethral passage of a cystoscope). The patient was transferred postoperatively to a urological unit. Gloria's daughter, who was a nurse on that unit, found the patient "filthy." Gloria was horrified. Her agitation was evident by her voice and eye movements. She broke her styrofoam coffee cup apart. She explained why it was so important for the patient to be clean. "A person's hygiene is the key function of the nurse. This patient has chronic renal failure, is not 'with it' mentally, and isn't moving that much. The patient being clean is important for infection control. It is worse if the patient goes to surgery. It's hard enough to keep the operative site clean."

Nurses knew that they were never to leave a patient lying in stool or urine. A nurse was labeled "a disgrace" if she were discovered by another nurse to be neglecting her patients' hygiene. Many nurses independently agreed with Gloria's statement that they would "always clean someone up, whether incontinent of urine or stool *even* after my shift ended. It's my responsibility. If I find it, I take care of it. It's part of caring for the patient. If I don't know about it, that's another thing."

At times the strong value that nurses placed on cleanliness conflicted with their patients' values. For example, a nurse from the medical unit adjacent to 7H insisted that a patient bathe herself. The patient refused and complained to her family that the nurse had "stripped and bathed her." The family reacted negatively and threatened to physically harm the nurse. The clinical nursing director, Kristen, moved the nurse to another unit to protect her. This incident confirmed the value that nurses held about the care of patients, even though some of their patients failed to see the importance of the frequent bathings that were scheduled throughout the nurses' twenty-four-hour work day. Other patients expected the nurses to bathe them, no matter how successfully they were recuperating, or how capable they were of bathing themselves.

Nurses seemed to follow the unwritten law, "Every patient must be bathed daily." Whether able to bathe themselves or needing the nurses caring for them to bathe them, 7H patients were unable to avoid the daily washings. Deidre thought that nurses in general are "rigid." She gave the bed bath as an example of this rigidity: "Nurses are great suppressors." Nurses are compelled to give complete bed baths to patients unable to bathe themselves even though at times a patient's hygiene does not require it.

An example of this "bed bath imperative" occurred when Deidre decided that a new bath policy was in order. Kate explained the change. "Deidre thinks that we are spending too much time on

baths and not enough on nursing care. We are going to start that
every other day [morning] bath. It would be better if we were teaching [patients] than giving baths." Sarah listened to Kate's explanation and replied in an amused tone, "If the patients who figure that
at $250 [cost per day in the hospital] they should have a bath, they'll
get a bath." Sarah disagreed with the policy change.

Deidre saw the daily bath as mechanical. "Who is doing it? If they
are using it for assessment, that's one thing. If not, it's mechanical."
Deidre instituted this policy change, supported in her conviction
by the fact that bathing elderly patients' skin too often resulted in
excessive dryness and skin lesions. However, six days later the 7H
nurses seemed to have abandoned the policy. Beth explained how
the "every other day" bath for complete patients was going. Beth
said that she gave "most everyone a complete bath." Most of the
patients were incontinent of urine, stool, or both and needed to be
bathed. "So, I did," she said. The other patients might expect a
bath. "Not to have one might negatively affect how the patient sees
his hospital stay." Beth indicated that she bathed "this type of patient." The resistance to this change in policy dramatized nurses'
internalization of the value of "good" personal hygiene for their
patients.

Bathing patients on the day shift marked the beginning of the
morning shift and the progression of the evening and night shifts.
The "washing up" of patients seemed to help the nurses feel a sense
of accomplishment about nursing duties. Nurses on the day shift
would comment, "I've got the two easiest ones done. Now comes
the hard one." A few patients already may have completed their
bathing by the time the day shift nurses arrived on 7H. Those going for diagnostic studies, those who were "on their feet," independent of the nurses' help for bathing, and those awaiting either
the next diagnostic test or discharge from the hospital were
checked off systematically by the night nurse during report or by
the day shift nurses in the district as being "done."

During the evening shift, P.M. care began between 8:00 and 8:30.
L.G.P.N.'s and R.N.'s straightened patients' wrinkled bed linens and
changed them if necessary. Incontinence of stool or urine was
"cleaned up." Skin soiled from urine or stool was washed, rinsed,
dried, and powdered or lotioned. New patient gowns were put on,

if the patient had soiled the old one. Back rubs were offered and given with the patient's consent. The patient was prepared for sleep and the night. Evening care incorporated washing the patient's skin, if needed, rubbing his back, straightening his sheets or changing them, helping him with mouth care, and working to have him "look good."

On the night shift, patients were kept free of soiled skin, clothes, and linens. Miriam admitted, "We are usually so busy on nights, that all we do is meds and keep people clean."

Nurses apologized during shift report if a patient's bath remained to be finished after noon of the day shift or after the end of the shift on which they worked. In the following example, the day shift nurse was upset that her patient's bath had not been completed during the day shift. The patient had severe, chronic pain from metastatic cancer. The nurses responded to the patient's wishes by delaying the completion of the bath until the patient agreed that he was ready. The nurse said:

> Sometimes he lets us do it later in the day. He hasn't had back care. And he's also lying on the sheets that he went down to X-ray therapy in, but he did not want us to move him. As soon as he got back, he got his morphine again and his fellow [nursing student] just gave him his Percocets. So I don't know if the pain's ever gonna go away enough for him to want, you know the sheets to be taken off. . . . But he's on a draw, two draw sheets and two bottom sheets. They're not soiled, though.

Nurses were embarrassed when they did not complete baths during their shifts. They apologized to other nursing staff in a manner that was almost confessional.

A nurse who worked occasionally in the ICU described her astounded reaction to the fact that ICU patients sometimes got one complete bath during each shift. She speculated that the causes for the high frequency of complete baths could include the fact that during shift report the nurses did not pass on the information that the patient had been bathed, or, that, finding a patient's bed was dirty, a nurse might have thought, "If I'm going to change the bed I might as well bathe the patient." She also thought that the frequency of baths was related to the need to have the patients look "tidy."

RECORDING THE BATH AND THE BATH PROCEDURE

After nurses finished bathing patients, they recorded this accomplishment on the nursing care flow sheet. This record was kept close to the patient, on a clipboard left in the patient's room. The bath was recorded on part of the flow sheet devoted to hygiene.

Under "Hygiene" were included the following subcategories: "complete bed bath; bed bath c [with] assistance; self: tub/shower/ or bathroom; mouth care; back care; perineal care; Foley catheter care; anti-embolism [moving clot] stockings." This flow sheet was developed to speed the recording of some of the details of nursing care. It also acknowledged in writing the nurses' major concern and responsibility for patient hygiene.

The details of the bath procedure were printed in the *Hospital Policy and Procedure Manual.* A step-by-step progression of actions was listed, along with a rationale for these actions. The nurses were never observed consulting the manual for the bath procedure. Instead, they relied on demonstrations and word-of-mouth directions when modifications of the bath procedure were required by patients with special hygienic needs. Seasoned nurses directed neophytes in all of the witnessed examples.

SHOWING GENTLENESS, RESPECT FOR PATIENT DECISIONS, AND
CONSIDERATION FOR PATIENT PRIVACY DURING THE BATH

Besides shortages in supplies, the only factor that seemed to hinder the nurses' progress with bathing was a patient's refusal. Refusal usually came from patients suffering from the pain of metastatic cancer. The pain sapped their strength. It was difficult for them to endure the mouth care, hair care, and other exertions of bathing. When nurses could avoid bathing patients, that is, if incontinence did not force them to clean the patient, they complied with the patient's request.

Chris provided an example of a patient who temporarily refused her bath. Chris carefully completed Amy White's mouth care. Mrs. White, emaciated with metastatic breast cancer, had barely been able to endure the mouth care. She was so weak that she swallowed her mouthwash, unable to expectorate it into the waiting emesis basin held by Chris. When Chris asked her if she wanted her bath, she said, "Wait." Chris went to get her pain medication. Later, with the help of the pain-dulling narcotic, Chris finished Mrs. White's complete bed bath.

Mrs. White did not often speak to her nurses, family, or friends about her pain. When the nurses moved her, she screamed. The patient moaned "quite a bit, frequently." Whenever the nurses discovered Mrs. White's incontinence, they had to bathe her, but they did this as gently as they could, "It's so hard. When you rub her, she screams," said Chris. The patient could never be left neglected and dirty, lying in her own urine and stool. So eventually Chris or another nurse bathed her.

Patients who required a complete bed bath were often very debilitated; some were near death. I found the gentleness with which the nurses bathed these patients to be universal. The following bath incident illustrates this gentleness and provides an example of how nurses combined the practicalities of clean and dirty work as they cared for their weak and comatose patients.

Marie was bathing a slowly dying comatose patient who was on a ventilator. The elderly woman had "coded and made it" over the weekend. Marie carefully bathed the anterior left side of the patient, her face, her neck, left arm, and left leg. The fact that she was connected to IV's and a ventilator and the fact that she was lyuing on her side necessitated this change in the progression of the bath procedure. The patient lay on her right side. As Marie bathed her patient with great care and a gentle touch, she talked to her about the next steps in her bathing. Marie shook her head disapprovingly to herself. The patient's skin was edematous and delicate. She had bed sores. Later Marie turned her to her back, bathed her right side, and proceeded to remove the dressings from her right foot. Marie did this with reluctance. An unpleasant odor of infection permeated the patient's room as she began to cut the old dressings off.

Marie walked out of the room to complain out of earshot of the comatose patient, "Did you smell it? I have a cold and I smell it." Returning to the room, Marie and Chris discussed how a blister had become necrotic and infected. Marie discarded the dirty dressings, put on sterile gloves, and redressed the foot with Betadine solution and 4 × 4 gauze dressings. She was worried about the patient's deteriorating condition. She completed the patient's bath, remaining gentle throughout.

Patients noticed nurses' gentleness. Two patients acknowledged their appreciation of Beth's gentleness and caring during their morning baths. Both told their roommates about this nurse, each predicting a similar experience for them since they were also Beth's patients.

The morning bath time was a private time for the nurse and her patients. G.N.'s, R.N.'s, L.G.P.N.'s, and nursing assistants seemed reluctant to share this time with me. Most often this reluctance was more obvious with the G.N.'s. On four occasions, Chris managed to evade my observations. Colleen put me off once by delaying the assignment of patients in her district, although a few minutes later I noticed that she was bathing her patient. Perhaps the new nurses were reminded of observations by their nursing instructors. The R.N.'s, the L.G.P.N.'s, and the nursing assistants were more secure in their bathing skills than were the G.N.'s, yet they too resisted observation.

The bath exposed both the nurse's skills and the patient's nudity. The nurse and the patient had to deal with violations of the usual personal space boundaries. The nurse had to be simultaneously adept and comforting. The patient needed reassurance that his nudity, his incontinence, and his bodily characteristics were private matters and would be kept private by the nurse.

Most of the nurses were careful to respect their patient's privacy by closing the curtains around the bed, closing the door to the room (if the patient's roommate was not in the room), and by draping various parts of the body with a towel, a patient gown, or a top sheet as the bath progressed. For example, Caroline, a nursing assistant, exemplified her respect for her patients' privacy by covering what are considered "private parts": breast for female patients and genitals and anal areas for male and female patients. On one occasion, Caroline was having a difficult time keeping the door closed to her patient's room. Different hospital personnel walked in and out. One left the door open. The curtain just managed to reach around the bed. Caroline closed the door and exposed the patient's genital area so she could wash around the Foley catheter. Her patient, Bertha Thomas, cried out when she was uncovered.

Caroline worked rapidly and efficiently to finish the bath so that her elderly patient who complained of being cold would not be upset or chilled. Her voice was quiet. She spoke to her patient in simple sentences, telling what she was doing at each step of the bath. Her respect for her patients was evident as she bathed them.

Only once did I observe one of the L.G.P.N.'s failing to cover a confused, elderly female patient's breasts and pubic area. This patient almost reflexively covered her breasts by crossing her arms over them. It was obvious during this bath that the L.G.P.N., Elsie, was in a hurry. While giving the bath, she talked over the patient to another L.G.P.N. about personal matters and opinions. The door of the patient's room was open. Her nakedness was visible to anyone who walked in the hall and looked into the room. This incident represented an exception to the usual maintenance of patient privacy by the nurses.

The nurses knew that patients were embarrassed when they had to be bathed. Colleen told Kate about an incident involving a patient who questioned her ability to bathe him. "Yesterday Mabel bathed me; I felt more comfortable, since she was an older woman. Have you ever seen a man naked before?" he asked Colleen. (Colleen looked like a teenager.) Colleen assured him that she had been bathing patients for five years. "I lied," Colleen said, "to make him feel more comfortable." The patient said, "Excellent job," to Colleen after she bathed him. This elderly Jewish man, who was diabetic, had been admitted because he had become disoriented suddenly, short of breath, and incontinent of urine, to the dismay of his attentive son. His embarrassment at being seen naked and bathed by a young woman in her mid-twenties caused him to procrastinate about his personal care. He wished aloud that he would be discharged so that he could get a shave and a haircut. As Colleen bathed the man, she talked to him and to his son, and promised to return after lunch to shave him.

Patients were embarrassed by their incontinence and the exposure of their genitals and by nurses' contact with their private parts. Their facial expressions changed or they groaned as their breasts, genitals, or anal area were washed. At times they apologized, wishing aloud that they could manage bathing themselves. The nurses often dealt with the embarrassment by carefully talking to the patient about other matters while efficiently and matter-of-factly bathing them.

Some patients managed their embarrassment by hiding for a time the fact that they could not bathe themselves. The nurses soon discovered that a patient had not been bathing, because the patient's body odor became evident.

BATH AS PURIFICATION

The nurses pursued unpleasant odors with a vengeance during the bath. Elsie demonstrated this. She bathed an elderly female patient with vigor, still trying to locate the source of odor on the second day of caring for the patient. She muttered to herself about the odor, wearing gloves throughout the bath.

> I wash them because they are dirty. It's common concern and care. I check them for lice and wash their hair. I guess you do it the way you were taught. I was taught to *wash* people. If they are dirty, you wash them with soap. Some parts of the body [private areas] you have to wash with the soap. With the elderly, after they are clean, you can use Keri soap. Sponge baths don't get people clean.

Following this bath, Elsie felt that the odor decreased. She admitted that the mysterious source of the odor had not been discovered nor totally eliminated.

Another example of a nurse's reaction to discovering a patient's body odor came in a change-of-shift report.

> Her last name is Krenski. She's 60 years old, [an] obese female. What I was told this morning, a very foul odor is coming from her. She sounds like she needs a good bath. She had a history of colon CA [cancer]. O.K. She's, from what I've been told, ambulatory.

The nurses had assumed that because the patient was ambulatory she could bathe herself. Apparently the nurses needed to help the patient with her bath. Her body odor suggested this, and her primary nurse helped her bathe. The noticeable odor disappeared after the nurses took charge.

Body odors, originating from urine, feces, or other sources, were systematically investigated and removed by bathing during each shift. Nurses went on "incontinence check" rounds, seeking to detect soil and the odors associated with soil. The nurses energetically bathed their patients, cleaning and purifying, keeping clean and dirty separate.

HANDLING CLEAN AND "DIRTY" BODY PARTS DURING THE BATH

Nurses classified their patients' body parts in various categories of clean and dirty. They always bathed the patient's face first and the perianal area last. They followed an unspoken rule when bathing patients: Always wash from the clean to the dirty. The face, the neck, the chest, the arms, the legs, and the back were among the clean body parts. The hands were less clean than these. Nurses often used more soap, more friction, and more frequent washing of the hands. While the feet were considered by some nurses to be dirty, they were treated the same way as the hands and were scrubbed with the same amount of soap and enthusiasm as the hands. The buttocks seemed a bit cleaner than the feet, but were dangerously close to the perianal region.

Some nurses wore disposable plastic gloves as they washed the genital and perianal regions of the body. It was difficult to determine which of these areas was considered the dirtiest. Deidre described her bathing of different parts of a patient's body: "I always wash the genital area. The feet are the dirtiest part of the body. A lot of people [nurses] have trouble washing the genitals because of sexuality. I have seen a lot of nurses use gloves with anal or Foley care, or refuse to wash the pubic [area] more [often] than the anal area. It's the sexual part."

In general, the genitals, including the perineal region, and the perianal area were considered the dirtiest body parts. Nurses signaled this difference by carefully changing the bath water in the basin after washing genitals and by washing the perianal area of the patient last. Nurses also discarded the disposable washcloths after washing the genitals and the perianal area. They were more vigorous in their cleansing of these parts and of hands and feet than of other body parts.

The nurses' bathing practices brought them into unavoidable contact with body parts that were explicitly and implicitly considered by them to be dirty. Checking on patients' hygiene and bathing patients made the nurses confront their own and their patients' feelings about exposure of the "private parts" of the body. Generally this was handled discreetly. However, when some aspect of a patient's behavior suggested to the nurses that the patient might be enjoying the exposure and the contact, the nurses reacted and aired the situation in discussion during change-of-shift report. At one level of meaning, "sexual" was equated with "dirty" by the nurses. The nurses had to keep genitals clean along with the peri-anal body area. They accepted that their work contained contact with the dirty or profane elements of human functioning.

The nurses knew that patients' ideas of clean varied. "Some patients want their hands clean after they urinate. Others can insert a [rectal] suppository and not worry about their hands. I take my cues from the patient," said Beth, who also asserted that she was careful to wash her hands. "I don't want to take infection home [to] either me or my children."

Excreta, Secretions, and Infection

The 7H nurses removed and washed away the traces of human soil on a daily basis. Their common experience with infected materials, excreta, such as urine and stool, and secretions, such as respiratory and wound drainage, was closely associated with the repeated washing of patients during each shift.

The nurses believed in the efficacy of hand washing in order to protect themselves from possible contamination and infection. Students were repeatedly reminded in nursing school that hand washing was the best protection against contamination from a patient's bodily products. On one occasion, Beth provided a scientific explanation for good hand washing techniques.

Beth's instructor in the isolation technique—that is, how to isolate a patient from contamination from other people or objects in the environment—said that very seldom did the nurse need to wear gloves for protection from contamination. Hand washing took care of cross-contamination. Beth believed this, as did other 7H nurses, but hand washing was not the only medical aseptic technique that they used to protect themselves and patients from contamination by contact with potentially infected materials.

More L.G.P.N.'s and nursing assistants than R.N.'s routinely used disposable gloves to protect themselves from infection. The gloves had magical qualities in providing protection from infection. They were used almost as a panacea, whether the patients were infected or not. If an R.N. suspected infection, she quickly donned the disposable plastic gloves as she cared for her patient. For example, Deidre, who seldom wore disposable gloves while bathing a patient and cleaning stool, explained her reason for wearing gloves on one particular occasion. "I smelled a foul odor. I expected infection [when she took decubitus dressings off]. Some people wear gloves, touch infected skin or material [drainage] and then touch everything [with the gloves still on]. That doesn't make sense to me."

Nursing students who spent time on 7H were advised by the seasoned nurses how to decrease direct contact with excreta. On one occasion, Rachel, a nursing assistant, advised a nursing student to wear disposable gloves as she obtained a "clean catch" urine specimen. (Obtaining the clean catch specimen meant giving instructions to the patient about cleaning the urethral area with an antibacterial solution, starting urination, interrupting urination, and restarting urination into a sterile plastic container so that later a laboratory examination of the specimen could determine if the urine was infected.) The nursing student had to help an elderly female patient with the collection and held the specimen container close to the urethral opening. To reinforce her advice about wearing gloves, Rachel added, "Afterwards the clean catch jar will be all peed on."

The plastic disposable gloves were an added protection against pathogenic microorganisms, but scientific theories of microbial transfer were not offered to explain their use. The use of gloves was ritualistic and, for some of the nurses, accompanied by magical thinking.

The nurses were fastidious in their handling of excreta. If a confused patient was incontinent of feces and managed to smear the stool on himself or his bed, some nurses used gloves to protect themselves from the uncontained soilage. They washed and dried the patient and changed the linens so that no trace of stool was evident.

If a patient was incontinent of urine or stool, the nurse who discovered this bathed the patient and changed the linens as soon as possible. All of the nurses were careful to separate the soiled bed linens from the soiled blue pads. These disposable blue pads were used to save linen and prevent skin breakdown. But it is questionable how much linen was saved, since the nurses had many individual preferences about ways to layer the pads with the linens to save work and to keep the clean and dirty separate.

When the blue pads were soiled by urine or stool, the nurse handled carefully as she left the patient's room and placed them in the covered utility room trash can. If the pads were not excessively soiled or odiferous, they were placed in the patient's trash can. Soiled linens were also handled carefully and placed in the linen hampers in the hall.

The nurses were often able to predict episodes of incontinence, since they knew most of their patients well. Miriam, for example, predicted that her patient would have diarrhea when she came back from the X-ray Department. Miriam "double sheeted" and "blue padded" the bed. When the patient returned, her diarrheal incontinence was rapidly taken care of. Miriam's ability to predict and her strategic preparations helped her to remove stool and maintain order.

Occasionally it was difficult to contain or eliminate soiling from stool. When stool accidentally got on a pelvic traction belt the nurse apologized, washed it, and asked the next shift to order another so that the patient would have an alternate.

The nurses' frequent contacts with patients' bodily products lulled them into a sense of complacency at times. Beth noticed that a confused, elderly man with organic brain syndrome was wandering out of his room without slippers. His two gangrenous toes were partially exposed through loose dressings. Beth rapidly helped to get him seated on a chair in the hall. She removed the loose dressings, after placing a clean blue pad under his feet. After applying Betadine liquid to his toes, she fitted sterile aseptic dressing and roller gauze on his foot. She did not use gloves but washed her hands thoroughly after the dressing change. Although she commented aloud that sterile dressings "would be right on the wound," her comment reflected a valid fear that the patient, not the nurse, might become infected. She wore no sterile gloves as she removed the soiled dressings or as she applied the new dressings. Such complacency was infrequent, however, and was the exception rather than the rule among the nursing staff.

The nurses also protected themselves, other patients, and their families from infection by hand-washing techniques and by wearing plastic gloves. They also wore disposable masks and cloth gowns when in direct contact with airborne pathogens and pathogens that spread to objects such as the nurses' clothing. The 7H nurses chose to wear the yellow gowns of isolation precautions despite the fact that at times the infecting microorganism and posted infection control signs indicated that gowns were unnecessary for safe contact with the patient.

The nurses used gloves, hand washing, and containment of excreta and secretions to reduce and eliminate the effects of soil and to return their patients and themselves to a clean state. If they were involved in a nursing function considered to be clean, such as administering medications, and discovered an incontinent patient, they avoided contact with the excreta. Another nurse was asked to clean the soiled patient, so that the nurse involved in the clean activity could keep the clean and dirty separate.

All of the nursing staff handled excreta, secretions, and infected materials. All of the nursing staff washed excreta and secretions from their patients' skin. If an R.N. or other staff earned the reputation of consistently avoiding contact with excreta, she was seen in a negative light. Nurses were expected to "clean it up" (it referred most often to stool).

CONTACTS WITH DIRTY BODILY PRODUCTS

Many patients were incontinent of stool and urine. While nurses did not welcome these products, they responded to stool and urine contact quietly and matter-of-factly. The following example illustrates typical reactions.

During report, Loretta described Maureen O'Day's difficulties with having a bowel movement. The patient could not have a bowel movement on the uncomfortable bedpan. The nurses helped her with some difficulty in and out of the bathroom several times. No luck. Eventually she was incontinent of stool in bed, "B.M. was wet," Pam told Loretta. Both Loretta and Pam were accepting of this and noncommittal. The patient continued to have problems with her bowels the next day. Every day 7H nurses made frequent checks on some of their patients' bowel functions.

It was particularly difficult for the nurses to collect a stool specimen to be tested for the presence of infection, such as ova and parasites. Ann stated her aversion to dealing with potentially infected stool during shift report. "He's on stool precautions. He got that nasty stool last night. I wrote 'done' on there." Ann responded to the fact that the patient's stool had to be handled carefully, for fear of infecting other patients and nurses. In addition to the stool precautions, which basically referred to disposal and careful hand-washing technique, Ann had to carefully collect potentially infected stool into a specimen container, so that the laboratory personnel could examine the specimen microscopically. Hand washing followed specimen collection.

Often collecting stool specimens was part of each nursing shift's unfinished business and the nurses could not mark "done" beside the specimen request on the Kardex. They acknowledged this during report. "She still needs stool for ova and parasite." Many times the patients were able to collect their own specimens. If they could not, the nurses were expected to do so.

The nurses found it difficult to collect specimens, whether potentially infected or not. On one occasion, a G.N. complained angrily about an attending physician's order to hematest (test for blood) a patient's stool. Pam said, "That was the attending's idea, 'cause he was convinced that she had blood in her stool the other day. . . . He wanted her stools hematested and checked her H & H's [hemoglobin and hematocrit—tests that would indicate bleeding and dehydration]. And if anything, they've been going up." The nurse questioned the necessity of collecting a stool specimen. The fact that the patient's hemoglobin level was increasing indicated to the nurse that the patient had no gastrointestinal bleeding. The nurse reacted to what she considered unnecessary exposure to excreta. In most instances doctors did not collect these specimens. It was the nurses' job.

Patients exhibited embarrassment about collecting of stool specimens and giving the specimen containers to the nurses. During shift report, two nurses discussed an incident:

Apparently she had a bowel movement this morning and she flushed it and we didn't test it.

No.

She always flushed it.

That's par for her. She always does.

I don't know why she does. I think she's embarrassed about it. I really do.

In another example, a male patient with pancreatitis and alcoholism failed to give the nurses a stool specimen.

He's hematest all stools. He had to be reminded of that. . . . I explained the whole thing to him twice now. And he keeps going in the bathroom and using the toilet. . . . I have a little hat [fits into the toilet seat to collect specimen] and everything back there and a sign up, but he. . . . I don't know, he's very personal. He thought that that was kind of gross when we asked him to do that.

The nurses were required to collect the stool specimens for diagnostic purposes. Their matter-of-fact and routine handling of specimens, fecal incontinence, and fecal impaction made public matters out of what were commonly private matters.

The nurses predicted urinary incontinence as they did fecal incontinence. They joked during shift report about incontinent patients they had recently washed and changed. The patient was "dry when lasted checked" and would be "incontinent, of course." Their attitudes toward these events were accepting, factual, and tolerant.

Urinary incontinence was treated in a more cavalier manner than fecal incontinence. Nurses knew that urine was not as abundant with microbes as stool. Contact with urine was treated with less concern about contamination. Nevertheless, nurses reacted to the possibility that certain patients' urine was infected. A nurse interrupted report once with the interjections, "Did you know that she had Pseudomonas [a microbial opportunistic infection] in her urine!" "Oh boy!" Another time, a patient's urine was described as "foul smelling and looks yucky."

The nurses checked on patients' urinary functions every eight hours. Intake and output of urine was monitored during every shift or more frequently. Bedpans were requested by patients more frequently for urination than for defecation. Nurses inserted urinary catheters into female patients and occasionally into male patients. They drained Foley catheter bags at the end of each shift.

During report, the nurses described urine specimens collected, gave reminders about those to be collected, and identified characteristics of patients' urine that alarmed them. For example, the nurses discussed a terminally ill patient who was worrying about dying. The nurses were documenting his vital signs and urinary output. One nurse said, "His output for us was about 200 [cc. or ml.] and the urine was almost a greenish color. Check his . . . look at his urine. . . . [It's] a little foul smelling." The nurses were concerned about the volume of urine of the patient's urinary output, since low-volume urine output was seen as a sign of impending death. Healthier patients were described by nurses as, "voiding copious amounts of urine in the bathroom." Obviously, nurses had frequent contact with this type of excreta.

Respiratory secretions were seen as more dangerous or potentially virulent than urine. In one example, 7H nurses cared for a patient with a tracheostomy for almost two months. The patient's trachea required frequent stimulation with a catheter, to encourage coughing so that secretions would be moved up to the surgically created tracheal opening. Miriam noted that "most of the time just by putting the catheter down to stimulate him enough that he's able to cough most of it up to the top of the trache. He's had trache care done twice. [He's] shooting that stuff [mucopurulent secretions] out of there." Miriam indicated that she was disturbed by the spray of secretions.

Nurses referred to respiratory secretions in a variety of ways, revealing their revulsion to this particular body product. However, they recognized the need to be clinically explicit when describing these secretions because of the importance of the airway in maintaining life.

Gloria and Beth discussed a stroke patient's respiratory status.

> When he was vomiting, a lot of the stuff that came up when he was vomiting was that really thick . . . mucus.

Mucousy kind of stuff.

Yeah.

So he's been coughing it up pretty nicely. Cause he sounds like a lot of
upper airway junk to me, boy.

Even though respiratory secretions were referred to as "junk," the
nurses were pleased at the patient's ability to clear his airway.

Miriam detailed her problems with cleaning a patient's tracheostomy tube. She estimated that she spent thirty-five minutes cleaning out the inner cannula. "It was so full of gunk [dried, tenacious
secretions]. It was . . . crusted in the inside." Miriam was concerned
that the removable metal inner cannula was cleaned adequately before being reinserted into the more permanent outer cannula. Otherwise the patient's airway would become obstructed.

The nurses were proud of their skill in removing respiratory secretions from patients. For example, an elderly female patient aspirated food and fluids easily. Beth reported her success with
suctioning the patient's respiratory tract secretions. "She does have
a lot of rales there [in her lungs] and is really gunky [in the upper
airway]. But she's bringing up a lot of that mucus on her own just
coughing. So I did suction her once. . . . She seems to feel better
when you go down her mouth. . . . And you do get mucus." Beth
was pleased with her ability to comfortably suction the patient.

The 7H nurses' descriptions during shift report of sputum or
respiratory secretions were similar to their descriptions of the characteristics of other excreta. Sharon reported, "We got all of the
sputums [specimens]. He's putting out this large amount of green
stuff. He just coughs it up." A question was asked about a patient's
sputum. "How was this sputum? How was it looking?" "It's still
thick." "Still thick?" "Horrible." The nurse's use of the word "horrible" most likely referred to her worry about being able to liquefy
and suction these secretions that could partially occlude the patient's airway and result in hypoxia (decreased oxygen).

The nurses frequently used the word "gunky" to refer to respiratory secretions. Gunky sputum was thick, tenacious, infected,
and dangerous if not expectorated or suctioned.

Nurses who had colds also reacted to their own respiratory secretions with repugnance. "I've got a runny nose," one nurse said dur-

ing report. "As long as it stays over on your side, I don't care," the other nurse replied.

Since 7H was a medical unit, not a surgical unit, the sight of frank blood was limited most often to venipuncture sites for IV's and laboratory tests, skin lesions, occult blood in the stool of patients with gastrointestinal bleeding, and blood transfusions. Frank blood required that nurses evaluate the source and amount. Evidence of bleeding was removed as soon as possible, such as by changing dressings and bed linens. When Miriam was unable to change a sheet that was soiled by "a small drop of blood," she apologized, saying the patient "didn't want us messing around."

The presence of blood was alarming. A long-staying patient's tracheostomy tube came out. The resident had difficulty reinserting the metal tube. Miriam and another nurse discussed the episode later.

> It was bleeding and we had the suction on and he kept trying.
>
> Oh, how, oh!
>
> Aye.
>
> It took him a good fifteen, twenty minutes getting it in. Bleeding all over. It's back in, and his trach care was done and that.
>
> Yuck!

The 7H nurses occasionally and accidentally received puncture wounds from contaminated IV and other needles. Their concern was apparent as they discussed such events with the other nurses. They worried aloud about developing hepatitis and talked themselves into reporting the puncture wound to the employee health nurse so that they would be protected.

The nurses were afraid of contact with parasites. On the one occasion observed, two G.N.'s carefully avoided close contact with a patient whose hairline looked suspicious of lice. A more seasoned nurse assessed the patient and found no lice, but instead, dandruff. The G.N.'s were relieved. If lice had been detected, the nurses would have applied a medicated shampoo to kill the parasites.

Common language and humor helped the nurses transcend their repugnance for secretions, excretions, infected patients, and parasites. For example, "She had a Fleets enema . . . for them [the evening shift nurses] last night and she pooped her brains out for me. . . . She had her hands all in it." As the nurses laughed, they did not seem to be laughing at the patient, but at their situation of having to handle the excreta. Fear of further embarrassment to patients held tongues in check, except in the vicinity of the utility room, the nurses' station, and the corridor.

The nurses seldom referred to feces, urine, blood, or respiratory secretions as excreta. They called feces "stool," "B.M." (bowel movement), "shit," "it," "present" and "poop." For urine, they used the verbs "urinated," "voided" or "peed." They referred to blood as "blood" or "hemorrhage." They referred to respiratory secretions most often as "gunk," "fungy," "funky," or "sputum." Their language reflected a tolerant and humorous reaction to dealing with profane or dirty substances.

RECORDING EXCRETORY AND SECRETORY FUNCTIONS

Nursing staff documented stool "output" on the bowel movement flow sheet, kept at the patient's bedside. The nurses knew that some patients would soon encounter difficulties with bowel functions because of disease or immobility. Certain elderly or confused patients would become constipated and later impacted. Since the nurses had to deal with both of these conditions, and since they caused patients distress, they worked to prevent them.

Early in the G.N.'s tenure on 7H, Sarah reminded the new nurses to "continue to keep up" the bowel movement flow sheet. "Do your 'shit' list every day," Sarah joked. Since the flow sheet was kept at the patient's bedside on a clipboard, it was easy for the nurses to rapidly document whether or not their patient had a bowel movement during their shift.

The nurses also discussed bowel function during change-of-shift report, with such comments as: "He had two large diarrheas twice today"; "She would not take her Per Diem [a laxative] because yesterday she had two B.M.'s and it was marked on her sheet"; "No B.M.'s"; and "She's [scheduled] for a sigmoid [sigmoidoscopy] this morning at bedside. She had her Fleets [small phosphosoda enema] enema with moderate results." It was important that the nurses mention the patients' status in relation to bowel function.

Similarly, urinary output, respiratory secretions, wound drainage, and bleeding were recorded on patient records and reported during change-of-shift report. Descriptions of the characteristics of these bodily products were graphic, and often accompanied with colorful language.

RESPONDING TO EXCRETA, SECRETIONS, AND INFECTED
SUBSTANCES: HUMOR AND FEAR

During shift report, nurses often joked about getting a stool specimen from a patient in order to hematest the stool in the utility room.

> Chris, are you taking care of Mrs. Zeller, too?
>
> Yeah.
>
> If she makes any stools, can you put a little dab on the old [hematest paper]—see if there's blood in it?
>
> Yeah, a little dab'll do you!
>
> A little dab'll do us!

In another example, the nurses had checked on an elderly woman once and found her dry. Later she was incontinent of urine. The patient was frequently incontinent of urine, so that nurses expected this.

> She was incontinent, of course, but she's clean and dry now. [Laughter.]
>
> Well, the last I saw she was, Beth! All right. She gets her insulin, too.

Humor about incontinence sometimes became insensitive. Jean, a laboratory technician working the evening shift, entered a patient's room to collect a blood specimen. She came out of the room abruptly, laughing. The patient was incontinent of feces. She had smeared it everywhere, on her hands and feet, all over the bed rails, everywhere. The laboratory technician obviously delighted in the fact that the nurses had to clean the stool so that the patient and the bed would be approachable for her.

Ann and Nancy ran down the hall to see the patient. The humor about the "shit" lasted at the nurses' station and in the hall for several minutes. Since the patient was in Ann and Betty's district, Betty cleaned the patient and the bed. Ann was administering medications, did not want to stop, and was happy to have Betty do it.

The following example illustrated one nurse's fear as she handled trash, potentially infected material. Aware that the trash in patients' rooms and in the utility room was potentially contaminated, 7H nurses were loathe to look for lost objects in the trash. Once Miriam put on disposable plastic gloves and purposely entered a patient's room. She dug around in the trash can, searching for a patient's reading glasses case that had money in it. Miriam admitted that she hated going into the trash; she was repulsed by the thought, but her patient was upset over the lost money and case. She found the glasses case, washed it off, and gave it to the patient. As the patient said, "Yuck," Miriam dried it off with a paper towel. The patient thanked Miriam, saying that it "wasn't just the money in the case" that made it important to retrieve.

Many times the R.N.'s seemed overtly unafraid of dealing with patients who were on isolation precautions because of infection. Beth, Deidre, Kate, Sarah, Tammy, and Miriam acted secure in their knowledge of what they were doing when caring for a patient with an infection. Fear of infection was hidden, and in most instances, not discussed during their daily work. Occasionally this fear surfaced. When they admitted fear, it was expressed as a hope that they would never bring "anything" home to their families or transmit it to other patients. Some of the L.G.P.N.'s and nursing assistants admitted fear more openly than did the R.N.'s.

In the following situation, evening shift nurses discovered during report that a patient was on stool precautions, to prevent others from contamination by infected stool, and had been for two days. After the day shift nurse reported "stool precautions," the evening nurses, Ann and Nancy reacted.

Why?!

Because he's got this fungus or some funky thing. We started a stool for . . . white count.

Well, did somebody tell us that!

It was just started Monday or Tuesday.

They didn't tell us that!

It was just started Monday or Tuesday.

They didn't tell us that!

Well, here it is [written on the Kardex]—"stool precautions." Was I here
Monday? [Laughter.] And he's still gonna have the diarrhea. They
[doctors] don't want to treat the diarrhea. . . . That's the only way to
let it [the infection] out or something.

Both Ann and Nancy were upset that they had handled the patient's diarrheal stool without prior knowledge of the fungal infection and the ordered stool precautions. While their hand washing
had most likely been meticulous, because nurses assume that all
stool is potentially infected and capable of contaminating them,
they wished that they had worn gloves.

The 7H nurses protected themselves from possible infection by
recognizing the changes in body secretions and excretions that
might cause them to be suspicious of infection and by taking precautions. For example, Miriam requested that the day shift nurses
culture a patient's respiratory secretions into a sterile Luken's col-
lector because she had noticed that the patient had "something
funky growing." Whenever secretions seemed infected, obtaining a
specimen for culture and sensitivity assured the nurses that pathogens would be identified, if present.

One nurse described her concern about a patient's tracheostomy
becoming infected, as well as her concern about a foul odor from a
gastrostomy tube insertion site. She added, "He was secreting this
gooky drainage . . . from his gastroscopy tube . . . and they [the
doctors] were aware of that." The nurses alerted other nurses and
the doctor of a possible infection. At times the doctors ordered a
culture and sensitivity of excretions or secretions when they suspected infections. These orders in turn alerted the nurses who
were responsible for obtaining the specimen. This practice required that nurses get closer to the source of potentially infected
material than doctors.

The nurses' proximity to infection elicited various reactions.
During change-of-shift report, for example, two nurses discussed a
doctor's order for caring for an infected toe. "Please place cotton
between the toes on the right foot. Culture any pus," read the order
as the nurse repeated it from the Kardex. "'Pus,' what a word!" she

exclaimed. The other nurse replied, "Pus!" The word itself suggested contamination and infection, evoking fear and revulsion.

Despite the fact that they did not welcome the exposure to infected materials, the nurses often expressed relief at sending a specimen to the laboratory. At least they would know what pathogen, if any, they were dealing with. This knowledge helped to dispel some fear.

Often the nurses' fear of potentially infected excreta became secondary to their concern about another problem of their patient. For example, an elderly woman with congestive heart failure, diabetes, and a recently healed fractured lower leg had problems with low blood sugar and with severe diarrhea. Miriam said, "The patient had diarrhea—well, loose stools three or four times" during the night shift and once during the day shift. The stool was irritating her perirectal skin, which was being treated with cleansing and Mycolog cream. "She gets Mycolog cream to her perirectal area and that is so gross. . . . Oh, it is terrible. It's worse and worse every day. Red, raw, the skin just peeling off of it." Despite the fact that the patient had diarrhea several times, the nurses' discussions focused on the patient's skin breakdown. Rather than discussing their contact with stool, they discussed the Mycolog cream, where to keep it, either at the bedside or in the medication cart, and the need to use it frequently because of the patient's skin problem.

Fear of AIDS and Herpes Zoster

It is noteworthy that 7H nurses feared contamination from the then unknown pathogen causing AIDS. For example, Gloria discussed a situation that had developed on a neighboring unit. A homosexual male patient had a "tentative, inconclusive" diagnosis of AIDS, a disease that engendered fear of epidemic in anyone who heard about it. Gloria felt that the behavior of this gay patient's primary nurse was "inappropriate." She refused to take care of him and discussed this openly in front of the medical clerks, L.G.P.N.'s, and nursing assistants at the nurses' station. Gloria was disgusted with the R.N. and labeled her behavior as "inflammatory."

The 7H nurses became alarmed when they learned that one of their patients was a homosexual. He received frequent injections for pain. The nurses expressed a fear of his having AIDS, automatically assuming that since he was gay, he had AIDS. "You know this man is homosexual?" Ann whispered. Pam replied, "Yeah, now they [the doctors] tell us. After we've been giving the guy injections. Now they tell us." These G.N.'s were openly afraid of AIDS and suspected that the patient had it merely on the basis of his homosexuality, without the support of clinical evidence.

Later, Kate, Sarah, and Deidre, all seasoned R.N.'s, discussed which 7H staff members would care for a 7H AIDS patient, should one be admitted. Deidre said, "You know who would be taking care of the AIDS patient. Kate and me." Sarah added that everyone panics when an AIDS patient is on a unit. Deidre commented, "On one floor, housekeeping personnel would not clean the [patient's] room, or even go into it." She suggested that the nurses were left with their usual responsibilities as well as those of Housekeeping. Nurses could not neglect any patients. If any R.N.'s, L.G.P.N.'s, or nursing assistants refused to care for an AIDS patient, the nurse manager and assistant nurse manager would.

Fear of herpes zoster infection also aroused fear in 7H nurses. A reporting nurse warned the oncoming staff:

> Mrs. Shaunessy. . . . Big thing on her—she's developing a rash. She's itching as she puts it [calamine lotion] on her right side and back. Apparently it had been noted by the doctor, and first they thought it was just some sort of macular, papular rash. Now the latest note I saw on there, it might be preeruption of herpes zoster, so use good hand washing with her. . . .
>
> I didn't see any rash . . . what do they call that?
>
> Shingles. Yeah, well you can actually feel it. You can't see it, but you can feel it.

The next day it was confirmed that Mrs. Shaunessy had herpes zoster on the skin over her abdomen. The nurses discussed their fear of this virus. They moaned as the reporting nurse said, "She also had herpes zoster on her back. Don't swallow your cigarette, Tammy."

Miriam discussed the skin precautions, or medical aseptic practices, with Tammy in detail.

Dermatology was in to see her yesterday. O.K. They said . . . what they told me is basically use the gloves when you're touching her. One of my questions, with Mrs. Becker in the same room and her being on so much prednisone, her immune system is down. Check with Epidemiology whether possibly Becker should be moved, you know, into another room, just for her own safety. It was also recommended by the night nursing supervisor that you have different people [nurses] do each of them, you know, try not to cross-contaminate between them.

After morning report, an R.N. warned Meredith to remember to call the Epidemiology Department about precautions from herpes zoster. The nurses wanted to be certain that they were carrying out correct medical aseptic practices so that they could protect themselves and their other patients.

When David Kuhn was admitted to 7H, the nurses were confronted with the dilemma of how to care for a patient when fear of a contagion interferes with their sense of responsibility toward patients. Mr. Kuhn, small in stature and elderly, had crusted lesions on his left eyelid and forehead. Both of his eyelids were swollen, almost closed. He periodically touched these lesions, apparently unconsciously thinking of them. His diagnosis of ophthalmic herpes zoster stimulated fear in the hospital staff. One of the evening shift nurses refused to care for Mr. Kuhn. Her reaction illustrated the depth of her fear about caring for infected patients.

On the wall behind Mr. Kuhn's bed was a sign made by one of the nurses: "Attention. Please use very good hand-washing technique. Handle linen and other soiled items with caution."

One morning, I observed Mr. Kuhn's A.M. care. Mr. Kuhn lay asleep in his bed. His breakfast waited on his overbed tray. A yellow laundry bag was on the floor, awaiting soiled linen. Chris was assigned to Mr. Kuhn. She spoke to this "pleasantly confused patient" about eating breakfast. She touched his pillowcase, near his herpes ophthalmic lesions. She next put on plastic, disposable gloves and straightened his pillow case. As she prepared his breakfast tray, she was annoyed by the gloves sticking to the utensils. She said, "Darn!" when she ripped the glove but did not change it. After she asked Mr. Kuhn if he was comfortable eating, she disposed of her gloves in a trash can. Chris muttered something about washing her hands and did so after walking down the hall to the sink in the rear section of the nurses' station. Chris returned, having washed her hands so that she would avoid carrying other pathogenic organisms to others.

Dotty had previously taken care of Mr. Kuhn and planned to help with his care. When asked about how she felt about taking care of patients with herpes zoster or herpes ophthalmic, she responded,

> I put my arm around him. I'm not afraid. I'm not afraid of taking care of anyone with AIDS, either. Some people refuse to take care of them. That's wrong. The patient won't get healthy as quick if you're afraid. The only thing is, I use gloves if I'm going to give him eye drops, and I use alcohol to wipe the phone before I dial, because he doesn't know what he has. You tell him not to scratch his face, and he does.

It was clear that Dotty and Chris did not avoid contact with Mr. Kuhn because of his herpes ophthalmic infection, although they did avoid contact with the infected lesions. They encouraged him to eat lunch, and when he refused, helped him to return to his bed from a chair. Neither the L.G.P.N. nor the G.N. had disposable gloves, despite the fact that they touched objects in the room that could have been and were in contact with secretions from skin lesions.

I asked Chris whether Mr. Kuhn's lunch tray should be isolated from the other patients', but she did not really know. She was concerned enough, however, to ask Dotty. Dotty in turn checked with nurses in the hospital's isolation unit. The nurses from the isolation unit told Dotty to isolate the tray and to have all visitors report to the nurses' station before entering Mr. Kuhn's room so they could receive instructions about avoiding contact with his skin lesions. Chris feared infection and grimaced as she and Dotty discussed the herpes situation. When Chris was told by Kate that people who had had chicken pox were resistant to herpes zoster, she was upset. Chris had not had chicken pox. Chris reassured herself and the other nurses in the utility room that she washed her hands every time she left the patient's room.

The 7H nurses were confused about medical aseptic practices for the containment of the herpes zoster virus. One of the hospital's infection control nurses gave an educational tape to the staff on the herpes zoster virus. The content of the tape was developed from an in-service education program for nurses. Most of the staff listened to the tape. The major points addressed were:

1. Herpes is a family of viruses; chicken pox virus is included.
2. Virus lodges at nerve endings after recovery; after decreased resistance or any disease that influences the immune system, you may have recurrence.
3. Virus reactivates: trigeminal nerve on the face or nerves in the belt or chest area. Usually one side of the body is involved.
4. If you touch herpes drainage you can get chicken pox or if you are immunosuppressed, and have decreased white blood count and had chicken pox you can get herpes in a localized fashion. Usually the virus is not airborne.
5. What to do with the patient: good hand washing technique or wearing gloves when in direct contact with the drainage from the lesions. If your patient's roommate has not had chicken pox and is alert, it is safe to leave both patients in the same room. If the roommates share candy, etc., change the roommate.
6. You can't get herpes simplex, that "other" herpes from a patient with herpes zoster. [That "other" herpes was genital herpes. People who contracted this herpes were equated with a promiscuous pariah.]
7. The herpes problem on the weekend on 7H was a panic and crazy. The patient wished she could have hidden her herpes. Her herpes zoster is pretty resolved.
8. If the patient's lesions are draining, use hand precautions. If the lesions are crusted, you don't have to worry about it.
9. Nurses have to be trend-setters. We need to interpret our signs to dietary, when taking the [food] tray in and out.
10. The attitude that was conveyed by the individuals [7H nurses on the weekend] was conveyed to the patient and perceived by the patient as not being cared for. The patient was like a leper because of the drainage on her forehead. Vital signs were not taken, [food] trays were not taken out, people [nurses] would open the door and say, "What do you want?" We need to look at how we respond to people. She's [the patient] skeptical about how she's been treated. . . .
11. Let's look at how we handle a patient on precautions as more sensitive. There's a policy in your manual for infectious diseases. Call us [infection control nurses] if you have any questions.

Although most of 7H nurses listened to the tape, they were not convinced by the scientific facts included in the program.

They remained fearful of contamination from the herpes zoster lesions of the patient. The few nurses who were unafraid, Sarah, Kate, Deidre, and Dotty, were outnumbered. In the utility room, Dotty explained the incident that had occurred during the previous weekend, the herpes crisis. The female patient in 752W was upset, as was the nurse assigned, since the nurse had never had chicken pox. The nurse limited her contact with the infected patient. Other hospital personnel, nursing staff, and dietary staff opened the door to the room and stood at the door and asked, "What do you want?" The patient felt that she had had no care. Dotty agreed, saying that the patient could not help feeling "uncared for." The nurse's reaction to and refusal to care for this herpes zoster patient was based on fear. The source of her fear could have been her connection or equation of herpes zoster virus with herpes simplex virus, or genital herpes. This fear was irrational, since these viruses are different.

Despite in-service education, fear of herpes zoster contamination continued. Staff's exposure to several herpes zoster patients without harmful effects did not allay the fears. Wound and skin precautions, the usual hand-washing precautions, and in-service education failed to reassure the nurses.

MEDICAL ASEPSIS AS PROTECTION AGAINST CONTAMINATION:
SCIENCE AND NONSCIENCE

The acute care hospital was the place where infected patients could be admitted for care. Rehabilitation hospitals and extended care facilities had the luxury of refusing admission to patients with open infected lesions or other infected bodily products.

The 7H nurses were careful to use plastic disposable gloves and other means to protect themselves and other patients from contamination. Some nurses relied on gloves for protection from contamination when thorough hand-washing would have been sufficient. Some nurses admitted that they always used gloves when bathing patients. Elsie admitted, "Now I just don't feel right if I don't wear gloves" when bathing patients. As nurses bathed patients they felt that they were in close proximity with bodily products that were potentially infected. Hand washing was considered to be scientifically effective, but gloves were sometimes used nevertheless as a magical added protection, "just in case." Gloves were required for protection against some infected materials. However, hand washing was sufficient protection in many contacts with potentially infected materials.

Numerous techniques of medical asepsis were contained in the hospital's *Infection Control Manual.* Available on the shelf of the nurses' station, the manual was a source of scientifically based techniques for protection against and control of pathogenic microorganisms. The broad topical areas of the manual included the following: the infection control program for the hospital; isolation precautions; policies and procedures for specific diseases requiring isolation; general services provided for concurrent isolation cleaning and terminal cleaning, linen handling, and waste disposal; other infection control policies for syphilis, gonorrhea, and pediculosis; and departmental policies such as those for coronary care unit, delivery room, dietary, emergency unit, employee health, general service (housekeeping), maintenance and engineering, maternity, newborn and neonatal intensive care nurseries, nursing service, operating room, outpatient department, pediatrics, physical medicine and rehabilitation, radiology services, recovery room, renal dialysis center, and respiratory therapy.

The content of the *Infection Control Manual* of greatest potential use to nurses was the section dealing with diseases requiring isolation precautions. Relevant topics included were the initiation of isolation or "precautions" on patient units, strict isolation, respiratory isolation, enteric precautions, modified protective precautions, and major and minor wound and skin precautions. Wound and skin precautions and enteric precautions were most often used on 7H.

Despite the wealth of information in the manual, the nurses did not consult it for protective techniques. I did not observe 7H nurses consulting it when patients were known to be infected and were placed on isolation precautions. Instead, the nurses relied on other nurses' word of mouth descriptions and demonstrations of how to handle the infected patient.

In the following typical example, a nurse gave detailed instructions about how to apply compresses to the skin lesions of a patient with ophthalmic herpes zoster.

He got the warm compresses to both eyes. He gets them [the compresses] twice for you. And now the area that's scabbing up on his forehead, that's to be washed with soap and water b.i.d. and lightly apply a gauze bandage. So what we did, we washed it and then we put Kling bandage around his head and then after we did that, we had to apply Neosporin ointment to affected areas where the scabbing is after washing it. So when you do it this evening, after you wash it with soap and water, the Neosporin ointment is to be applied and then the Kling.

Other warnings of infection were provided by the hospital's infection control nurses. A set of signs (Figure 9) were posted on doors to the rooms of infected patients. The signs were designed to warn and instruct nurses, other hospital personnel, and visitors about isolation techniques for infected patients. The signs did not identify the offending pathogen, but were printed in different colors: red, respiratory precautions; brown, enteric precautions; green print on light green, minor wound and skin precautions; white print on dark green, major wound and skin precautions; pink, secretion precautions; blue, modified protective precautions; red print on white, blood precautions; orange print on white, antibiotic resistant organisms; and brown print on cream, excretion precautions.

The infection control nurses also provided small cards, tiny reproductions of the door cards, to be used in the Kardex. I did not see these small cards inserted into district Kardexes.

Other warnings related to infection control were provided by the infection control agents throughout the hospital. When nurses or laboratory technicians obtained or were in close contact with specimens that were thought to be infected, the specimens were labeled with stickers. These stickers were printed with the following phrases: protective isolation; caution hepatitis; enteric precautions; strict isolation; stool and needle precautions; AIDS precautions; blood precautions; and respiratory isolation.

Bright colors alerted hospital personnel about infected linens and trash. Patient gowns and bed linens were placed in a yellow cloth bag, which was next inserted into another yellow cloth laundry bag. The color of the bags and the double bagging technique warned Laundry Service personnel that the bags contained laundry that had been in direct contact with infected patients. Nurses wore yellow gowns when in direct contact with certain infected patients or products.

Contaminated trash was placed in a special red trash receptacle in the utility room. Used needles contained in a securely taped box and trash from the rooms of infected patients were also placed in this receptacle. The contaminated trash was also double bagged and sealed in a red plastic bag. Contaminated trash was transported by the Housekeeping personnel in a "pathological trash" truck to a trash holding area. A biohazard symbol warned personnel that actual or potentially dangerous waste was contained in receptacles labeled with this symbol.

The 7H nurses responded to warnings about dangerous materials. They used hand washing, warning signs and labels, yellow laundry bags, red trash bags, and yellow protective gowns to contain the spread of infection. For extra protection against pathogenic organisms, some nurses used plastic disposable gloves and yellow isolation gowns despite the fact that specific infecting organisms were controlled by hand washing alone.

Nursing Rituals in Medical Aseptic Practices

The 7H nurses' hygienic care of patients centered on the techniques of medical asepsis. Hygienic practices pervaded nursing care.

As they bathed patients, nurses did more than remove bodily soil. They also gave comfort and a sense of well-being to their patients. The repeated bathings during the twenty-four-hour hospital day provided an opportunity for the laying-on-of-hands, for the intimate contact needed for healing.

Baths were therapeutic. After bathing, some patients' conditions improved. Nurses were convinced that bathing and associated activities helped. Symbolically, nurses washed away disease through bathing.

Respect for patients' bodies was conveyed through the vehicle of the bath. Nurse and patient relationships developed as patients talked and cried to their nurses during bathing activities about their personal situations.

Bathing patients was the nurses' domain and responsibility. The regularity of the times when bathing was done was important to

MINOR WOUND & SKIN PRECAUTIONS

Visitors - Report to Nurses' Station Before Entering Room

1. **Room** - single room not necessary.
2. **Gowns** - not necessary.
3. **Masks** - not necessary.
4. **Gloves** - necessary for contact with infected area.
5. **Hands** - must be washed before and after contact with the infected area.
6. **Articles** - articles in contact with or contaminated with drainage from the infected area must be disinfected or discarded. See Infection Control Manual.

MODIFIED PROTECTIVE PRECAUTIONS

Visitors – Report to Nurses' Station Before Entering Room

1. **Room** - single room necessary. Door should be closed.
2. **Gowns** - not necessary.
3. **Masks** - not necessary.
4. **Gloves** - not necessary.
5. **Hands** - must be washed prior to patient contact, before leaving the room and as indicated during patient care.
6. **Articles** - all articles that contact the patient must be disinfected or sterilized prior to patient contact. No special precautions after use.

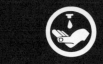

SECRETION PRECAUTIONS

Visitors - Report to Nurses' Station Before Entering Room

1. **Room** - single room not necessary.
2. **Gowns** - not necessary.
3. **Masks** - not necessary.
4. **Gloves** - must be worn for any contact with secretions or secretion contaminated articles.
5. **Hands** - must be washed after patient contact or after contact with secretions.
6. **Articles** - articles contaminated with secretions must be disinfected or discarded. See Infection Control Manual.

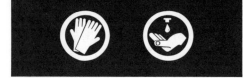

EXCRETION PRECAUTIONS

Visitors - Report to Nurses' Station Before Entering Room

1. **Room** - single room not necessary.
2. **Gowns** - not necessary.
3. **Masks** - not necessary.
4. **Gloves** - must be worn for any contact with urine, feces, or articles contaminated with urine or feces.
5. **Hands** - must be washed after patient contact, contact with excretions, or contact with articles contaminated with urine or feces.
6. **Articles** - articles contaminated with urine and feces must be disinfected or discarded. See Infection Control Manual.

Figure 9. Door signs for infection control precautions.

RESPIRATORY ISOLATION

Visitors - Report to Nurses' Station Before Entering Room

1. **Room** - single room necessary. Door must be closed.
2. **Gowns** - not necessary.
3. **Masks** - necessary for all persons entering the room. Patients should wear mask when leaving room.
4. **Gloves** - not necessary.
5. **Hands** - must be washed after patient contact or after contact with respiratory secretions.
6. **Articles** - articles contaminated with respiratory secretions must be disinfected or discarded. See Infection Control Manual.

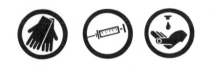

ENTERIC PRECAUTIONS

Visitors - Report to Nurses' Station Before Entering Room

1. **Room** - private room necessary only for children.
2. **Gowns** - must be worn by all persons having direct contact with patient.
3. **Masks** - not necessary.
4. **Gloves** - must be worn by all persons having direct contact with patient or with articles contaminated with fecal material.
5. **Hands** - must be washed on entering and leaving room and after patient contact.
6. **Articles** - articles contaminated with urine and feces must be disinfected or discarded. See Infection Control Manual.

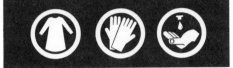

BLOOD PRECAUTIONS

Visitors - Report to Nurses' Station Before Entering Room

1. **Room** - single room not necessary.
2. **Gowns** - not necessary.
3. **Masks** - not necessary.
4. **Gloves** - must be worn for contact with patient's blood or secretions or with articles contaminated with blood or secretions.
5. **Hands** - must be washed before and after patient contact.
6. **Articles** - articles in contact with blood or secretions must be disinfected or discarded. See Infection Control Manual.

MAJOR WOUND & SKIN PRECAUTIONS

Visitors - Report to Nurses' Station Before Entering Room

1. **Room** - single room desirable.
2. **Gowns** - should be worn during direct patient contact.
3. **Masks** - should be worn during dressing changes *ONLY*.
4. **Gloves** - must be worn during contact with infected area.
5. **Hands** - must be washed before and after contact with infected area or with drainage from the infected area.
6. **Articles** - articles that have come in contact with the infected area or drainage must be disinfected or discarded. See Infection Control Manual.

"Antibiotic Resistant Organisms"

1. Private room necessary.
2. Good handwashing mandatory.
3. Gloves necessary when handling secretions and excretions.
4. Those articles contaminated with excretions and secretions must be disinfected or handled as pathological waste if disposable.
5. Specimens to lab must be double bagged and labeled.
6. No linen bagging is required.
7. No special tray is required.

the nurses. Getting baths finished gave the nurses a sense of accomplishment and symbolically imposed order over the events of the shift.

Bathing patients shortly after admission to the hospital represented a symbolic purification of the patient. One R.N.'s comments emphasized the importance of this ritualistic washing: "If a new patient comes in 'off the streets,' I use gloves for a few days, then I stop. I know they have been washed if they have been here for a few days." If a patient had been in the hospital for a few days and was not bathed, the nurses were horrified.

The nurses' guilty responses to unfinished bathing emphasized the ritual nature of bathing. As a therapeutic nursing ritual, the bathing of patients was performed to have a beneficial effect. The latent meaning of the bathing practices of nurses reveal "patterned, symbolic action that refers to the goals and values of a social group" (DeCraemer, Vansina, and Fox 1976). Healing, order, and cleanliness were important to 7H nurses.

As the nurses handled patients' excreta and secretions and were in direct contact with infected patients, their reactions ranged from tolerance to fear. It was evident that science alone did not protect the nurses from contamination from bodily products and infected patients.

The nurses used disposable gloves as almost magical protection even when gloves were unnecessary according to scientific rationale. In this manner, gloves provided symbolic protection for the nurses.

Throughout the study of medical aseptic practices of nurses it was evident that nurses relied on demonstration and word of mouth transmission to impart the knowledge, practices, and values of nursing to nursing staff.

V

The Nursing Ritual of
Change-of-Shift Report

Change-of-shift report holds moral significance for nurses. Nurses are unable to begin work formally without sharing this report.

For the 7H nurses, change-of-shift report served the explicit function of passing information, but it also served as implicit function. Time and facts were suspended or frozen, so that other nurses coming "on the floor" could begin work with an orderly perspective. Order was imposed on uncertainty as the nurses informed each other of patients' progress in relation to the signs and symptoms of disease.

Change-of-shift report also provided a forum where nurses could complain and express humor and concern. Nurses used report as an opportunity to diffuse some of the difficulties of the nursing role.

Shift report was used as a testing ground for G.N.'s. During report, G.N.'s were evaluated, shaped, and corrected. Change-of-shift report was clearly the domain of the R.N.'s, although the contributions of L.G.P.N.'s and nursing assistants were valued.

The nurses tolerated interruptions during the sacrosanct time when shift report was conducted. They tolerated interruptions directly related to the work of nursing and patients better than they tolerated the interruptions of doctors. Nurses' reactions to interruptions illustrated the ritual nature of change-of-shift report.

The nurses warned each other of situations in which error could take place and acknowledged errors as they occurred. In this way the nurses' responsibility toward their patients was kept before the whole nursing staff. Errors were to be avoided; after errors were made, they were scrutinized publicly.

As the nurses exchanged information and interacted during report, they communicated in a hospital-bound, nursing-specific language. The language kept the meaning of report somewhat secret and was intelligible only to those who were initiated into hospital nursing life.

The fact that nurses helped each other complete unfinished business after report emphasized the shared responsibility the nurses felt toward their work. The commitment to continuous coverage and the responsibility of the nurses toward their patients was symbolically portrayed during the transfer of patient ownership at change-of-shift report. While other mechanisms of coverage and responsibility were present, shift report was characterized as an occupational ritual of responsibility. Standards of care were set and reemphasized during report. Professional behavior was expected during report.

Dividing Patients for Coverage and Waiting for Change-of-Shift Report to Begin

The total patient capacity on 7H was thirty-two. The care of patients hospitalized in the unit was divided by nurses according to the staff available on each shift. During the day shift, assignments were divided into four districts with eight patients each. During the evening and night shifts, the number of districts was determined by the staff available. Assignments of staff to each district for all shifts was made by Deidre, the nurse manager, or Kate, the assistant nurse manager, in advance. This assignment was posted on a schedule adjacent to the primary board. On each shift, however, the most senior nurse on the unit adjusted the assignments after considering the numbers and status of patients, patient acuity and experience level of the staff, and events occurring on the unit.

The clearest signals to nurses coming on duty that change-of-shift report was about to begin was the completion of staff assignments to districts by an R.N. The R.N. wrote nurses' names on the primary board across from the nurses' station. Then the primary nurse for each district retrieved the Kardex for that district from the desk or the medication carts in the nurses' station.

The report was given by an R.N. or a G.N. Thus the responsibility for patients was transferred from professional to professional. The R.N. or G.N. accepted the primary responsibility for knowing and judging the facts thus shared. The associate nurses were not as directly responsible, although they assumed responsibility for the care they gave their patients.

Staff for the on-coming shift arrived early, signed in and awaited these signals for report to begin. Some staff sat in the utility room, smoked a cigarette, drank coffee or soda, and chatted. Usually there was much conversation. For example, one morning Marie, an L.G.P.N., discussed a code for a patient who had had a cardiac arrest and died the previous day on another nursing unit. Marie remembered the woman, since she had been a former 7H patient. Marie was fond of the patient and her son and recounted that as the patient had left 7H, her family stated that they knew she would be admitted to the hospital again.

Some of the social discussions while waiting for report to begin included: comments about a gift that was given to Miriam, a newly married R.N.; complaints about physical facilities for 7H staff; commiseration with a G.N. as she considered the unfinished work that she had to complete after report and before going home; the sharing of photographs of vacations and stories of family celebrations; complaints about the hard work of nursing; teasing about having the previous shift's nurses stay to help the current shift nurses; courteous greetings to the oncoming staff; solicitous questions about whether the assembled staff minded smoking; and joking about who would eat the most junk food, pretzels, or Tootsie Rolls when one of the nurses brought them to the unit.

Sometimes in conversations held before district reports the nurses discussed nursing business subjects such as the nursing care the G.N.'s had been involved in the previous evening. Sometimes they aired concerns about possibly becoming a pool night nurse who did not know so much about the patients. "It's hard to keep an eye on everybody. Thirty-two patients," one nurse worriedly stated.

While day shift nurses waited for their district reports to begin, they distributed linens for morning care, answered lights, and checked on patients. The nurse manager or assistant nurse manager sometimes had to remind the staff to distribute the linens.

While occupied with listening to report, nurses were still responsible for patient care. Often the L.G.P.N.'s and nursing assistants from the previous shift left the unit promptly at 8:00 A.M., 4:00 P.M., and 12:00 P.M., leaving the patients "uncovered" except for the staff of the on-coming shift, some of whom were listening to report. All 7H nurses realized that events were progressing on the unit during the time staff spend listening to shift report, but time was frozen for those in report. Staff from the reporting shift "kept an eye on the floor."

During change-of-shift report unit events were treated as suspended by those nurses involved in report. This suspension of time helped the nurses know how to begin their work, starting with a set of assumptions and facts about their patients, and working from that perspective throughout the shift, always comparing to those beginning notions of what was "going on."

When a staff member's assignment was inadvertently not posted on the primary board, confusion reigned. For example, Betty, a nursing assistant, interrupted Pam, a G.N., as she gave change-of-shift report.

> There's no assignment up there [on the primary board]. I don't . . . I have no idea where I'm working. There's no assignment there. Just give the numbers [patient room numbers] and I'll know where I'll work. The magic numbers.

After the assignment was made, Betty settled down and listened to report on the patients to whom she was assigned. Another time, report was interrupted and assignments changed midstream. One of the nurses requested clarification of the change of assignment. She seemed annoyed and asked, "Can we find out?" When nurses knew their patient assignments, they were able to concentrate on the facts shared during report that were specific to their patients.

The nurses extended courtesies to one another as the nurse giving report prepared the primary nurse worksheet on the patients of her district for the on-coming nurse listening to report. When shift report ended, the 7H nurses who had given the report frequently wished the on-coming nurses a good day, evening, or night. Another courtesy, almost universally extended, was the appreciation voiced by the nurse receiving report to the nurse going off duty. Often at the end of report a "thank you" was stated; this acknowledged the effort spent by the nurses after working the previous shift.

Generally, Miriam gave report promptly at 7:30 A.M. as the night shift ended and the day shift began. On rare occasions, when there were two R.N.'s on the night shift, two sites were used for different districts' morning report. The utility room, Deidre's office or the doctor on-call/laboratory room were the usual locations. Most of the time, Miriam gave report about patients on successive districts. Nurses assigned to a district listened only to the report of patients in their assigned district.

When the evening shift began, nurses listened to report most often in the utility room or Deidre's office. When the night report began, it was held most often in the utility room. One afternoon, doctors occupied the utility room at 3:30 P.M., change-of-shift time. This was surprising, since the 7H utility room seemed to be nursing's territory, although other hospital staff occasionally shared this space. Deidre was surprised at the occupation by the doctors, and mentioned that hospital building and renovation projects included plans for two conference rooms on each nursing unit. Once, on a quiet morning during the Christmas holiday season, Beth gave morning report at the nurses' station. The few staff present were surprised.

Typically the utility room was disorderly and crowded as Miriam gave morning report. Starting with District I's patients, she identified the room number, usually whether the bed was in the door or window location, and the patient's name. Interspersed with the medical diagnosis and other relevant information about a patient were facts such as the patient's blood level of Digoxin or how much IV fluid was left in a viaflex bag. In addition, Miriam told stories about encounters with patients during the night or reported stories that had been told by the evening nurse. One morning, for example, Miriam said, "Watch the schizophrenic patient [with arterial fibrillation]. She may have stolen cigarettes from the med drawer," and of another patient, "That woman's dying, it's sad," and of another patient, she said, "Did you know she had Pseudomonas in her urine. Oh boy!"

The nurses giving report often said, "You know these patients." If the nurse taking report did not know the patients, she elicited more information by stating, "I don't know these people" or "I don't know anyone in District I."

The nurses who listened to report responded to Miriam with questions, laughter, facts about the patient, and stories of their own. One morning, Miriam reported on Districts II, III, and IV, in order. On other mornings, Miriam asked the nurses coming on the day shift if they were "ready for report." District II's report preceded District I's at times. For a while Deidre insisted that the nurses from two districts listen to the reports of their own district and the adjacent district, so that they would be more knowledgeable about the patients in the more unfamiliar district while covering during lunch and breaks. The nurses gradually resumed their preferred pattern of listening solely to their own district's report.

Events on the unit sometimes disrupted report. One afternoon, Colleen, a G.N., gave report in the utility room in a matter-of-fact manner, emphasizing important points by her tone of voice. Pam, who was receiving the report, exchanged questions and answers with Colleen. Abruptly the pleasant interchange stopped, because there was a problem with staff assignments to districts. Pam, obviously annoyed, left abruptly but soon returned to the utility room. Apparently Deidre became upset with Pam's behavior. She also interrupted report to tell Pam, "I want to see you right now." Pam left again, returning in a more temperate mood. Since Pam was known to be "short" or angry from time to time, Deidre felt that her behavior had to be confronted, dealt with, and modified. This rare deviant behavior and Deidre's reaction to it demonstrated that Deidre expected that a professional code of conduct be observed during change-of-shift report.

Nurses shared much information during report, sometimes in a disjointed manner. For example, during one report, Sharon, an R.N., asked Ann, also an R.N., about specimens that needed to be collected; Ann expressed concern that a patient was too fearful to signal for a nurse when Ann was in another room and was not able to respond rapidly; someone reported that a patient was having difficulty not swallowing a medication that was to be kept under his tongue; both Sharon and Ann agreed that a patient had a "weird affect"; Sharon worried aloud about laboratory study results that were not recorded; a nurse stated that an "ornery" patient did not like to eat and another had an "attitude" problem—she did not think that the nurses were doing anything for her; another nurse advised to "just be extra nice" to a cancer patient; a nurse commented that a patient who had a Texas catheter "gets a charge out of it and likes to look under the covers"; Ann forgot to record giving narcotics and the nurses laughed when she remembered; someone described a new admission, an elderly woman, as "cute as a button"; and someone else reported that a doctor's writing was described as a scribble. The nurses had difficulty transcribing his order.

The nurses were purposeful about shift report. They wanted to end their work or begin it promptly. The agenda was serious and the delivery and reception of information was thoughtful overall. Report usually started as close to the designated times of 7:30 A.M., 3:30 P.M., and 12:00 P.M. as possible, unless a crisis such as a cardiac arrest or death occurred. Report for the district involved might be delayed up to fifteen minutes.

After change-of-shift report 7H nurses continued to discuss the business of nursing. For example, one morning Kate reminded Sarah of a hospital policy change; both nurses discussed the transfer of a patient from 7H to the Intensive Care Unit and then to a rehabilitation hospital; and a nurse mentioned that a confused patient was transferred to another room after he tried to pull out his roommate's indwelling Foley catheter.

Another day after morning report, the R.N.'s discussed how to collect a stool specimen for fecal fat. They asked each other if a stool specimen contaminated by urine changed the results of this laboratory test. They eventually decided to call the laboratory for information.

The nurses also used the time after report to answer questions that had been partially explained during report:

O.K. Now do we have to take her blood pressure in another hour?

Yeah. At 4:30 it has to be taken again. 'Cause that's when the hydralazine works and I gave it at 3:30. So at 4:30. . . . It [blood pressure] . . . it'll be down.

O.K., when I do my rounds.

Mr. Feldman's IV is infiltrated again so I have to wait for them [an IV nurse] to come up. . . . Did he get flowers for his wife today?

Yes, he did.

Oh, good.

Um hm! He was real excited about that.

Change-of-shift report was a scheduled, three-times-a-day opportunity for nurses to come together to discuss nursing care and patient progress. It marked the twenty-four-hour cycle of events on the unit with a temporal structure imposed by nursing.

Patterns and Progression of Change-of-Shift Report

Nurses gave report in sequence, from the lowest numbered patient room within a district to the highest numbered patient room in a district. Although the nurses followed Kardexes that were also arranged in this order, they found it necessary to apologize somewhat profusely when they stopped report and returned to previously reported-on patients.

Characteristically, each of the three change-of-shift reports differed little in content during each twenty-four-hour period. Morning report seemed to set the stage for each twenty-four-hour cycle. Details of patient events during the night, including pain medications administered, patients' disorientation or confusion, preparations for diagnostic tests, and discharges planned for the day shift were frequently mentioned.

The content of report on two patients is included in the following typical example. The patients' names were omitted from these examples.

741D ———. [Nurses sigh. This is a chronic patient who has been in the hospital for many months.] He's better, Beth. Vital signs ———. He's on the respirator 10 P.M., to 8 A.M. daily. The Gortex trach [tracheostomy tube] is in. What does it look like? It's white and blue plastic. He gets treatments with mini nebs. the respiratory therapist gave him a treatment. He's been having a lot of plugs [mucus]. He says something is in his throat. [All laugh at Beth's comment.] It's the trach. His IV is aminophylline in 210 cc. He is suctioned every one to two hours. He was suctioned two to three tonight. He took some juices. Some discussion about his glottis and problems with swallowing when one has a tracheostomy.

654D ————. The "difficult patient." She has stump edema [is an amputee] and vulva edema. Her abdomen is distended. I know from the progress notes that they are talking to her but not really assessing her. I wrote them a nice note, about [abdominal] girths. Maybe they'll notice. Do you think they'll do something about the edema? BUN and protein are elevated. I asked them about a code status. She's been talking about death. She was straight cathed on evenings. Can they order ointment for excoriation of the vulva? Her lungs had an infiltrate. She won't say it [complain about anything] when the [doctors] come in; let's get Deidre in on this. [Chris comments,] "She's hard to cath."

The nurses often reported matter-of-factly. For example:

The reason that he has so much bleeding, too, is he was on Coumadin at home until about maybe two or three days prior to admission. His PT—or his PTT—is—and both are really elevated.

Right.

So he's going to be getting Vitamin K for three days.

O.K.

In this example, the patient's bleeding problem was being taken care of by vitamin K injections. The nurses were aware of the problem and reassured by the actions of prescribed medication.

For the most part, the exchange of information during report was quiet and uneventful. When problems existed and persisted, however, the nurses' reactions covered a range of emotional expression: anger, sarcasm, humor, impatience, sadness, pity, criticism, hopelessness, and exasperation. During one report, two nurses commented, "We have a lot of CA on this floor." "Yeah, I know. . . . It's so depressing."

Since there were many points of discussion during report, and many details to be addressed, nurses relied heavily on the nursing Kardexes to structure the report. Kardex information included the patient's room number, door or window location, medical diagnosis, surgical procedure, private physician and physician team, IV fluids currently ordered, laboratory and scheduled diagnostic tests, medications, treatments, known allergies, and nursing care plan. In addition, index cards or notes were added to the Kardex when additional or special information was needed, such as the specific activities of a "cardiac rehab #5" regimen. Nurses often used the Kardex to help them recall important facts. For example, during report Ann could not remember a detail and flipped the Kardex back, reading it carefully. She muttered that there was something forgotten, "something about him," about which she was unsure.

Kardexes were quick references for those nurses who did not have time to search for information in the more detailed, cumbersome patient charts. If nurses remembered a detail about a patient after moving on to another patient's report, they would apologetically flip the Kardex back and tell the listening nurses the omitted information. For example, Beth said, "Ann, can you back up for one minute?" and then asked for a specific IV order and flow rate.

The nurses were upset when details were forgotten. The G.N.'s were especially shaken. "All right, Pam, what was I supposed to be doing? And I gotta call Chemistry. . . . And I gotta take the Holter [monitor] off."

In addition to the Kardex information, the nurses receiving reports recorded facts about the patients in their districts which they considered important on the "primary nurse worksheet." Usually the nurse giving report had filled in the patients' names and room numbers and a few other facts on the worksheet as a courtesy to the primary nurses of 7H's districts. If the previous shift's nurse or nurses were unable to do this, they apologized, usually citing a crisis or problem that prevented them from preparing it. All of the primary nurses used this worksheet as a written reminder of their work. Some of the nurses used a red pen to alert them to a critical detail such as IV's, insulin dosages, and DNR status of a patient. This worksheet helped the nurses to plan and thus control some of their workday, some events of which were sure to be uncontrollable. Both the Kardex and the primary nurse worksheet also helped the nurses to order their thoughts and actions as they transferred responsibility from one nurse to another during change-of-shift report.

Functions of Change-of-Shift Report

The fact that 7H nurses added information and asked questions at the end of report was an example of the continuous nature of their information exchange throughout each shift.

The amount of factual material shared by the reporting nurse increased when critically ill patients resided in 7H rooms. When George Bowers was in 741 Door, with his tracheostomy connected to a respirator, the facts were abundant.

> He had a "trach" inserted yesterday. Big thing with that. He's losing a lot of blood around it. His stoma [surgically created opening] is fairly large and it looks like the trach is almost being sucked in. We have it hooked as best we could. It has Vaseline gauze around it. . . . Bilaterally his breathing is equal. He's not in any sort of respiratory distress. Stat ABG's [arterial blood gases] on him, which are down from what they had been earlier. These reports just came back. He's [the doctor] aware of them. His PO [arterial oxygen] dropped from like 96 to 69. So what Respiratory [Respiratory Therapy] just did, they increased his FI [fraction of inspired oxygen] about 10 [minutes] after 7 [A.M.] to 40 percent. Increased it from 35. They ordered a stat portable chest [X-ray]. . . . What else on him? He's running a temp this morning of 40.2°[C].

These facts were only part of the report Miriam gave on Mr. Bowers that morning.

Information commonly provided on all patients included IV's, bowel movements, and laboratory studies, those recently or routinely ordered, and the results of these studies. For example:

> Mr. Flowers with his abdominal pain. He had a Foley in. Um, he had IV #2 hanging, D5 1/2 normal saline, it's running O.K., 100 cc. an hour, and you have a full thousand credit there until 1700. He did have a nice size B.M. . . . He's out for CBC with diff [complete blood count with differential] today.

More detailed information was given on recently admitted patients. For example:

> Ernestine Zachs. She's in with rule out MI. She has a history of unstable angina. O.K. Initially came in with severe substernal chest pain which awoke her from sleep at home. Was not relieved by 3 nitros. She had no chest pain when she came into the E.R. Her enzymes were negative. She also has a permanent pacemaker which is set at 70. O.K., And she also

has a history of chronic anemia. When she came in she was running 8.7 [hemoglobin]. Yesterday she was running 7.7 [hemoglobin] over 24.8 [hematocrit].

In unusual circumstances, different information was added to the report, a change from the usual custom of giving just the patient's name, medical diagnosis, brief history, and factual information. For example, a report might include the following information: a patient's family stayed the whole shift; a patient was told to tell the nurse when she administered her own eye drops; a patient was classified as DNR, Category III (a fact almost always reported); how much IV fluid was left in the bag hanging at the patient's bedside and how many hours that fluid was to run into the patient; a patient who walked with a cane required assistance; a patient may not have had an EEG—the nurse receiving report would have to check; a patient was incontinent of urine; a patient was discovered to be mute, as formerly suspected; two roommates were not able to get along with one another, so one was transferred to another room; a patient's daughter was taught how to do a gastrostomy tube feeding; and a patient had left the unit to go to Physical Therapy.

Problems were often mentioned during change-of-shift report. Once Kate and Colleen discussed the options of an elderly man who was going home the next day.

> Look, he's never going to be any better, though. He's got left ventricular hypertrophy and he needs a new heart, you know. What can you do? . . .
>
> He doesn't want the surgery. [He said] that he didn't care if it took his life. He'd be willing to go through it to get a new . . . but then I heard another story, that everyone was saying that the doctor came in to talk to him about it and he refused it, so. I don't know what the true story really is. They wanted to replace his valve. . . . The valves are messed up, the ones they [already] replaced. They wanted to replace them again to try to see if that would help, but I don't know.

Kate left the situation at that.

Technical difficulties were also discussed. In one example, a patient's nasogastric feeding tube became clogged. Pam described in detail the problems she had flushing the tube. Problems with nasogastric feeding tubes occurred fairly often.

The tube has been clogged so many times. . . . I had to give him water. How much water? 75 cc.? I was giving him 300 cc. Whatever it takes to flush that thing through, because we can't go by this [the doctor's order].

Patients' or their families' decisions about signing for or against resuscitation permission were often discussed at length during shift report. For example, a nurse said of her patient:

The husband decided not to make her a no code . . . to make her, you know, no code; to do everything possible but if she has a cardiac or respiratory [arrest] to just let her go. But everything short of that.

Cancer patients' problems also stimulated discussions. "Yeah, it's . . . it is a malignancy," said Kate, "but it's mets, they don't know where the primary site is. She is not aware of it yet. She has not been told." Another example revealed a problem with feeding a cancer patient Sustacal, a nutrition supplement. The nurses agreed with the doctor's order, but because the patient was increasingly anorexic, at times he refused to take his Sustacal liquid supplement. The nurses pleaded with each other for release from the obligation to give the feeding to the refusing patient, saying, "We don't have to give it to him tonight, do we?" Colleen answered, "No, we can't force it on him." Another cancer patient, Ina Smith, had lung cancer and pericardial effusion. The reporting nurse noted that the patient "feels that this Demerol is not doing anything for her." The nurses wondered if the cancer was far advanced or not and speculated why the doctors were not ordering morphine or methadone.

When patients were diagnosed with cancer, the nurses were upset. Shift report about Mr. Griffiths contained evidence of their concern.

Does he have CA of the what?

Esophageal.

Nicest guy, but that's the way it goes. Did you hear anything about that theory. . . . Cancer and the types of personality types [sic] of people who develop it?

Suppressed anger.

That, and they're usually the type person, you know, they're usually real giving people.

Cancer personality.

The nurses were pleased by the fact that Mr. Griffiths did not have metastasis. They knew also that he would suffer from his disease.

Often the problems discussed by the nurses within the context of a patient's report were partially resolved or unresolved. It seemed to take time, a few shifts of days, for some of these issues to be resolved or abandoned.

When doctors and nurses disagreed about policy, there was a thorough airing of the issue by the nurses within shift report. After reporting briefly on Jerome Kane's status after his prostatectomy surgery, Miriam described a situation where an unpremedicated patient was sent to surgery:

> Feldman [the attending physician] was pissed because we called him at home at six in the morning. He refused to come in that early and medically clear him. He said, "I'll write it later in the day, just send him down" [to the Operating Room]. I said, "Well, we can't medically send him down." Then he hung up on us. Called back and bawled Ann out on the phone and said, "I'm holding you personally responsible." . . . The other surgeon came up and he says, "Oh, the heck with it."

Miriam and Ann were using hospital policy to guide their actions. The doctors were bending the rules; one was offended that the nurses would question his judgment. This example was typical of confrontations on 7H between nurses and doctors.

The information exchanged during change-of-shift report served both explicit and implicit functions. The following sections include examples of specific functions of change-of-shift report.

Explicit Functions of Change-of-Shift Report

Change-of-shift report served many functions for nurses. These functions displayed the practical, day-to-day work of nurses.

ACKNOWLEDGING SIGNS AND SYMPTOMS OF DISEASE DURING REPORT

The 7H nurses valued report as a means of sharing their clinical acumen through the identification of patient signs and symptoms. They offered patient signs and symptoms to on-coming nurses as data to investigate on the next shift. The nurses who listened to report were alerted to the trends in their patients' statuses.

Both the presence and the absence of signs and symptoms were significant to the nurses. When they reported that a patient did not have expected signs and symptoms, it was often a relief, such as in the following example:

> Mr. Moore. He's in with syncope [fainting]. He's a seventy-year-old-male. . . . He's been passing out for the last two weeks. He's alert, lungs are clear, he had no complaints of nausea, dizziness, or vomiting.

When signs and symptoms persisted despite hospitalization and treatment, the nurses noted this with misgivings. One nurse reported, for example:

> He came in initially with urgency, burning on urination. After urination he's had a feeling of fullness, pulling down his bladder type of feeling. . . . He says he has a burning sensation still. Not as bad as it has been since he's been here. But still has this like pulling down feeling in his bladder.

The nurses were concerned with the persistence of these problems, despite treatment, and were attentive to this part of report.

Pain was described in the many ways it was manifest in 7H's patients. Chest pain or "chest tightness . . . not actually a pain—a tightening" made the nurses anxious. Questions were asked to determine how this symptom was treated. "Did Elsie increase her Nifedipine?" asked Pam. Sharon described the symptoms and the nursing care.

> During the period [of chest tightening] her major complaint is she feels like she's not getting enough air. And she keeps saying throughout the whole thing that she can't take a deep breath. . . . I gave her three nitros. She didn't get any relief. At one point she had pain in her right shoulder. I turned the oxygen up to 3 liters. I put her in high Fowlers.

The patient's symptoms did not go away. They resisted different medications, oxygen, and a semi-sitting position change. It worried the nurses. They discussed the pain characteristics, the patient's behavior, and the different therapies to relieve it. The nurses were accustomed to the patient's having this type of pain periodically, but they wished that they could relieve her.

Chest pain always captured the nurses' attention during report.

Other pain such as from an abdominal aneurysm, a "pulsating mass," that Mr. Andrew Bond reported in his "left, right lower part [abdomen], radiating to his upper abdomen" also was cause for concern. Pain and medication for its relief were frequently mentioned during shift reports.

The pain of 7H's cancer patients evoked sorrow in the nurses. When a patient's treatment by analgesic, radiation, or other means, was labeled palliative, the nurses knew that their job was to make the patient comfortable by whatever means possible. Ann reported that Mrs. Audrey Hillman was told that day that she had cervical cancer. Her "leg pain is because she's got a growth that's pressing against a nerve which is causing the pain." Ann stated that her prognosis was "not all that grand." Ann was genuinely sad as she described her patient's pain and situation.

The symptoms reported during change-of-shift report ranged in severity. Pain, especially chest pain and cancer pain, received more emphasis during report than constipation or urinary incontinence. The inability to determine a logical explanation for a patient's symptom, such as how it related to a patient's disease or the events of hospitalization, would cause a nurse to ponder the symptoms with her colleagues until an explanation or temporary solution was reached.

Symptoms of imminent death were emphasized in report. "[The] woman's not getting any better, I'll say that," said Miriam. In another report on a dying patient, Kate said, "You know, she's just . . . I mean, the woman's not gonna live that much longer. She's very old, her face is all sunken, you know, she looks dehydrated . . . Her ears are back" (a sign to some 7H nurses of death).

When a recovering patient suddenly became acutely ill, the 7H nurses documented such a change during report. For example, Ann reported:

> She went back into coma. . . . Her pupils are sluggish to react; she had no voluntary movement. She doesn't talk; she opens her eyes once in a while and that's about it. Her blood pressure shoots up and down like crazy. The last one was 160/92. But like, sometimes it shoots up to 200/110.

The nurses reviewed the events leading to the change so that those listening to report were well advised.

When a patient was progressing, such as a patient with resolving spinal cord compression, the nurses discussed the improvement. The pain sensation in a patient's legs improved, and Kate reported: "Neuro check on the legs is fine. He can stand up himself." The nurses were gratified when patients began to recover.

The nurses also noted symptoms of psychological dysfunction. When patients were confused, they were labeled "out of it." When the nurses reported unusual behavior, they provided examples to support the conclusion. "This lady also has a very strange affect. After she drinks a cup of tea every morning, she comes up and asks, 'Was I allowed to have it?' I mean, like after the fact," said Colleen. Another patient seemed depressed. The reporting nurse described him: "Last night he was in bed all night. He just seemed real lethargic. I was getting kind of worried and thought maybe they [the doctors] should draw gases [arterial blood gases], but I think it's mostly mental. I'd be depressed, too, if they told me for two days I was going for a [cardiac] cath [catherization] and biopsy and didn't go."

Reports of physiological signs and symptoms predominated during change-of-shift report. Vital signs including temperature, pulse (or heart rate), respiration, and blood pressure were frequently identified. If a patient's blood pressure was unstable, or a respiratory rate rapid and irregular, the nurses worried until those signs stabilized. A patient's blood pressure was noticeably different in each arm, so the nurses emphasized this discrepancy. "Mr. Stones. His blood pressure is different on his both arms. Left is 156/100 and right is 138/100."

Temperature was not usually mentioned during report unless a patient's temperature was elevated during or before that shift. The same situation was apparent in the cases of pulse or heart rate, respirations, and blood pressure. Abnormalities and fluctuations were identified, by such statements as Ann's: "His blood pressure is doing a little bit weird [sic] things tonight."

The characteristics of patients' excretions and secretions were described, and the presence of blood provoked concern, whether a small or large amount. After one patient had a tracheostomy tube inserted, blood oozed around the stoma and tracheostomy tube. Miriam was upset and called the doctors. "He's losing a lot of blood around it. . . . He's oozing quite a lot of blood," she reiterated, "not as much this morning as earlier when I came in. It was running down the side of his throat."

Another patient bled from his colon after a sigmoidoscopy. The suture line from his colon resection of the year before might have been bleeding. The nurses discussed the patient's frank bleeding at length. Miriam stated, "He's been having frank blood clots." "A lot, Miriam?" asked Kate. "Um hum. It was just blood," replied Miriam. The nurses passed descriptions about the characteristics of the patient's bleeding along from shift to shift and acknowledged their discomfort about it. As she reported about the bleeding of a patient with pulmonary embolus, Loretta said, "I just don't like the way he's coughing up blood. I consider it to be a lot, but he [the doctor] is aware of it." Loretta and the nurses who took responsibility for the patient on the next shift continued to watch and worry about his bleeding.

Respiratory secretions were described in some detail. "How was this sputum?" asked a nurse. "It's still thick and . . . horrible. Not as much though," replied another. In addition to secretions, the excretions of urine and stool were detailed. "They [her bowels] finally stopped going all over the place;" and "His stools were dark stools," commented Miriam.

Other signs of disease were identified through the results of diagnostic tests. Both normal and abnormal results either confirmed the effectiveness of therapy or alerted the nurses to illness. Extremely abnormal findings, such as a blood sugar of 1072, were greeted with amazement.

REPORTING ON LABORATORY STUDIES, SPECIMEN COLLECTION AND DIAGNOSTIC TESTS

The 7H nurses reported specific laboratory studies ordered for their patients. "What's he out for today?" a reporting nurse asked herself. She immediately answered, "CBC, BUN, creatinine, K, phosphorus, calcium, magnesium." Most 7H patients had laboratory studies of some type ordered daily. Fasting blood sugars and serum K (potassium) levels were the most frequently mentioned during change-of-shift report.

It was an unusual day that a 7H patient did not have a laboratory study ordered. On such a day, the reporting nurse stated, "He's not out for anything today."

In addition, the nurses noted during report if blood specimens had been collected by the laboratory technicians. Nurses awaited the results of the studies and predicted when they would receive them. Results were identified and discussed during shift report, as, "His H & H last night was 14 and 44;" "Her fasting [blood sugar] was 138, BUN was 42 and Creat 3.3. The lytes [serum electrolytes] were all within normal limits. K is 3.7." When laboratory study results were abnormal, the nurses discussed the related doctors' orders and nursing care of the patient. The actions of both nurses and doctors were directed to minimize or eliminate the problem indicated by abnormal laboratory findings.

The 7H nurses occasionally disagreed with residents about excessive ordering of laboratory studies. They saw how often the patients were "stuck" to obtain venous blood specimens. Some of their patients had so many venipunctures that the nurses were angry when they thought that the doctor was ordering tests unnecessarily. Once Sharon complained, "If she has to be typed and crossed again, I'm gonna make him [the doctor] pay for it."

The 7H nurses thought that completing forms for laboratory studies, monitoring lab slips that were "out," noting when the technicians collected specimens, and reporting and following up the results of the studies was their domain. This territory was well marked. A conversation between Sarah, who ignored the nurse manager's decision that 7H nurses were not to check on "bloods" (the results of hematologic laboratory studies), and Sharon reveals the nurses' understanding of what was their responsibility.

> SHARON: We were in meetings today and I'm not supposed to check on bloods.
>
> SARAH: You're not supposed to, but when someone's on q. 6 hours, I don't care what they say. I want to know [the results].
>
> SHARON: It's not in our job description.
>
> SARAH: Well, I don't care. Check it anyway. Like last night there was a problem with Blazeck's H & H. He [the doctor] wanted to know the result. I went through the slips. They lost the blood or something, so

I made specifically sure that H & H was out there for this morning. . . .
Just for your own peace of mind, you know . . . I don't want to look
like a fool.

Despite Deidre's wish, 7H nurses continued to be concerned with
the results of blood studies. Knowledge of these data alerted them
to imminent or actual patient problems, which they proceeded to
deal with and about which they alerted the doctors so they too
could respond therapeutically. Often medications were prescribed
on the basis of abnormal blood studies. For example, need for potassium chloride replacement was identified by the nurses during
report on the basis of lab studies, although this treatment for low
serum potassium levels required a doctor's order.

Nurses, not laboratory technicians, were responsible for collecting urine, stool, sputum, and other potentially infected secretion
specimens. Nurses reported with relief, and sometimes with sarcasm, that a specimen had been obtained from a patient thought
to be uncooperative: several nurses commented, "She actually gave
us a sputum specimen today." Collected specimens were noted on
the patient's Kardex as "done." Nurses reported their collections
during report. "We did all that last night. I got all my samples. I
was really proud of that." When a specimen was missed, 7H nurses
reported it as nearly obtained, regretting the fact that they were
unable to get it. "I told him that we need to test his stools. He had
a stool tonight and he flushed it away."

Sometimes the patients were embarrassed by requests to save
urine, stool, and sputum specimens. The nurses knew this and discussed it during report. Nevertheless, they complained when unable to get these specimens and finish some of their work.

The nurses occasionally were able to collect specimens rapidly
and to obtain blood glucose levels after a glucometer, requiring
only a blood specimen, was introduced to the unit. Although the
use of the device was not widespread initially, the nurses knew that
it would upset the laboratory technicians' sphere of responsibility
in the hospital. The nurses became upset when they realized that
there was a discrepancy between the glucometer reading and the
traditional laboratory measured blood glucose level. The nurses
demonstrated that they relied on the laboratory results as absolute
facts, even for a brief time, during shift report. The discrepancy

between both methods of collection of blood glucose studies was upsetting.

Diagnostic studies included laboratory studies, as well as endoscopies, CT (coaxial tomography) scans, barium enemas, EKG's, ultrasounds, and others. After the doctors ordered these tests, the nurses or the clerks sent request slips and scheduled them through various hospital departments and prepared the patient for the study. The preparations were described during report, along with any patient signs, symptoms, or reactions to the preparations.

The nurses were sympathetic to patients who had many diagnostic tests and to elderly patients having tests. "He is getting impatient with all of these tests, I'll tell you. . . . He's had everything. I don't blame him," said Sharon. An eighty-eight-year-old woman with congestive heart failure was scheduled for a cardiac catheterization. Sharon asked during report, "Why do they do cardiac caths on eighty-eight-year-old ladies?"

During change-of-shift report, 7H nurses described nursing care including observation of patients after diagnostics tests, such as barium enema or arteriogram. "His arteriogram was through the right groin. That site looks real good. There's no oozing; it's dry, pulses are good," said Colleen.

Implicit Functions of Change-of-Shift Report

The hidden functions of change-of-shift report illustrate the importance of the report in socializing new nurses into their role, upholding nursing standards, and maintaining nurses' responsibility for the care of patients.

COMPLAINING

The complaining of 7H nurses about their work on the unit was a form of release. In the safe forum of change-of-shift report, nurses complained about patients, hospital staff, each other, and their work. Thus their anger, hostility, powerlessness, and frustration was diverted from seemingly fruitless and possibly harmful confrontations.

Often the nurses' complaints focused on doctors. They criticized doctors' skill, doctors' interpersonal relationships with patients and nursing staff, doctors' decisions about patient care, and doctors' inaction in response to patient situations.

On one occasion, Miriam joked about a doctor who planned to teach a difficult patient, saying, "The house officer [the resident] will show him the inhaler." The nurses listening to report laughed. "You can't tell him about IV's. How do they [the doctors] expect him to understand the inhaler?" 7H nurses considered themselves to be better than doctors at teaching patients. Miriam thought that this patient would have difficulty learning to use the inhaler. "Are they going to sit over him?"

Pam worried about another patient's tachycardia (rapid heart rate). She thought that the doctor's count of her patient's heart rate was inaccurate. She described the patient's heart sounds as "racing away." Her count was 20 points higher than the doctor's.

As nurses criticized doctors' interpersonal relationships, they indirectly asked for support from their peers during report. Often the nurse describing the unpleasant interaction between a nurse and a doctor had been the target of a doctor's anger or rudeness. For example, Colleen and Kate were caring for a patient experiencing a life-threatening cardiac tamponade (accumulation of fluid in sac surrounding the heart with subsequent cardiac compression). Colleen described a doctor's treatment of Kate as the doctors inserted chest tubes in the patient. "I wanted to tell one of them to shut up. He was so obnoxious to Kate, I just felt like saying to him, 'you know, why don't you shut up.' He was so mean. . . . He was so obnoxious I couldn't believe it."

Ann questioned a doctor because a patient did not have medical clearance for his scheduled surgery, a TURP (transurethral prostatectomy). The doctor angrily said, "I'm holding you personally responsible if this man doesn't get his TURP done." "He was very rude to me," Ann said. The patient was sent to the Operating Room without medical clearance. Ann worried about the doctor's threat, saying "I don't want him retaliating against me."

A doctor shouted at the nurses listening to report in the utility room, that he wanted to do "that lumbar puncture now." The night nurse had been waiting to help him but he had delayed. When he was ready his demand could not be instantly gratified.

A nurse giving report complained about a doctor's bluntness when he told a patient that he needed a leg amputation. Colleen was critical of another doctor when he failed to order blood gases for a dying patient: "Dr. James said they don't want to do blood gases. They don't care. . . . She's going to die anyway. What difference does it make? What an attitude to take."

The 7H nurses evaluated doctor's decisions about patients and commented critically among themselves about doctors' orders when they disagreed. An elderly man with healing herpes ophthalmic skin lesions was taken off wound and skin isolation precautions by the residents' orders. Sharon sarcastically questioned this order. The extended care facility to which the patient would be discharged would not admit any patient with open skin lesions. Sharon thought the doctor's haste was related to his desire for the patient to have a rapid discharge.

It was common for 7H nurses to mock certain doctor's orders that did not fit their expectations. One doctor ordered electrocardiograms before and after the patient had chest pain. The nurses laughed; it was customary for doctors to order electrocardiograms during chest pains. Another doctor ordered that a patient's stools be hematested and given hemoglobin and hematocrit blood tests. The nurses thought it foolish to continue after the third day of this testing, since the patient's stools failed to contain occult blood and her hemoglobin and hematocrit results had been improving.

At times nurses preferred their own solutions to patients' problems over those of doctors. In one example, an aphasic patient was constipated with hardened barium after a barium enema. The nurses wanted to give the patient mineral oil by the oral route. The doctor ordered an enema. The doctor's order prevailed as the nurses complained among themselves.

The 7H nurses sometimes felt that the doctors' treatment of terminally ill patients was too aggressive. "I wonder what they'll try on him next," was an unanswered query of Sharon. A graduate nurse identified her concern about a dying patient. "I just wish they would let him go. It's so sad." Sarah agreed and commented on the poor results of the aggressive therapy: "All the salt poor albumin (IV) and Lasix is not pulling anything out. It's just not working."

During shift report nurses also criticized inaction by doctors. A doctor was unable to come to 7H to change a patient's leaking Foley catheter. The nurses resented this, though the doctor may have been legitimately busy. When a dying patient's respirations rose to forty per minute, Colleen complained that the doctors did not do anything. Some of the 7H nurses' complaints about doctors seemed to be related to the futility that nurses and doctors experience when their therapies have no positive effect on dying patients. Other criticisms reflected the nurses' desire to be treated as co-equals of doctors. At the very least, the nurses thought the doctors could be more courteous in their communications despite the stresses of patient care. Some of the nurses seemed to be afraid of threat and reprisal by doctors.

The nurses thought they knew certain areas of health care better than doctors, other hospital personnel, family members, and patients. However, nurses' defensive response to the behaviors of those who invaded their turf remained largely rhetorical. Although they dealt daily with those "invaders," they seldom confronted them face-to-face. Their complaining helped to diffuse their anger and frustration, so that patients were protected by the nurses' very complaints.

Doctors were not the sole target of nurses' complaints. Other hospital personnel were mentioned critically during report. Some of these complaints, as well as several of the criticism of doctors, were related to territorial prerogatives. If another health professional transgressed on what was perceived to be the nurse's domain, a reaction was forthcoming. For example, a speech therapist came to 7H to evaluate a patient's eating behavior. For several weeks the nurses had been feeding the patient successfully. The patient began to wear ill-fitting dentures and had difficulty eating and speaking. When the doctor noticed that "all of a sudden, he couldn't eat," he asked a speech therapist to assess the situation. The nurses, critical of the speech therapist's efforts, alluded that "Nurses know more about patients than speech therapists."

The pharmacy was a frequent recipient of negative comments. A G.N. left the unit to get IV ampicillin from the pharmacy. The pharmacy staff insisted that they had already sent two bottles of the

IV. Kate said "They didn't want to give it to her, so they charged it to the floor rather than to the patient because they said they sent two bottles." The nurses disagreed and complained about the pharmacy decision. Often the nurses were impatient with the pharmacy because medications did not arrive as rapidly as they would have liked. This was a daily problem, so the nurses' complaints about pharmacy services were frequent.

The X-ray Department was another object of complaints by nurses during shift report. "The chest X-ray I called about again for the fifth time now and they should do it today. . . . They better do it . . . for the fifth day in a row," said Sharon. This graduate nurse had sent chest X-ray requests for one of her patients on five successive days. While this number of requests for an X-ray was unusual, problems with scheduling radiologic studies were regularly aired in shift report.

The 7H nurses were critical of private duty nurses and nurses from other hospital units who "floated" to 7H or transferred patients there. An ICU nurse transferred a patient to 7H. During report, Kate criticized the nurse's knowledge of the patient, saying, "She doesn't know when the last time he had a bowel movement was." "Hm, that's good . . . ICU," another nurse replied. During another change-of-shift report, Chris criticized a private duty nurse who cared for a patient in Room 741. "There was some bloody mucus that she was getting out today, but I'll tell you I wasn't too crazy about the nurse. She made me nervous all day. She went in this far when she went to suction [the patient's tracheostomy]. What are you going to get with that?" In the example of the critical care nurse, the 7H nurse hinted that the critical care nurses, no matter how skilled, were unable to keep track of a simple but important detail, the patient's bowel movements.

The private duty nurses were generally distrusted by the 7H nurses, although there were exceptions. Some of the private duty nurses did not have the skills that 7H nurses thought they should possess. Most of their complaints about private duty nurses appeared related to invasion of territorial rights to their unit and their patients, despite the fact that the private duty nurses provided care for some 7H patients.

Occasionally nurses criticized the directives of the nurse manager during report. Deidre did not want her 7H nurses checking on the patient's blood study results. She felt that the doctors who ordered these studies bore this responsibility. It was not in the nurses' job description.

Sarah may have told Deidre that she resisted her decision. However, it was clear that the nurses continued to share the responsibility with the doctors. They continued to check the "bloods" and alerted the doctors to abnormal results.

Criticisms of 7H patients and family members were also aired during report. A patient's sister called the Nursing Office and told the evening supervisor that her sister had a cold and wanted a 7H nurse to go into her room. Ann was enraged. Instead of the patient calling for her nurse, the patient's sister notified the evening nursing supervisor. Ann checked the patient, who admitted, "My sister gets on my nerves. I don't have a cold." In another example, a nurse sarcastically commented on a patient's demanding family, "We were graced by Mary's children today. . . . It's the same old thing. She wants to know what's going on with her mother."

When relatives acted as advocates for their hospitalized family members, 7H nurses reacted with annoyance. An elderly man had a small skin lesion. Nurses, doctors, and family were aware. Pam became upset with the patient's granddaughter who questioned about the patient's skin lesion. Pam said, "He's got this skinny granddaughter that's a pharmacist. . . . She had a fit [about the lesion] yesterday. And I had a fit with her." Pam's sense of possession of 7H and its patients caused her to reject the granddaughter's justified questions on her grandfather's behalf.

The nurses reacted, again asserting their domain, when a cancer patient's wife requested a stool softener for her husband. Colleen said, "She said he uses a stool softener at home. She's a pain. She doesn't know what he needs." The nurse's reaction emphasized the fact that they considered drugs, especially laxatives, their territory and responsibility, not the family's.

Positive comments about patient's family members also were shared during report. Sharon said, "Her daughter's really good back there. She comes in and walks her . . . to the commode and takes her out of bed and stuff like that." Another positive comment about family was made by Ann: "Whoever her children are, they really wait on that women. They come in and really take care of her. They're really good." The "good" families did not complain, asked safe questions, and competently assisted with nursing care.

The nurses also complained about their patients during change-of-shift report. Most of these patients were labeled "demanding." Jenny Fister, an elderly patient with advanced heart disease, was dying slowly. Known as a demanding or complaining patient, she engendered anger and frustration in the nurses who cared for her. Mrs. Fister had been a patient on 7H for over a month; her outlook was grim and her nursing care a challenge. She never claimed to feel better. Her nurses felt encouraged that what they did for Mrs. Fister made a difference. Although they cared for Mrs. Fister daily, she never acknowledged their care. One morning during report, Miriam, an R.N. and the night nurse, explained in an agitated manner,

> I refuse to deal with this lady any more. I absolutely refuse. I mean, when she starts spitting that's it. . . . She's screaming at the top of her lungs and I told her to shut up. . . . She worked herself up to such a frenzy this morning. she says, "I'm vomiting nurse! I'm choking! I'm choking!" . . . I said, "Jenny," I said, "If you'd just shut the heck up, you're gonna . . . you'll feel a little better. If you keep screaming like this, of course you're not going to feel well. You're going to be tired too fast." So that's what's going on with her. She just has me totally miffed.

Mrs. Fister spent some of her nights screaming "for hours" by Miriam's account.

Another patient, James Baker, was criticized by Ann because he was "on the button," waiting for his pain medication. "Nothing new on him except he stays awake all night waiting for his . . . he lives for his next pain medication." Nurses openly expressed their concern about possible patient addition to narcotics. By acknowledging their concern, other nurses would scrutinize the patient's analgesic use.

Patients with organic brain syndrome, such as Michael Bennett, tried the nurses' patience. He wandered and spat, sleeping few hours during the nights. "This man, when does he sleep? . . . He's just a mess! He spits everywhere. . . . He's got B.M. on the toilet, all in the sink. Everywhere," exclaimed Miriam.

Patients who stepped out of the role of the compliant patient and took their care into their own hands aroused the nurses' ire. Sharon said that a patient "insisted he needed Dilantin. Nothing was wrong." The doctors decided to give it to him to keep him happy, despite the nurses' disapproval. Another patient took charge of his IV when the nurses were not in his room. "I went in and made rounds and he was purging it himself. 'Cause they'd [the doctors] been in there all day purging it. . . . He had the needle out, purged it, put it back in." The nurses laughed, yet realized the danger to the patient from air embolism. The patient did not know the safety measures for IV's. IV's were part of the nurses' territory.

Patients, variously labeled "a pain," "demanding" or "complaining," succeeded in "driving me nuts," one nurse admitted. Each nurse, by getting her frustration out in the open during change-of-shift report, informed the nurses at large about her reaction to specific patients and defused her own response. This sharing of personal frustration provided a safe route of ventilation for the 7H nurses. It protected the patient from the nurse's anger and gave the other nurses information about patients. A patient was difficult to deal with, and the nurse needed help in distancing herself. She would recognize a bit more objectively that the patient was ill and not coping successfully. Her peers helped her.

The nurses complained in general about how hard they worked on certain days. "We like less IV's," Ann admitted. Nurses wished aloud for fewer incontinent patients and medications.

Shift report also provided a forum for airing disappointments. Sharon had never seen kidney stones. She was upset with a nursing student's instructor: "Neither one of them thought it important enough to tell me or let me see it [a kidney stone] until after they flushed it down the toilet." "Par," one nurse commented. "Are these your first stones?" "Yeah," Sharon replied, disappointed.

Complaining was a natural reaction to the nurses' work. Shift report allowed the nurses to air their complaints so that negative effects could be diverted from patients, families, and hospital staff.

EXPRESSING HUMOR

The 7H nurses had to deal with death and other human tragedies daily. The chronically ill and terminally ill patients drained their emotional and physical resources. Although they expressed sorrow during shift report, more commonly they used jokes and sarcastic humor to help them manage the crises, the sorrow and death, the insolubility of their patients' problems, and the powerlessness of their position as nurses. Humor, like complaining, served a positive purpose.

The 7H nurses joked about doctors during report. After five months, a new resident already had a reputation with the nurses for not knowing what he should. When he ordered an insufficient dose of laxative, one nurse asked, "Whoever ordered mag [magnesium] citrate, two tablespoons p.r.n.?" a nurse asked. "You want to guess who did that?" another replied. Other unusual orders were pointed out during shift report, as the nurses joked about the doctors. "All new residents today. . . . We don't even know who they are. They don't know who they are yet. . . . Oh boy, this is the dumbest order," as she referred to the resident's nasogastric tube feeding order. Both the G.N.'s and the residents were new to their work in July, August, and September of the first year of their professional practice.

When doctors tentatively diagnosed medical diseases that the nurses thought obvious, the nurses used sarcastic humor to reveal their thoughts: "I can't understand why they think she might have diabetes." "Isador Strecker with his rule out organic brain syndrome." "Rule it out?" The nurses laughed. They were dealing with these patients constantly and could not believe the doctor's tentativeness.

When for practical as well as for scientific reasons, Stuart Cohen's doctors stopped his wound and skin precautions, the 7H nurses laughed. They knew that the skin lesions were drying and crusty, yet their fear of contracting herpes ophthalmic infection caused them to resent the doctors who wanted the patient discharged. At least the skin and wound precautions protected the nurses from pathogens. Their laughter contained traces of fear.

During report, 7H nurses laughed at themselves and their work. Loretta and Beth laughed about how difficult it was to write care plans. At the end of another report Ann jokingly asked Sharon to stay with her to help her during her shift. Sharon smilingly replied, "I can't." Ann was serious on one level but humorous on another.

The nurses often joked about their work that dealt with excreta such as testing patient's stool for blood. They laughed but were pleased for a happy patient who was thrilled that he had passed gas for the first time in months. Colleen said, "Yeah, that is good, I guess, . . . considering the way his bowels are." They joked about possible codes or cardiopulmonary arrests. Kate commented, "He also has extended wear contacts in and he had the saline solution by his bedside, but in case of an emergency . . ." Another nurse interrupted, "Whip them out before we code them." The nurses laughed.

When anticipating a patient's death, a G.N. joked nervously, "He's a little apneic. Oh, God, he's gonna go!" Her laughter was shaky. She feared her patient's death, the code that would most likely precede it, and her ability to handle her responsibilities.

When 7H nurses laughed about patient situations, they laughed at their own human frailty and at the intimate mixture of the sacred and the profane in their work. The 7H nurses' expressions of humor was a way of coping with the daily crises and the suffering of their patients. Whether joyful or tinged with sarcasm or fear, their humor provided a safe release during report for their restrained emotions.

When Meredith threatened to "plug up" a screaming patient, she merely emphasized with her humor how difficult it had been to listen to her patient's screaming for hours during the night shift. Nurses were amused by patients who lied about their age by stating that they were younger than they were. They were amused by ornery patients; by patients such as the one who "pulled out her Foley again"; by long-staying patients described as "your pal and mine"; and once by a patient's daughter who "talked her father into having chest pain" by repeatedly asking, "Daddy, you having chest pain? You sure you're not hurting in your chest?"

Patients' behavior brought humor to the nurses' report. A very ill patient got himself back in bed when the nurses were not looking. Their amazement and admiration at this determination was grudging but full of warm humor. "Do you believe him?" one nurse asked. When patients were repeatedly incontinent, the nurses laughed at each other as the report described the patient as clean and "dry for now." When two patients with skin lesions were admitted to 7H at the same time, the nurses laughingly speculated at how it would be to have them as roommates, "scratching together." They joked about an elderly woman who bounced on and off the bedpan, causing her nurse to laugh and report that she cautioned the patient to "take your time."

At times the nurses' humor was mixed with fear. An alcoholic patient had a history of DT's. The nurses laughed during report as one said, "So by the time he beats you up tonight, they'll give him some Librium." The nurses feared the violence of the patient in DT's. Another male patient was a hairdresser, and although he was married, the nurses laughed at his occupation. In fact they feared he was homosexual and possibly infected with AIDS. Although this patient had metastatic adenocarcinoma (a malignant tumor), and not AIDS, the nurses laughed in response to their fear of becoming infected.

A primary nurse reported that her patient with pleural effusion and chest tubes would likely sleep throughout the evening shift. He had been scheduled for a bronchoscopy and had received Thorazine, Demerol, and Valium at different times during the day shift. The nurse reported his last vital signs and laughed. She was glad that he would sleep, yet she was concerned about the effects of these medications on her patient's status.

Loretta laughed at her own concern as she tried to console a patient's wife. The patient had "passed out," scaring the nurses and his wife. Loretta said she was doing her "nursing duty" by providing support for this shaken woman. The patient's problem stimulated Loretta's fear that he was "coding."

The nurses' ability to joke during shift report enabled them to release some of the tension that their work engendered. Fear was sometimes mixed with humor as the nurses considered dealing with combative or infected patients. Dark humor or gallows humor was expressed nervously as 7H nurses contemplated their patients' plights and their own handling of human bodily products. Sarcastic humor was directed at hospital personnel, patients, and family members who seemed to encroach on the territory of the nurses.

EXPRESSING WORRIES

The nurses worried about their patients and themselves. When surgical patients were admitted to 7H because surgical beds were not available in the hospital, the 7H nurses repeatedly voiced their concern. Sharon asked, about a patient who had had a prostatectomy, "Why did the surgical patient come back to this floor?" A G.N. echoed her concern: "I don't think that it's all that safe for him to be here, urinating blood and whatever."

The 7H nurses knew the limits of their knowledge and skills. The nursing care of medical patients was central to their practice. Surgical patients caused them anxious moments. Sharon wished that a patient going to the Operating Room for a coronary artery by-pass graft would not return to 7H after surgery: "He better not come back here." Whether a patient had had a simple inguinal hernia repair or more complex surgery, 7H nurses, especially the G.N.'s, feared the limits of their knowledge and expertise as they cared for surgical patients.

The nurses were concerned about their patients' symptoms of disease and disability. As vital signs became unstable and abnormal, nurses who were reporting off their shift told the nurses on the incoming shift when the next measurement was due. The possibility of a fractured rib in a comatose patient and an unstable fractured hip in an elderly woman resulted in discussion with nurses and doctors so that careful, injury-preventing nursing care could be given after these problems were resolved. As nurses mentioned the possibilities of a patient's narcotic addiction or infection in a diabetic's toe, they alerted their peers to their concerns.

Colleen's worry was evident, for example, when she described her patient's perirectal skin. "It is terrible. It's worse and worse every day. Red, raw, the skin [is] just peeling off." Nurses sitting in report listened carefully to her suggestions about how to care for this patient's problems. In another example, Miriam feared that a patient who had been attacked and beaten may have been abused

by her family. Her concern was reiterated in morning report for
several days.

The suffering of cancer patients elicited sympathy from the
nurses. Ann described how a doctor had informed a patient of the
diagnosis of lung cancer when the patient's sister was present. The
elderly patient was unable to talk with Ann about her reaction even
though Ann encouraged her. Another cancer patient's situation
caused Deidre to express her anguish during report as she realized
the patient had not received the correct analgesic for his pain.
"Well that is just great. He came in for pain control and we didn't
give him anything until three o'clock." Deidre worried that the confusion in the patient's medications resulted in unnecessary patient
suffering.

The appropriateness of an anemic patient's signing one permit
for three different diagnostic procedures was discussed by Kate
during report. She worried aloud about informed consent. "All in
one permit . . . he [the doctor] wrote for the sigmoid with the co-
lonoscopy and a gastroscope and she signed it as of the third [day
of the month]. I don't know if that's still any good for her now."
Kate reassured herself and Miriam that the patient would be awake
when she "gets down there anyway." Kate was concerned about
whether the patient understood her diagnostic tests and was relieved that the doctor would have to explain the steps of the procedures to her while she was still alert.

The nurses worried about their own performance at work.
Whether evaluating their skill and efficiency at a code or their
ability to calculate and time IV fluids, 7H nurses exposed their own
vulnerabilities during shift report. At afternoon report, Chris explained her performance during the day shift by saying that she
was ill. "I probably could have done more, but I . . . I'm a little out
of it." Her virus got the best of her that day. However, she felt
compelled to work in spite of her illness because staffing was poor.

The worries that nurses had about their patients at times took
the form of premonitions. Miriam carefully explained that she had
checked a patient during the night and warned Sharon to do the
same. She recalled that she had "checked the rest of his [vital] signs
which were fine for him. . . . He's just . . . something in me . . . just
a weird feeling."

Another patient, John Sendak, was being transferred to CCU. Deidre explained her premonitions to Sharon during report.

> I'll tell you he was fine all night, but I had a funny sensation something was going to happen. Well, I took his vital signs and something was irregular. And I listened and . . . he was tachycardic. We got Dig. IV .125 [mg.]. He's got nitroglycerine. It just started all of a sudden this morning. He was nauseous. He had no specific pain. Just achy all over the chest area. . . . It was scary.

The premonitions described in report occasionally were not substantiated when patients failed to take a turn for the worse. However, when the nurses' fears were confirmed by changes in patients, these confirmations supported their taking premonitions seriously. Premonitions were reported most often by the most experienced nurses, Beth, Miriam, Kate, and Deidre. Their clinical premonitions were addressed openly in report and reminded the G.N.'s to pay attention to intuitions of this sort.

The nurses worried aloud during change-of-shift report. They worried about the conditions of patients, technical difficulties with procedures, violations of hospital policy, and repercussions from doctors. They worried about not knowing enough to help their patients and measured their own performance against the high standards of the more expert nurses.

The nurses also expressed their fears about their own safety while caring for 7H patients. They were afraid of being injured by combative patients such as alcoholic patients who might have delirium tremens or by "rammy combative" patients who "took swings" at the nurses. Two nurses had been slightly injured by two combative, confused patients, and thus fears were realistic. The 7H nurses were also afraid of becoming infected by patients with herpes zoster, tuberculosis, hepatitis, AIDS, and other communicable diseases and by patients with lice. Radiation exposure elicited similar fears. The nurses' open expressions of worry during shift report helped alert the nursing staff to these concerns.

TELLING "WAR" STORIES ABOUT PATIENTS

The 7H nurses told "war" stories about their patients. These stories were interspersed with other aspects of change-of-shift report and represented a special kind of nursing lore. More than the other aspects of report, they were shaped with the nurses' personal perspectives.

The nurses talked about their patients' lives, their tragedies, and their independent acts with enthusiasm and embellishment. These stories added relish to the discussion of facts in shift report and revealed the sympathies and compassions, as well as the tolerances, intolerances, and acceptant responses of 7H nurses toward their patients.

The nurses told stories of "what I put up with this weekend" or "what I put up with this shift" as a means of reporting to the incoming nurses of perils they had recently experienced. Kate reported one day that the unit had been "bananas" over the weekend: a confused patient hit his roommate; an elderly, confused male patient wandered into women patients' rooms and touched their breasts and genitals; and a confused man repeatedly insisted he should have certain medications.

War stories about roommates were common. Roommates were a fact of life on 7H because of the two-bed construction of the sixteen rooms. When roommates failed to get along with each other, if they quarreled, for example, over whether to watch television or listen to the radio, the nurses planned to move them as soon as possible. At times patients fought verbally about the use of the television in their room. "One of these guys has to be moved eventually," said Kate. Another example of roommate conflict emerged as "Joe got jealous yesterday. Sam got too much [nursing] attention."

One roommate delayed requesting a room change. Her chronically ill, slowly dying roommate screamed throughout the night. "She really wants a new roommate . . . but she said she's going home tomorrow and she said, 'Oh what's one more night.'" The patient endured the problem but had little rest or sleep during her hospital stay.

Roommates disagreed about the temperature of the room. Mabel Fanish was so disturbed by a cool room that she insisted that she wanted the air conditioner off. Beth talked about her during report:

> She called her roommate a crazy, confused lady. She really hurt Mrs. Stern's feelings. . . . I talked to Mrs. Fanish and told her if she would like

a private room procured, to let us know. . . . She had to understand that she had a roommate and she can't fool around like this.

When roommate situations became difficult, 7H nurses told these stories and eventually separated the parties. In this previous example, both patients were separated and slept overnight in the ADU in another part of the hospital. One patient was moved to another room the next day.

Often, complaining and demanding patients were described in nurses' stories during shift report. For example, a chronically ill and dying patient was perceived by 7H nurses as a complaining, demanding, "difficult" patient. "She won't say it [complain about anything] when they [the doctors] come in." She complained consistently to the nurses. Her diabetes, congestive heart failure, abdominal pain, and urinary tract infection continued to make her miserable. The patient's screaming during the night, and her complaints about "belly pain" and not being able to urinate upset her nurses. They could do little to effectively help her become more comfortable. "[The] woman's not getting any better, I'll say that," Miriam stated as she told the story of her patient's eventful night. When she was quieter and seemed more comfortable the nurses were pleased. She spent a quiet morning. "You can hear her now, but for the morning she was relatively quiet," said Miriam. As the patient was heard calling, "Nurse, nurse," she seemed the prototype of the complaining, demanding patient, very ill, afraid of dying and talking of death, and frequently asking the nurses for attention. The attention and comforting often seemed futile to the nurses, since only temporary periods of relief and sleep resulted. The nurses needed to tell their story of the patient and her nursing care.

Confused patients required nursing attention and warranted storytelling. They wandered out of their rooms and caught the nurses' attention. The nurses described one elderly man as confused and paranoid. The patient was on "low key suicide precautions" and had to be checked every thirty minutes by his nurses. He wandered often and escaped from the unit three times but was found by the hospital security guard. "He ran us ragged!" said Beth. The nurses placed him in restraints for his protection and so they could care for their other patients. This man also refused to take his medications. "He says that we're trying to kill him," stated Beth. Another confused man plugged the toilet in his room with paper towels. The nurse telling this story voiced her concern about what he would do next.

Patients who acted assertively or independently were sometimes praised by their nurses in stories about their behavior during report. A postoperative patient refused to take her Demerol and Vistaril. The nurses, seeming always to fear narcotic addiction, agreed with her decision. A terminally ill patient with congestive heart failure who was on fluid restriction asserted that he was watching his fluid intake yet was seen drinking a large glass of water. While the nurses disagreed with his action, they praised his independence.

Another patient with weight loss, depression, and dehydration physically resisted having a feeding tube. A nurse described her actions during report: "She had a feeding tube put in and she ripped it right out. . . . So they decided not to put another one back in because she makes such a . . . she called three of her family members." The patient put too much food into her mouth at once, "So she almost choked to death." The 7H nurses embellished their account of this determined patient.

Some patients, despite their debility, surprised the nurses with their independence and determination. Carl Sander, hospitalized with a CVA (stroke) and chest pain, was described as "weak, but he's able to stand up to his bedside commode." Chris expressed her amazement at this small victory. Mara Williams, a frequent patient in this hospital, astounded the nurses with her determination to die without heroic measures. "On the twenty-seventh she arrested. She extubated herself on the thirtieth," said Chris. Mrs. Williams removed her endotracheal tube, thus separating her connection to the respirator. Later she signed a "do not resuscitate" consent. The 7H nurses approved of Mrs. Williams's independence during their story of her situation at change-of-shift report.

There were patients whose antics 7H nurses took delight in describing during change-of-shift report. Miriam was amazed that a confused patient chewed through cloth restraints. She related in detail how another patient tried to pull out his roommate's Foley catheter.

When an elderly woman's restlessness and confusion resulted in her arm being caught between the mattress and the side rails, the nurse reported the situation calmly. Since the patient frequently challenged the nurses' ingenuity, they tended to react complacently to the newest episode in her story. Confused elderly patients often called out or "yelled" during the night and tried to get to the bathroom by climbing over their side rails.

At times the nurses disapproved of patients' behavior that they interpreted as sexually overt. They related this type of situation openly during change-of-shift report. Their stories often reflected their amusement with the situation and brought the uncomfortable matter out in the open. In one example, a patient had a scrotal suspensory ordered by his doctor. The nurses had to check that the suspensory was in place and had to order a second suspensory so that one could be washed while the other was worn. Two nurses discussed the patient:

FIRST NURSE: Does he flirt with you?

SECOND NURSE: I avoid him.

FIRST NURSE: Yeah, you have to. . . . Someone [one of the 7H nurses] came in to look at . . . the gentleman's scrotum, and he said no. But yet he seems like he's always willing for you to peek under the covers.

The nurses were uncertain how to interpret the patient's behavior. The fact that the scrotal support was ordered, that they had to check on it, and they had to keep the patient (and his genitals) clean, meant that they had to acknowledge the unavoidable sexual nature of some of their work. They handled their reactions in part by sharing an account of their experiences during report.

Another war story was stimulated by a thief who threatened the nurses and patients of 7H. During the evening shift, a thief entered a patient's room. Betty discovered the thief searching through a patient's bedside belongings. Sarah, the R.N. covering that district, chased the thief down the stairway. Both the nurses and the patients were upset, according to Meredith's account during the following morning shift report. The tale of the intruder was repeated for several days.

The nurses discussed dying patients and care of these patients during shift report. Miriam nervously described irregular breathing patterns, to convince the listening nurses of her observations, stating, "She did stop breathing momentarily. I yelled . . . you know I yelled for help and she . . . started right back up." Nurses told of patients who had been recently transferred to CCU after they "coded" during their shift. Those nurses present were told the story of the previous shift's stressful experience. A dying patient was described: "He doesn't look real good, but he doesn't look bad, you know."

The nurses predicted when patients "might not make it out of here." Colleen stated:

> I mean, this lady was not being able to breathe all morning long. And they didn't want to code her. . . . She was going out. Finally somebody decided that they were going to intubate her. . . . She was gone to-day. . . . God it was pathetic sitting there and watching somebody who can't . . . not being able to breathe.

Colleen's exaggeration emphasized her discomfiture with the patient's struggle to breathe and her suffering, and acknowledged her limited ability to help.

The nursing stories told during shift report were important enough to the nurse who was reporting that she needed to share the account with several nursing staff. Based on fact, the nursing lore contained in these stories helped both seasoned and neophyte nurses learn about patients, their nursing care, and other hospital situations that a nurse might experience. Telling these stories gave the nurses an opportunity to teach each other and to socialize.

INITIATING NEW GRADUATE NURSES TO THE ROLE OF R.N.

Change-of-shift report reflected the serious as well as the friendly nature of the 7H nurses' working and social relationships. For the new graduate, particularly the new graduate who was weak and having difficulty adjusting to the complex role of the hospital R.N., that shift report functioned as a mechanism whereby the graduate was tested, shaped, sanctioned, and accepted or rejected.

Early in the data collection period, Meredith's shortcomings became apparent. Ann questioned her in an abrupt manner about her pronunciation of the word "angina." Pam chimed in with sarcasm, criticizing the pronunciation. These episodes of criticism were frequent among these G.N.'s. Most of the nurses were gentler in their comments. Examples of Meredith's shortcomings emerged in public during report and included her confusion about where to feel pulses after a renal arteriogram, her ignorance of the abbreviation E.O.D. (every other day), her failure to report sufficient information about many of the patients for whom she cared, her confusion about which IV fluids were infusing, her insecurities about the meanings of patients' diagnoses (such as postprandial pain), and her slowness in reporting. These incidents alerted the nursing staff to her weaknesses. Meredith's reports were tension-ridden and emotionally exhausting for participants in report. While most of the R.N.'s and G.N.'s were supportive, even though somewhat impatient with Meredith, Pam and Ann, the other G.N.'s permanently staffing the evening shift, ridiculed her.

Meredith tried strenuously to adjust to the rigors of being a 7H nurse. She was preceptored and shadowed by R.N.'s and helped by Gloria, but her insecurities prevailed. She eventually agreed with Deidre that she should leave 7H and the hospital and continue her nursing career by seeking employment in a less demanding hospital.

The other G.N.'s skills and knowledge also became public during change-of-shift report. Colleen and Sharon were obviously the most skilled G.N.'s. Their performance during shift report served as some evidence of their competence. Even the seemingly most confident G.N.'s lacked confidence. They prompted each other with information such as, "They ruled out an MI on her." They laughed at each other when they had difficulty pronouncing a medical diagnosis, they tolerated a G.N.'s forgetting the anatomic location of the pubic ramus, and whether the patient's IV had 200 or 250 cc. of fluid remaining in the bag that was hanging. G.N.'s were embarrassed when their reports were long and there was confusion about facts important to their patients' welfare. Few surgical patients were admitted to 7H, but their admission stimulated fear in the G.N.'s. During one shift report, Pam's fear was obvious. A surgical patient with left pleural effusion (fluid in the intrapleural space of the left lung) was admitted to 753 Door. Pam was upset; she exclaimed, "Lord, help me." She commented that the patient's Pleur-Evac drainage system connected to an Emerson pump was bubbling more than usual. Pam asked the nurse giving report,

"Can you have both?" that is, both a hemothorax and a pneumo-thorax (blood collecting in the intrapleural space and air collection in the intrapleural space). Pam's question showed her ignorance of this fact. She may have learned this during her nursing education program but had not cared for many 7H patients with chest tubes since working as a graduate nurse. Had she worked instead on a surgical unit, she would have been more familiar with them. Her lack of experience and knowledge was revealed.

Sharon, a more confident and competent G.N. than Pam, was upset that a surgical patient was readmitted to 7H after his trans-urethral prostatectomy. During report, after several attempts to identify her discomfiture, she stated, "I don't think it's all that safe for him to be here, urinating blood or whatever." Another example of Sharon's uneasiness was evident during report. James Cannon had left 7H for the Operating Room, where he was to have a femo-ral popliteal by-pass graft (a vein graft to improve arterial circula-tion). Sharon said, "He better not come back here [to a medical unit after surgery]." She knew that her lack of knowledge about and skill with surgical patients was dangerous to those few surgical pa-tients who stayed on 7H.

The G.N.'s frequently asked questions when they were unaware of certain details of their functions. Loretta asked Miriam one morning whom she should call to request a diagnostic study. Mir-iam told her to notify Nuclear Medicine. The R.N.'s gave informa-tion and guidance freely to the G.N.'s. They were aware of the adjustment difficulties the new nurses encountered. Kate and Beth were the most supportive R.N.'s. On one occasion, Kate teased Sharon about delaying the times a patient received his medication, saying, "You and your staggers!" (Staggering a medication meant that the medication was delayed, given not at the usual time but with appropriate and safe intervals between doses.) "I want to tell you what they did to us last night, Sharon!" Sharon asked Kate whether the confusion the previous evening was her fault. Kate assured her that it was not, that she was kidding. But the unwritten message was there. It was acceptable to stagger medications occa-sionally, but making it routine disrupted the timed flow of events during subsequent shifts.

The stressful aspect of the G.N.'s adjustment to the nurse's role emerged during an incident of cardiac tamponade one evening when Kate and Colleen were on the evening shift. Kate and Colleen reported this during their district report. Luckily Kate had listened to the patient's heart sounds, and as they became duller and duller, this experienced R.N. alerted Colleen and called a doctor. The patient soon was pulseless as his pericardial sac filled and compressed his heart. Colleen ran, but had difficulty finding equipment. Kate stayed with the patient and the doctor. The patient was helped and sent to ICU. Colleen was so upset that she reviewed the event twice during report. She said that she had difficulty sleeping and looked up information about cardiac tamponade and chest tubes in the middle of the night.

An experienced R.N. who was curt with a young G.N. during report apologized after report, since she knew the young nurse had had a difficult time during her shift. The stresses of the job were obvious. Colleen once summarized a shift as she finished report and her work for the day by stating, "I hope to God that you have a nice night because today was the pits."

The R.N.'s frequently used change-of-shift report and the time immediately after report as an opportunity to teach the G.N.'s many of the details of their nursing role. The first example of this instruction occurred as Beth, an R.N. preceptor, advised Chris how to manage her patients. I'll be available for you. You'll have the preop [preoperative patient who was to receive his medications and other care immediately before surgery]. I'd like you to pick up with the primary nursing. Set a goal for each patient today." Beth and Chris reviewed the patients and their problems. Beth took the lead in the discussion and guided Chris.

Gloria gave information to Colleen about the effects of erythromycin, an antibiotic, on patients' gastrointestinal tracts. "Sometimes the patients get diarrhea and sometimes they vomit from it. . . . It's a humongous number of very upsetting pills to the GI tract." An R.N. explained how to give Imferon, an irritating parenteral iron medication, by the infrequently used Z-tract method of injection. The seasoned nurse discussed the technique in depth, identifying the specific steps of the technique.

Additional examples of this teaching of G.N.'s included the following: Kate explained to Sharon how to reorder a fasting blood sugar since the patient was "off the unit"; Beth explained to Ann the differences between a Salem sump nasogastric tube and the vita feed tubes used for nasogastric feedings; Sarah discussed with Ann the timing of intravenous ampicillin to be administered every eight hours for two doses, not every twelve hours; Kate teased Chris about remembering to write a patient's breakfast preference (oatmeal with artificial sweetener) on the Kardex. She wanted Chris to be careful with this detail as well as others; Tammy gave Pam specific instructions in the technique and amount for a patient's tube feeding; Sarah instructed Chris to add potassium chloride to an IV bag—Chris required help with the calculation of the dosage as well as with the technique; Colleen asked for and received from Beth an explanation of crescendo angina; Miriam told Colleen that a doctor gives the IV digoxin while a nurse prepares the medication, adding, "You'll have to grab one [a doctor] and [he'll] 'push' it"; Deidre corrected Sharon who said that an anxious family would "be all over here if there isn't a CCU bed," saying that more problems would arise if the patient was transferred to CCU without the family's being notified; Deidre explained to Sharon her precise method of recording absorbed intravenous fluids; and Beth described to Chris the "drift" phenomenon as patients are cooled on hypothermia blankets.

During all of these incidents of R.N.'s teaching G.N.'s, the information was given factually, kindly, and at times with gentle teasing. The G.N.'s often asked the R.N.'s, for this direction. Otherwise, it was given spontaneously and freely by the R.N.'s, who wanted to ease the new nurses into their roles.

When report moved slowly, during times that nursing students needed greater detail or G.N.'s were slowly learning their role, the seasoned nursing staff was patient. Usually the primary nurses coming on the shift listened to the previous shift's report and repeated it with expanded information for the nursing students. In this way the associate nurse could more rapidly begin her work.

One example of a report that moved slowly involved a new graduate nurse who was being oriented to the night shift. That morning, report lasted from 7:30 A.M. to 8:45 A.M. Nursing staff of Districts III and IV were upset at this, but understood that Cecile was being oriented to the night shift and had to report on all the patients. Marie, a long-tenured 7H L.G.P.N., was impatient with Cecile, as evident in her words and gestures. She asserted her need to get a fast report and stated her expectations of R.N.'s giving report. Ann, another graduate nurse, and Camille, an L.G.P.N., were verbally supportive of Cecile. Cecile was obviously fatigued. She became confused about a few facts, yet was able to correct this. Some of Cecile's inaccuracies were corrected by the R.N.'s receiving report. Both Beth and Tammy, seasoned R.N.'s, corrected Cecile kindly yet firmly. They were understanding and supportive. Yet there was an unspoken "You'd better meet our expectations" present in their manner. Clearly there was an acceptable time limit for reports at change-of-shift. About forty-five minutes was the unspoken, acceptable time limit for report on all four districts. While nursing students and G.N.'s were given more latitude with this rule, the ability to give a concise, factual report was a highly valued R.N. behavior. Using more time than acceptable upset the staff and disrupted their care during the shift. Change-of-shift report provided an opportunity for the seasoned nursing staff, R.N.'s, L.G.P.N.'S and nursing assistants to communicate their expectations to the G.N.'s and for the G.N.'s to expose their skills before a critical but sympathetic audience.

WARNINGS AND ACKNOWLEDGMENTS OF ERRORS

Nurses used change-of-shift report to review potential patient problems, to warn about problem situations, to air lack of knowledge, and to acknowledge errors.

The following are examples of warnings about potential patient problems: the spinal precautions needed for a postoperative patient who had spinal anesthesia; a medication that had to be given at 10 P.M.; and a dosage change of Slow K, a potassium replacement medication, because a patient's serum potassium level was decreased. In these instances, the nurses were alerted so that appropriate and therapeutic action could be taken. These warnings further helped to prevent confusion and error. Similarly, the nurses used reminders to alert other nurses that a patient who was not eating well had to be fed, that Kardex care plans and medication Kardexes needed to be written, and that another dose of medication had to be given.

During report nurses openly acknowledged their ignorance. Often questions were asked; nurses contributed information or admitted their lack of it. An example of this involved a question about an unfamiliar drug. The discussion that followed alerted the nurses to the fact that most knew little about this drug and served as a warning that they needed to be cautious and learn more about it.

Warning, reminding, and airing lack of knowledge helped the nurses avoid errors. Nevertheless, errors happened. Nurses were careful to correct inaccurate information as they recognized it during report. They also acknowledged their own errors and those of other nurses, so that the nurses of each shift could help them correct a situation if possible, or at best help to minimize any harmful effects on patients. Report also provided the nurses with the opportunity to check the accuracy of those sections of the Kardex related to tests, medications, and nursing care. The nurses were able to check the information that they obtained about patients against what was written on the Kardex. When doubts or conflicts arose, they checked the doctor's order sheets after report or discussed the facts as they knew them during report.

Report helped the nurses to take stock of the work they had in store in the next shift as well as to review the work of the previous shift. In fact, after report on a patient, one of the G.N.'s declared, "See how I pick all these things up when I'm kind of settled down? That's why I hate to rush—the hustle and bustle—and take all these people [patients] when everything's going on at one time." Her comments emphasized the respite or freezing of time that shift report provided. Report also helped nurses audit the nursing care given during the shift.

Change-of-shift reports contained many acknowledgments of error. Report was like an open confessional that enabled them to receive the support of their peers and to confront the fact that sometimes they did harm to patients, although unintentionally. Accidents and errors happened and flew in the face of the unspoken warning of nursing learned as nursing students: Never make mistakes; your mistakes take their toll in human terms—you deal with vulnerable people."

Incidents that happened despite the nurses' vigilance were treated as error. Although a nurse may not have been able to stop the event from occurring, she was responsible and therefore culpable. "Joe's been wandering, up and walking. He fell last night," was reported. It was stated almost matter-of-factly that another patient had fallen four times despite nursing watchfulness. Some of the elderly patients fell as they became disoriented. If the nurse did not anticipate the fall and restrain the patient, she was to blame. An incident report documented the error in writing. But the nurse's acknowledgment during report made public her responsibility and blame.

Some errors were due to inaccurate transcription or interpretation of orders or other mishandling of records. This type of error was discovered in the abundant hospital records that tracked a patient's hospital experience. They were frequently identified during shift report. Camille, an L.G.P.N., discovered that a medical clerk had incorrectly transcribed an order for compresses from the doctors' order sheet to the nursing care Kardex. "Warm" compresses was mistakenly transcribed and carried out. The original order had specified room temperature compresses. Ann acknowledged during report that she had assumed a patient's "daily PT" was for physical therapy. The patient went to physical therapy. Instead, the PT was prothrombin time, a laboratory blood study. Sarah suddenly realized during report that she had thrown out an intake and output sheet, thus making accurate recording of a patient's IV's difficult. Her disgust with herself was obvious as she considered the ramifications of her action. Sarah's warning to those nurses listening to report alerted them not to repeat her mistake.

Medication errors, with drugs as well as intravenous fluids, were highlighted during shift report. When a patient's IV ran out, it was seen by the nurses as error. "My shift, my fault, my responsibility," Beth admitted. Another example of an error involving IV fluids involved the hanging of the incorrect percentage of saline. Miriam stated, "Last night when we came in she had D5 1/4 [saline hanging] instead of D5 1/2, so just so you know. We changed it and we wrote out an incident report on it."

Errors also happened because nurses were not sure of specific information. A patient had a collapsed lung. The doctors inserted a chest tube to help reinflate his lung. The chest tube was connected to underwater seal drainage, which was connected to suction. A G.N. failed to question why the suction was turned off. Later the patient's lung deflated again. There was an additional problem with the underwater seal tube. The G.N., insecure in her knowledge about chest suction and drainage, had failed to question the other nurses. She did not know what to recognize as incorrect in relation to the chest tube drainage system as she cared for the patient. Her error was described in detail during report.

When Sarah, a seasoned R.N., canceled a doctor's order for neurological checks on a patient, another seasoned R.N. discussed this during report. Miriam asked critically "Who gave you the order to D/C the neuro checks?" "Sarah," one of the nurses replied. Miriam explained that the patient's condition warranted continuation of the neurological checks. Her doctor had ordered these checks to help evaluate her status. Sarah made an error by overstepping her domain into that of medicine. She was challenged and gently criticized by her peers during shift report.

MONITORING NURSING CARE

The 7H nurses used change-of-shift report as a means to set standards and maintain standards of nursing care. During shift report, negative criticism prevailed, not praise for work well done.

A hearing aid was lost. The owner was a terminally ill patient whose private duty nurse reported it missing. Two days and several shifts later, another private duty nurse discovered it in his room. The 7H staff nurses criticized the private duty nurses' failure to keep track of the hearing aid.

During one report Pam incorrectly reported that a patient's right arm should be checked after an arterial catheterization. The patient's arterial puncture site was in the right groin. One shift report later, Tammy divulged Pam's error. Pam could not have correctly checked the arterial site the previous evening. She had reported unsubstantiated information.

There was competition evident among the three shifts as the

nurses reported. If one shift was more skillful than another, this was proclaimed during report. Sarah stated with pride that the day shift nurses had no problem with one patient's tracheostomy tube. The night nurses had to call the supervisor and the respiratory therapist for assistance with the tube. The night nurses were unable to get the troublesome inner cannula out for cleaning. When the day shift nurses came, "Mabel went in there this morning and zip, zap she got it out." The day nurses reveled in their success.

The nurses occasionally criticized the techniques of the nurses working other shifts. For a few days the night nurses wasted Isocal, a nutritional supplement, for a patient's tube feeding. They poured too much liquid supplement into the bag that dripped into the patient's tube. "Do me a favor with the Isocal," said Ann. "Don't put so much up, and ice it. We throw it out." The nurses were tired of wasting the supplement and considered it important to correct the other nurses' technique. Failing to ice the feeding tube could have resulted in the patient's getting diarrhea from bacterial growth in the bag and tubing.

The nurses also sanctioned other nurses when safe patient care was violated. Beth questioned the previous shift as she listened to report on one of her patients. Her patient's casted arm had been restrained a few days before. After the cast was removed, Beth worried. "They didn't restrain the arm that was casted, did they?" As she checked on the previous two shifts, she was most interested in the protection of her patient and in the maintenance of safe nursing care.

The 7H nurses alerted those listening to report to the fact that certain information had not been passed from shift to shift. Two examples show how the nurses brought omissions to each other's attention. The day nurses were not notified that a patient refused to accept an Imferon injection. The primary nurse on the day shift complained. "No. It wasn't passed on to me. So this morning it took me half an hour to figure out why . . . it wasn't signed out." Time was wasted and worry prolonged because information about a medication had not been shared during shift report.

The evening shift nurses forgot to report that a patient did not urinate during the shift. The night nurse criticized this. "They didn't tell me that she didn't void all night on their shift. I didn't know until I looked at the I & O sheet." Both examples served as reminders to staff, including those who eventually heard the reminder through the "grapevine" of shift report, that important details were not to be omitted during report.

When the nurses who listened to report later found their patients' situations to be noticeably different from what had been described, they were critical. Ann criticized Meredith during report: "See, Meredith's report today, on her IV's, they were a little screwy." When Ann checked on her patient's IV bag, she had found a discrepancy in the amount of fluid remaining. She had to bring this information to the attention of the next shift. Otherwise, the IV intake would continue to be inaccurate, along with the patient's intake and output record.

The most frequent criticism involved those nurses whose patients required respiratory suctioning. Beth found a patient to be full of "gunk." "Why don't they [the night nurses, specifically the L.G.P.N.'s] suction?" she asked. Mabel observed that her patient with a tracheostomy had crusted secretions blocking the inner cannula. "It was like crusted in the inside. I don't know how long it was sitting there. It's ridiculous."

Through the mechanism of shift report, concerns made their way to the nurse manager and assistant nurse manager and also to those nurses who were directly responsible. One nurse, criticized for her failure to suction a patient, responded to this allegation during report, saying, "I suctioned him. I mean I cleaned it [the inner cannula of tracheatomy tube]! 'Cause somebody said I wasn't cleaning it [tube] and I was. . . . I might've missed last night, though."

Interruptions During Shift Report

Change-of-shift report progressed despite the many distractions and interruptions of 7H unit life. The most obvious distraction during report was noise. For example, a nurse flushed the utility room hopper beside the table where the nurses sat; a nurse in the hall called to a confused and wandering patient: "Sam, don't go away"; a patient sang a few lines of a song; another patient called, "Nurse, please help me"; and a Housekeeping employee removed trash from the utility room trash receptacle. Aside from frowns, no comments were made to these distractions, except to the patient's request for help as a nurse listening to report expressed the hope someone would attend to the patient. On occasion the level of noise was so loud in the utility room from staff's voices, moving equipment, and running water that the reporting stopped for a few seconds until it became quieter.

As shift report flowed, patient after patient, district after district, 7H nurses permitted certain interruptions. The most frequent interruptions were associated with questions or problems with controlled drugs or narcotics. For example, Miriam forgot to "sign out" a narcotic. The "count was off," so that the nurses counting the drugs were forced to interrupt report. In addition, searches were frequently conducted for narcotic keys to unlock the controlled drug drawer of the medication cart. Comments such as, "Keys, keys!" "Who has the keys?" or "Excuse me, can I have the keys, please?" stopped report as the nurses in the utility room searched themselves or thought about which nurse had the keys last.

When the narcotic count was off, it was imperative that the nurses doing the count intercept those nurses going off the shift so that the count could be corrected. When Kate discovered two Percocets and ten morphine sulfate tablets missing, she was quick to get an answer for this outrageous discrepancy. The nurses giving report were responsible. If they had left the unit before this was settled, the serious discrepancy in the narcotic count would be compounded.

Patient signs and symptoms were the second most frequent reason that shift report was interrupted. Often this interruption was a fact-giving or fact-receiving incident. Sarah commented, "Colleen, excuse me. The new patient's got diarrhea. They just cleaned her up. . . . So I went back to take her vital signs and she had the chills really bad—she was shaking and sweating. . . . So I called Dr. Thomas. He is aware of it." Another example concerned a patient's extraordinarily high blood sugar level. "Mary Crowley's 3 P.M. [blood sugar]?" asked Colleen. "688," replied Sharon. "Oh definitely 688. No wonder the woman doesn't feel well," said Colleen. Another interruption was provided by Dotty, an L.G.P.N. "He's holding steady, his vital signs. . . . He's still groggy."

These interruptions had a sense of urgency about them. The nurses giving report were relieved to have the information about a patient with whom they had been concerned. One of the 7H nurses was "covering" these unstable patients as others attended report.

The most dramatic interruption occurred as the nurses reacted to a patient's chest pain. Sarah, who was giving report, stopped abruptly and left the utility room to check on her patient.

When doctors interrupted report, the nurses weighed the importance of their interruption. Was the request or reason for disrupting the nurses' sacrosanct time worthy of the nurses' attention? Miriam was noncommittal as a resident asked her for the medication Kardex during morning shift report. She matter-of-factly tolerated the disruption. He stopped Miriam again for another Kardex, telling the nurses he would return it. Later as he casually dropped the Kardexes on the utility room table during report, Miriam commented disapprovingly. "That resident, see where he throws the Kardexes." Apparently this medical interruption was unjustified.

Another example of an interruption by a doctor occurred when a doctor inquired about a patient's medication dosage. The doctor's voice was controlled but angry. The nurses, Meredith and Ann, were embarrassed and upset. A patient was not receiving as much Lasix as he had ordered. The nurses admitted the medication error to the doctor and discussed the problem after he left the utility room. They agreed that he had a right to interrupt and to be angry.

A doctor was looking for Chris. Chris had been caring for a patient when this doctor had inserted a subclavian catheter. An accidental pneumothorax resulted from this catheter insertion, so the doctor's interruption was tolerated by the nurses. The incident report had to be completed.

If a nurse coming on duty was unable to find where her assigned district's report was taking place, she felt free to interrupt report. "What? Are we [having our district report] in here?" was a common question during this interruption. "They're down the hall" (in Deidre's office or less commonly in an empty patient room) was the usual reply. After these interruptions, report flowed on, seemingly undisturbed.

When Escort Service personnel interrupted report, the nurses accepted the interruption as legitimate since it concerned their patients, yet they often acted annoyed, since nurses not listening to report would have been found to receive the patient and help the Escort Staff get the patient back into bed. "D'Amico," the Escort Staff announced at the door of the utility room. "O.K., we're giving report now. Is anybody at the desk?" Sarah answered. The Escort Staff replied, "I don't see anybody out here." Since the nurses in report were not ready to stop report and help him, he searched for and found another nurse.

When a nurse giving report omitted a fact about a patient, she interrupted report and asked permission to go back to a patient who had already been discussed. Going out of order was somehow a flaw in report giving, yet it was tolerated. The nurses apologized to each other at this interruption as they requested permission to go back.

Other interruptions were also tolerated and seemed to be considered inevitable by the nurses. Patients who walked into the utility room to weigh themselves were greeted and helped briefly. "I was a hundred pounds when I came here," one patient announced. Report resumed. Telephone calls stopped report abruptly as nurses dealt with receiving patient information they had been awaiting. A laboratory technician interrupted during morning report to inquire whether a patient had anything to eat: "Excuse me. Evans, did she have anything to eat?" "What room?" asked Miriam. "749." "Not that I know of," Miriam replied. The nurses did not resent interruptions dealing with laboratory studies or other diagnostic studies. They saw these interruptions as acceptable and part of their responsibility.

Nurses, doctors, medical clerks, escort staff, and other hospital personnel always seemed to be looking for elusive patient charts. Since the chart was the chief source of important patient data, interruptions for charts were accceptable and seldom treated with annoyance. Other interruptions involved inquiries about equipment, such as where a Gomco machine was located, and by a family member, such as a daughter who wanted to know whether her father could have juice to drink.

Rarely did Deidre interrupt report. On one occasion when she did it was to set standards about the quality of nursing care on 7H. Deidre took a strong position as she chastised Ann in the presence of the other nurses. The previous evening shift had been busy. Ann delayed answering a patient's call light. The patient had urinary frequency and often needed help with a bedpan.

> ANN: Well, I told her that there was a possibility that the light may be on and we may not be able to answer right away.
>
> DEIDRE: But it doesn't mean that when you go in, you get nasty with her. I just want you to know where I stand on it. I don't want anyone on the floor becoming nasty to a patient.
>
> ANN: Yeah, we're not.
>
> DEIDRE: . . . and just get that across to your staff, too.

Deidre's controlled anger was obvious as she used the open forum of report to focus on a patient care issue and to put the evening staff on notice that their performance was being scrutinized and criticized. Another example involved Deidre's interrupting report because Pam's behavior was "short." Pam left the utility room in response to Deidre's request. "I want to see you right now." Standards of nursing behavior were again set straightforwardly by Deidre.

Seldom did the nurse's personal needs interrupt report. When Chris became ill, report stopped briefly, then resumed.

One report was interrupted by an R.N.'s giving support to a G.N. Miriam, about to give report, offered to help Suzanne finish her night shift work.

> MIRIAM: Is there anything else I can do for you? I'm just giving out the eight o'clocks [medications].
>
> SUZANNE: I just have to hang this D5 and water.
>
> MIRIAM: O.K. I'll hang it.

These nurse-initiated interruptions were more acceptable than interruptions by doctors or escort staff.

Other justified interruptions were those concerning patient welfare and details of the nurses' work. Unjustified interruptions, such as those by doctors, were associated with the nurses' unspoken need to maintain shift report as their forum and domain, sacrosanct and separate from outsiders.

Shift Report—The Domain of the R.N.

The R.N. or G.N. giving report sat at the table or desk with the staff taking report. While L.G.P.N.'s also sat at the small table, the direction of report information was distinctly R.N. to R.N. The R.N.'s shared the Kardex, as the R.N. giving report moved through it, patient by patient.

L.G.P.N.'s and nursing assistants once complained that the R.N.'s failed to ask them whether they knew the patients. Instead, R.N. asked R.N. or G.N. and disregarded the fact that the other nursing staff might be able to make contributions. The L.G.P.N.'s and nursing assistants asserted their right to be present at report and share in the information exchange. When Caroline, a nursing assistant, missed part of report because Meredith became confused about who her "ancillary" was, Meredith was questioned. "Didn't you . . . you already knew I was working with you," said Caroline. Meredith admitted, "I forgot."

In this instance, report stopped and the patient who had already been discussed was reviewed. This type of assertion by L.G.P.N.'s and nursing assistants was infrequent.

L.G.P.N.'s and nursing assistants occasionally offered information during report, such as whether a patient had had a diagnostic test or the recent appearance of a bedsore. Most often they quietly listened as the R.N.'s exchanged facts and thoughts.

Report demonstrated that the R.N. held a higher status than the L.G.P.N. and was a main actor among the nursing staff. When an L.G.P.N. initiated a suggestion to move a patient to a Clinitron bed, an R.N. abruptly discarded the idea, as she offered her reasons. The suggestions stopped there. Giving shift report was a test of proficiency for the R.N. For example, one afternoon Sarah became upset when she had to report on the patients in her own district as well as Colleen's, since Colleen had gone to a meeting. Sarah did not feel knowledgeable about Colleen's patients. She apologized at report for not knowing Colleen's patients as well as those in her district. After that, she proceeded to give an extremely detailed report.

Kristen, the clinical director of 7H and Deidre's immediate superior, explained the importance of change-of-shift report.

> Vital. If you have true primary nursing—the ideal, an every sixteen hour report would be sufficient. But patients change so rapidly here. And we have a lot of per diems, so. . . .
>
> The change-of-shift report is like a relay race where the flag is passed to the next person before she starts running. Change-of-shift reports *have* to be. . . . Before we had trouble here. There was one hour before the end of shift when people [nurses] geared down. No one [patient] was transferred. . . . We have changed that. During change-of-shift I want things to go on. The floor's patients should have nurses covering more districts while other nurses listen to report. The patient's lights need to be answered. Their needs should be met.
>
> Change-of-shift means, well, it's their patient. They "own" the patient. Change-of-shift report is a transfer of ownership. It's a chance to affiliate with the person they share the patient with. It's mutual sharing. . . .
>
> Certain people don't like to follow others [from one shift to another]. There are subtle attempts to modify behavior. A nurse might say "be sure to do—" in a subtle attempt to keep the nurse receiving report accountable and maintaining a standard for the patient. A "stake" in the patient for what should continue, and if the standard does not continue, to "call" that person on it.

Kristen emphasized the nonverbal ways nurses kept their less skilled peers accountable for high standards of patient care. An example of overt standard setting emerged during shift report. "Great. They changed this. . . . I don't know who the hell's taking off these orders. Excuse me," Miriam exclaimed. "She recopied the Lasix when it's right here and she didn't yellow out [strike out with magic marker when medication is canceled] the Phospho-soda," replied Sarah. Whether subtle or overt, it was evident that the R.N.'s kept high standards of practice before each other through the vehicle of shift report.

Change-of-shift report was clearly "owned" by the professional nurses, R.N.'s and G.N.'s soon to be R.N.'s.

The Language of Change-of-Shift Report

The 7H nurses used a hospital-bound and nursing-specific language during report. This language defied comprehension by uninitiated nursing students. Incorrect grammar was blended with this language and further confused the uninitiated. Confusion was apparent among the beginning nursing students listening to change-of-shift report together with the nurses of a district. The nursing instructor accompanying the students often translated the meanings of the alien terms. In fact, after regular shift report ended, the primary nurses of each district sat in the utility room with the nursing students and carefully pored over the details about the patients for whom the students would care during that shift.

While the doctors might understand and share with the nurses some common terms and abbreviations, it was obvious that the nurses used their own terms and meanings.

Among the phrases used by the nurses as they referred to diagnostic studies were: "out for lytes"—the patient had blood electrolytes; "going for an echo"—the patient was scheduled for an echocardiogram that day; "having an H & H"—the patient was scheduled for hemoglobin and hematocrit blood studies; "We need a UA and C & S on him"—the nurses had to obtain urine specimens so that a routine urinalysis and a culture and sensitivity could be done by the laboratory personnel after the specimens were picked up; "She went into SVT [supraventricular tachycardia], so they stopped the test. They're going to do a resting stress today"—the patient would have a resting cardiac stress test; and "He's for nothing today"—the patient had neither laboratory studies nor other diagnostic tests scheduled that day. "He's for a lot today"—the patient has many diagnostic tests.

Words were omitted as the nurses rapidly exchanged the messages of change-of-shift report. Abbreviations were the rule, not the exception. Patients were often introduced during report by name and room number, and medical diagnosis such as "Rule out P/E"—rule out, or eliminate through diagnostic tests, pulmonary embolus: "This man has a history of CABG [pronounced "cabbage"—coronary artery bypass graft] times two," said Beth. This demonstrated how acronyms became hospital neologisms. Another example was Sharon's statement that, "Mr. Adams went for a 'fem pop' bypass," indicating to the nurses that the patient had vascular surgery, a femoral popliteal bypass graft. "Fem pop" meant nothing to those uninitiated to hospital language. If a patient had "bag #3 hanging," the nurses understood that they had to check the Kardex to confirm the IV order. Usually the reporting nurse identified the exact IV hanging, including added medications, drop rate or amount of cubic centimeters per hour to be infused, and the remaining amount of fluid "credited" or left hanging in the patient's IV bag at the start of a new shift. Beth reported, "It's #3. D_5W [5 percent dextrose in water] with 12,500 units of heparin going at 28 [drops per minute] on the pump. And your credit is 200."

Some phrases used by the nurses had their roots in Latin and have been used in hospitals for many years. "OOB ad lib," that is, out of bed as libitum, combined an abbreviation with truncated Latin.

Other examples of uncommon language used during shift report and also shared with doctors included, "Push some Lasix on her tonight"—the patient was going to receive IV Lasix in a bolus or concentrated dosage; "She scarfed down a Jello and a tapioca"— ate food rapidly and voraciously; and "He's a little tacky"— the patient had tachycardia, or rapid heart rate.

Language more characteristic of nurses was also used in report. Being an initiated nurse guaranteed comprehension of this language. "A walkie-talkie" meant the patient was well enough to walk without the help of the nurses and held conversations with ease; "I tore the drawer down looking" meant the nurse took everything out of the patient's medication drawer as she looked for a missing medication; and "She gets decube care and a donut to the rear" meant that the patient had a decubitus ulcer over the sacrum, a treatment was ordered and pressure on the ulcerated area was to be relieved by positioning with an air-inflated, doughnut-shaped, rubber ring.

The use of the word "out," as in "He's out for lytes today," was used to communicate that the nurses had checked on ordered diagnostic studies, scheduled some of these by telephone, and sent slips to specific hospital departments.

When nurses reported "screening" or "blocking" a patient's room during report, the nurses understood that only one patient occupied the two-bed, semi-private room. "Screening" or "blocking" a room was a nursing comment on a patient's degree of mental confusion, or on the seriously ill, ventilator-dependent patient who needed more space for the life-maintaining equipment next to him. The Admissions Department would not schedule a patient admission or transfer to that room.

Two verbatim transcriptions of shift report confirmed the subcultural language of report.

> The new bag is up and it's hanging there on the pole ready for you to hang. O.K. She's out just for the daily PT and PTT. We don't have yesterday's results there. She's on hematest stools and I have not seen anything done. She's had a dose of Coumadin last night, 7.5 mg.
>
> Sternberg in the window with her rule out syncope and severe headaches. Out of bed with assistance. Routine signs. She's been fine as far as her vital signs. She's out for fasting enzymes this morning, lytes. Still need a UA on her, EKG, chest [X-ray] and she has to be scheduled for a twenty-four-hour Holter. She was going absolutely buggy from her roommate in there this morning and asked for a Valium, which she does not have ordered. I spoke to Dr. Small about it. He doesn't want to give her anything that might have a central nervous system depression.

The terminology learned by 7H nurses as students was too lengthy for shift report. Efficiency stimulated creative abbreviation. The special in-group language kept report confusing to the uninitiated. A nurse translator who understood this special language gradually initiated neophytes to the nursing subculture.

Completing Unfinished Business and Passing on Responsibility: Nursing Ritual

During shift report, 7H nurses frequently identified unfinished work. Nurses felt responsible for work begun or work they were "aware of" but had not completed, and they asked each other for help. When a primary nurse was unable to remove a patient's INT

(IV access), she asked the incoming primary nurse to take it out. The nurse on the next shift agreed.

A nurse reporting off occasionally offered to complete work, even if the work had begun close to the time of shift report. For example, Loretta told Pam that she would finish taking off recently written doctor's orders, saying "He has a new IV order. I'll take these off when I go back out." The nurses felt responsible for work begun on their shift.

When a patient's Theodur blood level was not at a therapeutic level, the night nurse emphasized this during report so that the day nurse would talk to the doctors about increasing the patient's Theodur medication. The day shift nurse shared her concern and informed the doctor.

Another example of unfinished business that involved nurses and doctors was unclear orders about bed rest and the activity status of patients. A nurse questioned the reason for a bed-rest order since her patient was "alert and oriented." She or the nurse on the next shift planned to question the doctor about his intent. Another patient needed to be continued on her nightly dose of Tranxene, a nervous system depressant drug. Beth repeated, "And we need an order for Tranxene. She used to take it at home and they wrote an order, but they wrote it for 10 A.M. which wasn't the brightest thing. She's to get it at bedtime."

The nurses anxiously awaited other reports of unfinished business, such as unreported laboratory study results, and told the incoming shift's nurses of their concern. When waiting for a 3 P.M. blood sugar result, the reporting nurse stated, "It [fasting blood sugar] was 396 and she was out for a 3 [P.M.]. Since the blood sugar was elevated there was some concern about the 3 P.M. result." Laboratory studies were always a part of the nurses shift-to-shift unfinished business.

On a symbolic level, change-of-shift report represented the nurses' taking on the responsibility for their patients. Patients were "owned" by the nurses and ownership was passed from shift to shift. It was shared or corporate in the sense that several nurses "owned" a patient during his or her hospitalization. Nurses spoke of "my patients" as they described their specific domain of responsibility.

Change-of-shift report emphasized the continuous, temporal nature of the hospital and the nursing unit. Patients were "covered" by means of reports and by the nursing staff's need to protect patients with a blanket of twenty-four-hour responsibility and accountability. The nurses of 7H took their responsibility of caring for patients seriously and transferred this responsibility from shift to shift by the vehicle of the change-of-shift report. Shift report helped the nurses to freeze or suspend time, so that they were able to focus on events and facts specific to their patients.

As an occupational ritual, change-of-shift report was a stage where nurses learned what it meant to be a nurse. Here the goals and values of nursing were taught and reemphasized.

Appendix 1: Post-Mortem Notification, Documentation, and Care: *Hospital Policy and Procedure Manual*

DEPARTMENT/DIVISION:	SUBJECT:
Nursing, Pathology Unit Management	Post-Mortem Notification, Documentation & Care

I. PURPOSE

To establish guidelines to be followed in the event of a patient's death.

II. GOAL

To insure that in the event of a patient's death, all the appropriate people are notified, all necessary forms and medical record documentation is completed, authorization for autopsy is obtained when applicable, and the body is cared for appropriately.

III. DEFINITION OF TERMS

Next of kin in order of survival:

1. Spouse
2. Adult children
3. Adult grandchildren
4. Parents
5. Brothers or sisters
6. Nephews or nieces
7. Grandparents
8. Uncles or aunts
9. Cousins
10. Stepchildren
11. Relatives or next of kin of previously deceased spouse

IV. GENERAL DESCRIPTION OF SCOPE AND PROCESS

A. The physician is responsible for:

1. Examining a patient and pronouncing death.

2. Notifying next of kin and, if they are not present at the hospital at that time, determining if they wish to view the body.

3. Obtaining next of kin's permission for post-mortem care when appropriate. (See "Authorization for Autopsy" in memo entitled, "Deaths Reportable to Medical Examiner's Office" contained in Nursing Service Policy Manual, Vol. II, Section V.)

4. Determining if death should be reported to the Medical Examiner's Office. (See memo entitled, "Deaths Reportable to Medical Examiner's Office," Nursing Service Manual, Vol. II, Section V.)

5. Completing the following forms:

   a. Certificate of Death (original and one copy)

   OR

   Medical Examiner's Notice *and* Pronouncement of Death (original and copy). (NOTE: A Certificate of Death is not completed if the Medical Examiner takes jurisdiction.)

   b. Undertaker/Coroner Release Receipt (one copy) (C-356).

   c. Post-mortem Examination Permit Form (C-255). (NOTE: This form is not complete unless signed by the next of kin and the physician who witnessed the signature.)

B. The RN is responsible for:

1. The disposition of the patient's valuables/belongings (see policy #A01-020 *Valuables Bag*).

2. Providing post-mortem care for the body or delegating this responsibility to an associate (RN, LPN, NA or supervised SN).

3. Verifying the patient's identity before the body is removed from the unit.

4. Insuring that the required information is documented in the medical chart (Post-mortem stamp—see appendix).

5. Notifying the clergy when appropriate.

6. Carrying out responsibilities of unit clerk when he/she is absent.

C. The Medical Clerk (or nurse in the absence of a clerk) is responsible for:

1. Notifying:

    a. The information desk (ext. 1416) (0800–2000, Mon.–Sat.; 1100–2000, Sun.)

    b. The telephone operator (ext. 2060).

    c. Admissions (ext. 3056).

    d. Unit Management

        (1) During the week

            (a) 0800–1700 Unit Management Office (ext. 8016).

            (b) 1700–2400 Unit Management evening clerk (beeper 7514).

        (2) Weekends/Holidays

            (a) 8088–1630 Unit Manager on duty.

            (b) 1630–2400 Unit Management evening clerk (beeper 7514).

    e. Night Patient Care Coordinator 2400–0800.

    f. The Department of Radiation Physics (ext. 2571, 3462) for patients who have been treated with radiopharmaceuticals or sealed sources of radioisotopes.

  2. Stamping the Nurses' Notes/Integrated Process Notes with the "Post-Mortem Stamp."

  3. Insuring that the completed medical chart is hand carried to:

    a. Unit Management Office (0800–2400)

    b. Nursing Office (2400–0800)

D. Responsibilities for the care of Fetal/Infant Remains are delineated in Policy #A01-068.0 *Fetal Infant Remains*.

V. EQUIPMENT
Valuables Bag

Shroud Pack

  Plastic shroud sheet
  Chin strap
  Cellulose pads
  3 identification tags
  3 36″ ties
  2 60″ ties

Bath Equipment

ABD pads

VI. PROCEDURE: POST-MORTEM CARE OF THE BODY
   A. Screen bed and place patient in dorsal recumbent position.
   B. Remove jewelry whenever possible, label and place in valuables envelope.
   C. Close eyelids and wash body.
   D. Insert dentures in mouth or label, place in cup, and send with patient.
   E. Place a rolled towel under the chin to prop the mouth closed (remove towel before body is viewed by family) and cover with a body sheet.
   F. After the family has viewed the body:
      1. Rolling patient side to side, place shroud beneath the body leaving enough room at head and foot to fold over. Apply cellulose pad or ABD pad.
      2. Apply chin strap.
      3. Fold arms over abdomen, pad wrists with ABD pad, and tie together.
   G. Verify identity with patient's ID bracelet and attach addressographed ID tag to toe.
   H. Fold and secure shroud sheet around body with ties.
   I. Fasten second addressographed tag on outer tie at wrist.
   J. Notify escort to remove the body to the morgue.

VII. SAFETY, CARE AND MAINTENANCE
   A. If the patient died in Isolation, follow appropriate Isolation precautions. (Policy #A40-412.1 *Care of the Body after Death Isolation Precautions.*)
   B. If the patient has been treated with radiopharmaceuticals or sealed sources of radioisotopes, the "Radiation Precautions" chart label will be fixed onto the outside of the wrapped body. Fasten a second addressographed tag on the outer tie at waist that states "body must not be released to the funeral director or pathologist until the radiation safety office is notified for instructions."

VIII. DOCUMENTATION
   A. To be completed by physician:
      1. Certificate of Death
                  OR
         Medical Examiner's Notice and Pronouncement of Death.

    2. Undertaker/Coroner Release and Receipt Form.

    3. When applicable, Post-Mortem Examination Permit Form.

  B. To be completed by Nursing personnel:

    1. The "Post-Mortem Stamp" on the Nurses Notes/Integrated Progress Notes (see appendix).

IX. POINTS OF EMPHASIS

  A. Verify identity of deceased and double check ID tag.

  B. After family members have viewed the body, tie chin, wrists, and ankles. Tie shroud around deceased.

  C. Fasten second addressographed tag on outer tie at waist.

  D. Notify all appropriate hospital departments of the patient's death. (See Section IV. C 1.)

  E. The completed Medical Chart must be *hand* carried to Unit Management Office (0800–2400) or the Nurses' Office (2400–0800).

X. RESOURCES

Approved by: _____ Date: _____

Approved by: _____ Date: _____

Approved by: _____ Date: _____

To be reviewed: Every two years

Distribution: *Nursing Procedure and Technique Manual*

Appendix 2: Medication Kardex

INSULIN MEDICATION SCALE

SUGAR (Blood or Urine)

ORDER DATE:

REVISED DATE:

DISCONTINUED DATE

PRE-OPERATIVE AND SCHEDULED ONE DOSE MEDICATIONS

Date Ordered	MEDICATION	DOSE	Directions (include date to be given)	Time Given	SITE	INIT.

STAT AND SLIDING SCALE MEDICATIONS

DATE	MEDICATION	DOSE	DIRECTIONS	Time Given	SITE	INIT.

——— of ———

P.R.N.
STAT AND SLIDING SCALE
PRE-OPERATIVE AND SCHEDULED ONE DOSE
MEDICATION ADMINISTRATION RECORD

(F # 571-A REV 2/84)

ALLERGIES.

The Patient's Need For And Response To PRN Medication Must Be Documented In The Nurses Notes/Integrated Progress Notes

Year 19 ———

P.R.N. MEDICATIONS

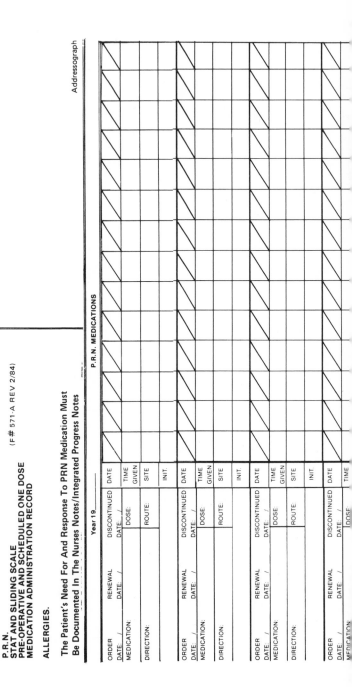

ORDER DATE: /	RENEWAL DATE: /	DISCONTINUED DATE: /	DATE
MEDICATION:		DOSE:	TIME GIVEN
DIRECTION:		ROUTE:	SITE
			INIT.

ORDER DATE: /	RENEWAL DATE: /	DISCONTINUED DATE: /	DATE
MEDICATION:		DOSE:	TIME GIVEN
DIRECTION:		ROUTE:	SITE
			INIT.

ORDER DATE: /	RENEWAL DATE: /	DISCONTINUED DATE: /	DATE
MEDICATION:		DOSE:	TIME GIVEN
DIRECTION:		ROUTE:	SITE
			INIT.

ORDER DATE: /	RENEWAL DATE: /	DISCONTINUED DATE: /	DATE
MEDICATION:		DOSE:	TIME

INIT.

ORDER DATE: /	RENEWAL DATE: /	DISCONTINUED DATE: /	DATE
MEDICATION:		DOSE:	TIME GIVEN
		ROUTE:	SITE
DIRECTION:			INIT.

ORDER DATE: /	RENEWAL DATE: /	DISCONTINUED DATE: /	DATE
MEDICATION:		DOSE:	TIME GIVEN
		ROUTE:	SITE
DIRECTION:			INIT.

ORDER DATE: /	RENEWAL DATE: /	DISCONTINUED DATE: /	DATE
MEDICATION:		DOSE:	TIME GIVEN
		ROUTE:	SITE
DIRECTION:			INIT.

ORDER DATE: /	RENEWAL DATE: /	DISCONTINUED DATE: /	DATE
MEDICATION:		DOSE:	TIME GIVEN
		ROUTE:	SITE
DIRECTION:			INIT.

INITIAL | SIGNATURE & STATUS | INITIAL | SIGNATURE & STATUS | INITIAL | SIGNATURE & STATUS | INITIAL | SIGNATURE & STATUS

Addressograph

ROUTINE MEDICATIONS

Initials	Signature & Status	Initials	Signature & Status

Year: 19___

ORDER	RENEWAL	DISCONTINUED
DATE: /	DATE: /	DATE: /

MEDICATION _____ DOSE

DIRECTION _____ ROUTE

ORDER	RENEWAL	DISCONTINUED
DATE: /	DATE: /	DATE: /

MEDICATION _____ DOSE

DIRECTION _____ ROUTE

ORDER	RENEWAL	DISCONTINUED
DATE: /	DATE:	DATE

MEDICATION _____ DOSE

DATE: /			DATE: /			DATE: /			DATE: /			DATE: /			DATE: /		
Time			Time			Time			Time			Time			Time		
Time	Site	Init.	Given	Site	Init.	Given	Site	Init.	Given	Site	Init.	Given	Site	Init.	Given	Site	Init.

ORDER	RENEWAL	DISCONTINUED
DATE /	DATE /	DATE /
MEDICATION:		DOSE
DIRECTION		ROUTE

ORDER	RENEWAL	DISCONTINUED
DATE /	DATE /	DATE /
MEDICATION:		DOSE
DIRECTION		ROUTE

ORDER	RENEWAL	DISCONTINUED
DATE /	DATE /	DATE /
MEDICATION:		DOSE
DIRECTION		ROUTE

ORDER	RENEWAL	DISCONTINUED
DATE /	DATE /	DATE /
MEDICATION:		DOSE
DIRECTION		ROUTE

ORDER	RENEWAL	DISCONTINUED
DATE /	DATE /	DATE /
MEDICATION		DOSE
DIRECTION		ROUTE

ALLERGIES:

DIAGNOSIS

NAME:

ROOM

INJECTION SITE DIAGRAM

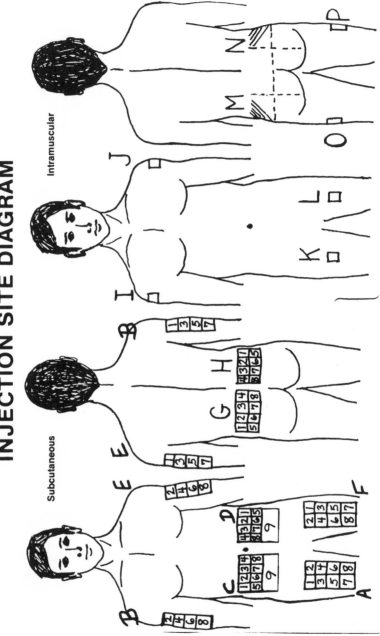

Subcutaneous

Intramuscular

ROUTINE MEDICATION ADMINISTRATION RECORD

ROUTINE MEDICATIONS	Year: 19___ Time	DATE: / Time Given	Site	Init.	DATE: / Time Given	Site	Init.	DATE: / Time Given	Site	Init.	DATE: / Time Given	Site	Init.	DATE: / Time Given	Site	Init.	DATE: / Time Given	Site	Init.
ORDER RENEWAL DISCONTINUED																			
DATE: / DATE: / DATE: /																			
MEDICATION: Heparin Flush DOSE:																			
DIRECTION: ROUTE:																			
ORDER RENEWAL DISCONTINUED																			
DATE: / DATE: / DATE: /																			
MEDICATION: DOSE:																			
DIRECTION: ROUTE:																			
ORDER RENEWAL DISCONTINUED																			
DATE: / DATE: / DATE: /																			
MEDICATION: DOSE:																			
DIRECTION: ROUTE:																			
ORDER RENEWAL DISCONTINUED																			
DATE: / DATE: / DATE: /																			
MEDICATION: DOSE:																			
DIRECTION: ROUTE:																			

Appendix 3: General Administration of Medication: *Hospital Policy and Procedure Manual*

DEPARTMENT/DIVISION: SUBJECT:
Nursing Service   General Administration of Medication

I. PURPOSE
   To establish a written procedure for the administration of medication.

II. DEFINITION OF TERMS
   Medication error—deviation from the physician's orders as written on the chart (i.e., omission, wrong dose, extra dose, unordered drug given, or wrong route).

III. GENERAL DESCRIPTION OF SCOPE AND PROCESS INVOLVED
   A. A physician will write an order specifying the drug, strength, dosage, route and frequency of administration.
   B. The R.N./G.N. or Medical Clerk will transcribe the order onto the medication Kardex.
   C. The R.N./G.N. will verify the transcription of the order.
   D. The R.N./G.N. or L.P.N. who meets the requirements in the

policy "Prerequisite for Administration of Medication" may administer medication.

E. The R.N./G.N. or L.P.N. will observe the patient for side effects and possible adverse reactions.

F. The R.N./G.N. or L.P.N. who prepares the medication should administer the medication.

G. Restrictions:
1) The Licensed Practical Nurse *will not:*
   a. administer medications to patients in critical care areas (Intensive Care Unit, Recovery Room, Coronary Care Unit and Neonatology).
   b. perform intradermal injections (P.P.D. skin test).
   c. prepare or administer intravenous medications or intravenous fluids.
2) The R.N./G.N., with the exception of the nurses in the critical care areas and delivery room, will not administer direct push intravenous medications except for heparin.

IV. EQUIPMENT

Medication keys
Medication Kardex
Medication
Hospital Formulary and Regulations Governing Drugs

Medication Cart

medicine cups	tongue depressors
syringes	lubricant
needles	paper cups
alcohol wipes	finger cots
paper towels	stethoscope
straws	water pitcher
narcotic record	juices

V. PROCEDURE	RATIONALE
A. Check that medication cart is stocked with the proper supplies.	Saves time.
B. Patient's Kardex will be stamped with addressograph plate and will list current medication.	Aids in identifying patient, room number and drugs.
C. Read the patient's name, room number, name of drug, dosage, frequency and route of each medication.	

D. Select the correct drug and read the label three times:

1. when selecting the drug.
2. when comparing the label with the data on the Kardex.
3. before returning the drug to the patient's drawer.

(Only use drugs that are clearly labeled from the hospital pharmacy.)

Verifies medication selected with medication ordered.

E. Check the expiration date on all packaged medications. Return any outdated medications to the pharmacy.

F. Check all medications against patient's drug allergies.

G. Prepare the medication (see procedure "Preparation and Administration of oral, parenteral and rectal medications" C01-057.1).

H. Before leaving the cart:

1. make sure narcotic drawer is locked.
2. place the cart in the doorway so that the drawers will face into the room.

State requirement for the control of narcotics.

I. Identify the patient by name and ID bracelet.

J. Perform special nursing action, e.g., apical rate, digoxin.

K. Remain with patient until medication is taken.

Verifies that patient has taken the drug.

L. Lock the outer door of the cart when the cart is left unattended.

Prevents free access to all drugs.

M. Wear keys around the waist so that they are visibly on your person while on the unit.

VI. CHARTING
   A. Medication Kardex—refer to Medication Kardex Guidelines.
   B. Narcotic Sheet

All narcotics must be signed out on the narcotic sheet when removed from the narcotic drawer.

C. Nurse Note
1. when p.r.n. medications are given chart the reason for giving and whether the medication was effective.
2. medications not given and the reason except NPO and REF.

VIII. SAFETY, CARE AND MAINTENANCE
A. Narcotic count is done at the beginning and end of each shift by two nursing personnel qualified to administer medication. One nurse will be from the shift coming on duty, the other nurse will be from the shift going off duty.

B. If unfamiliar with the drug, dose, frequency, route, trade name, reorder date or generic name refer to the *Hospital Formulary and Regulations Governing Drugs.*

C. If a medication error occurs, report it immediately to the charge nurse, the physician and Patient Care Coordinator. Complete an incident report.

D. Clean and restock the medication cart after every shift.

E. Keys will be carried by employed nursing personnel who have been supervised in administering medications. At no time are the keys to be taken off the floor.

VIII. POINTS OF EMPHASIS
A. Select the correct drug and read the label three times.

B. Check all medications against patient's drug allergies.

C. Check expiration date on all packaged medications.

D. Identify the patient by name and ID bracelet.

E. Remain with the patient until all medications are taken.

F. The narcotic box must be locked at all times.

G. When leaving the medication cart unattended lock the outer doors.

References:

Performance Checklist for Clinical Evaluation—Administration of Medications, Staff Development.

Hospital Formulary and Regulations Governing Drugs.

Approved by: _____   Date: _____

Approved by: _____   Date: _____

Approved by: _____   Date: _____

To be reviewed:　　　Every two years

Distribution:　　*Nursing Procedure and Technical Manual Administration*

References

Bosk, C. 1979. *Forgive and Remember*. Chicago: University of Chicago Press.

Bosk, C. 1980. Occupational rituals in patient management. *New England Journal of Medicine* 302 (2): 71–76.

DeCraemer, W., Vansina, J., and Fox, R. 1976. Religious movements in central Africa. *Comparative Studies in Society and History* 18: 458–75.

Douglas, M. 1963. *The Lele of the Kasai*. London: Oxford University Press.

Douglas, M. 1966. *Purity and danger*. London: Routledge & Kegan Paul.

Douglas, M. 1970. The healing rite. *Man* 5: 302–8.

Douglas, M. 1975. *Implicit meanings: Essays in anthropology*. London: Routledge & Kegan Paul.

Groff, J. 1896. Hand-book of materia medica for trained nurses. *The Trained Nurse* 16 (12): 635–40.

Hospital Nurse. 1890. Some notes on how to nurse the dying. *The Trained Nurse* 5 (1): 17–21.

Malinowski, B. 1954. *Magic, science and religion and other essays*. Garden City, N.Y.: Doubleday.

L. M. M. 1899. Laying out the dead. *The Trained Nurse* 3 (5): 169–71.

The Night Nurse. 1890. *The Nightingale* 5 (28): 217–18.

Tudor, J. 1890. After death. *The Trained Nurse* 5 (5): 225–26.

Turner, V. 1957. *Schism and continuity in an African society*. New York: Humanistic Press.

Turner, V. 1967. Symbol in Ndembu ritual. In V. Turner, *The forest of symbols aspects of Ndembu ritual*. Ithaca, N.Y.: Cornell University Press.

Turner, V. 1969. *The ritual process*. Ithaca, N.Y.: Cornell University Press.

Van Gennep, A. 1960. *The rites of passage*. Chicago: University of Chicago Press.

Walker, V. 1967. *Nursing and ritualistic practice*. New York: Macmillan.

Zerubavel, E. 1979. *Patterns of time in hospital life*. Chicago: University of Chicago Press.

Index

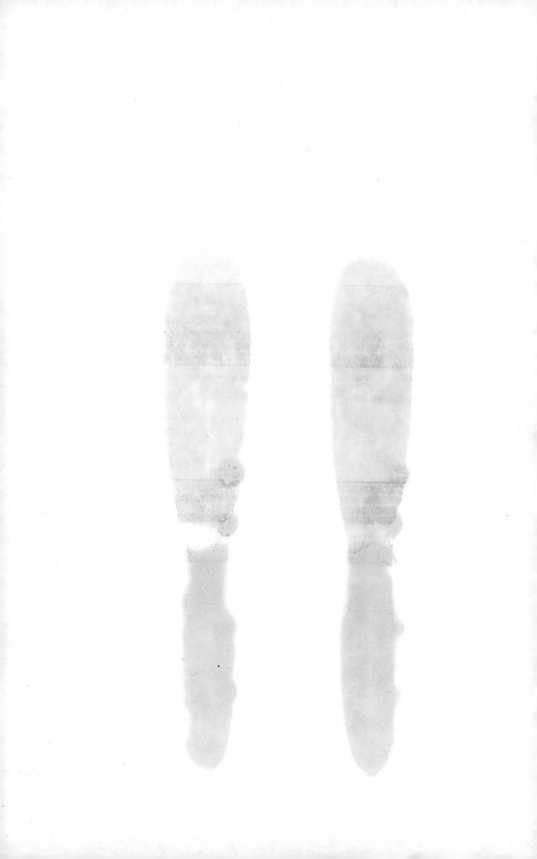